Asbestiform Fibers

Nonoccupational Health Risks

Committee on Nonoccupational Health Risks of Asbestiform Fibers
Board on Toxicology and Environmental Health Hazards
Commission on life Sciences
National Research Council

NATIONAL ACADEMY PRESS
Washington, D.C. 1984

National Academy Press 2101 Constitution Avenue, NW Washington, DC 20418

NOTICE: The project that is the subject of this report was approved by the Governing Board of the National Research Council, whose members are drawn from the councils of the National Academy of Sciences, the National Academy of Engineering, and the Institute of Medicine. The members of the committee responsible for the report were chosen for their special competences and with regard for appropriate balance.

This report has been reviewed by a group other than the authors according to procedures approved by a Report Review Committee consisting of members of the National Academy of Sciences, the National Academy of Engineering, and the Institute of Medicine.

The National Research Council was established by the National Academy of Sciences in 1916 to associate the broad community of science and technology with the Academy's purposes of furthering knowledge and of advising the federal government. The Council operates in accordance with general policies determined by the Academy under the authority of its congressional charter of 1863, which establishes the Academy as a private, nonprofit, self-governing membership corporation. The Council has become the principal operating agency of both the National Academy of Sciences and the National Academy of Engineering in the conduct of their services to the government, the public, and the scientific and engineering communities. It is administered jointly by both Academies and the Institute of Medicine. The National Academy of Engineering and the Institute of Medicine were established in 1964 and 1970, respectively, under the charter of the National Academy of Sciences.

The study reported here was supported by Contract EPA 68-01-4655 between the National Academy of Sciences and the Environmental Protection Agency.

Library of Congress Catalog Card Number 84-60249
International Standard Book Number 0-309-03446-9

Printed in the United States of America

Committee on Nonoccupational Health Risks of Asbestiform Fibers

Lester Breslow, Chairman School of Public Health University of California Los Angeles, Calif.
Richard Bates Health Effects Institute Cambridge, Mass.
Henrik Bendixen Department of Anesthesiology Columbia University College of Physicians and Surgeons New York, N.Y.
Strephen L. Brown Independent Consultant Portola Valley, Calif.
Patricia A. Buffler University of Texas Health Science Center School of Public Health University of Texas at Houston Houston, Texas
Arthur M. Langer Department of Community Medicine Environmental Sciences Laboratory Mt. Sinai School of Medicine New York, N.Y.
Jeremiah Lynch Exxon Chemical Company East Millstone, N.J.
James A. Merchant Department of Preventive Medicine and Environmental Health and the Department of Internal Medicine College of Medicine University of Iowa Iowa City, Ia.
Richard Monson Department of Epidemiology Harvard School of Public Health Boston, Mass.
Brooke T. Mossman Department of Pathology College of Medicine University of Vermont Burlington, Vt.
James E. Trosko Department of Pediatrics and Human Development College of Human Medicine Michigan State University East Lansing, Mich.
John Van Ryzin Division of Biostatistics School of Public Health Columbia University New York, N.Y.
Tibor Zoltai Department of Geology and Geophysics University of Minnesota Minneapolis, Minn.

Consultant

Warren Muir Department of Environmental Health Sciences School of Hygiene and Public Health The Johns Hopkins University Baltimore, Md.

National Research Council Staff

Barbara Mandula, Study Director
Frances M. Peter, Editor
Pamela Smith, Research Assistant
Waldena Banks, Administrative Secretary

Board on Toxicology and Environmental Health Hazards

Gerald N. Wogan, Chairman Department of Nutrition and Food Science Massachusetts Institute of Technology Cambridge, Mass.
Philip Landrigan, Co-Vice-Chairman National institute for Occupational Safety and Health Robert Taft laboratories Cincinnati, Ohio
Donald Hornig, Co-Vice-Chairman School of Public Health Harvard University Boston, Mass.
Edward Bresnick Eppley Institute for Cancer Research University of Nebraska Medical Center Omaha, Nebraska
Herman N. Eisen Department of Biology Massachusetts Institute of Technology Cambridge, Mass.
Ronald Estabrook Department of Biochemistry University of Texas Medical School Dallas, Texas
Emmanuel Farber Department of Pathology University of Toronto Toronto, Ontario
David G. Hoel Biometry and Risk Assessment Program National Institute of Environmental Health Sciences Research Triangle Park, N.C.
Michael W. Lieberman Department of Pathology Washington University School of Medicine St. Louis, Missouri
Abraham M. Lilienfeld School of Hygiene and Public health The Johns Hopkins University Baltimore, Maryland

Richard Merrill School of Law University of Virginia Charlottesville, Virginia
Vaun A. Newill Exxon Corporation Medicine and Environmental Health Department New York, New York
John Peters Department of Family and Preventive Medicine University of Southern California School of Medicine Los Angeles, California

Ex Officio Members

Gary P. Carlson Purdue University School of Pharmacy and Pharmacal Science Department of Pharmacology and Toxicology Lafayette, Indiana
Maureen Henderson School of Public Health and Community Medicine Department of Epidemiology University of Washington Seattle, Washington

National Research Council Staff

Robert G. Tardiff, Executive Director, until June 1983
Devra L. Davis, Executive Director, September 1983 to present
Jacqueline K. Prince, Staff Assistant
Joseph V. Rodricks Environ Corporation Washington, D.C.
Liane B. Russell Biology Division Oak Ridge National Laboratory Oak Ridge, Tennessee
Ellen Silbergeld Toxics Program Environmental Defense Fund Washington, D.C.
Roger O. McClellan Lovelace Inhalation Toxicology Research Institute Albuquerque, New Mexico
Daniel B. Menzel Department of Pharmacology Duke University Medical Center Durham, North Carolina
Norton Nelson Institute of Environmental Medicine New York University Medical Center New York, New York

Preface

Industrial progress during the twentieth century has contributed to our well-being, but has also resulted in environmental changes that have increased risks to human health. Not only are greater quantities and varieties of hazardous materials being taken from the earth and used in many ways, but the use of synthetic materials with similar physical and chemical properties has also been growing.

Adverse health effects from many of these new exposures have been receiving considerable attention. Radioactive substances, cigarette smoke, petrochemicals, and asbestos, for example, are well known for their potential to harm health.

The health risks from exposure to these and other materials are provoking some alarm because of several characteristics that they have in common. Relatively small, sometimes minute, amounts may cause severe damage to health. People are often not aware of their exposure at the time it occurs. Cancer, a particularly feared disease, can result. Cancer and other adverse health effects typically occur many years after exposure began. Evidence linking the particular substance to subsequent disease may appear—and be accepted—only decades after millions of people have been exposed. Asbestiform fibers, which for purposes of this report include both natural materials such as asbestos and synthetic materials such as fibrous glass, typify the problem.

Although asbestos and some of its uses had been known for centuries, twentieth century industry brought a vast increase in mining and distribution of that material. Then, some years after hundreds of thousands of workers had been exposed, it became apparent that considerable damage to health, including cancer, was occurring as a result. Ascertaining the harm precisely was complicated because other factors, especially cigarette smoking, often contributed to the same effects. As the hazard became more widely known in recent years, annual use of asbestos in the United States has dropped. However, asbestos had already been widely distributed in schools and other buildings, in the general outdoor air, and in some water supplies. Thus, tens of millions of people are still being exposed—although usually to very small amounts.

The usefulness of asbestos was so great that substitutes with some similar physical properties were developed for commercial purposes. Do these synthetic materials carry the same, or some, health risk because of the characteristics they share with the naturally occurring asbestos?

Given the widespread occurrence of these materials, concerned federal agencies commissioned studies to examine the potential health risk from nonoccupational exposure to asbestos. In one such study, the Safe Drinking Water Committee of the National Research Council sought to determine whether health damage was occurring because drinking water was contaminated with asbestos fibers. The committee found that the epidemiological studies of asbestos in drinking water had major limitations in design, but that the committee's risk estimates were compatible with the results of the epidemiological studies (National Research Council, 1983). Generally, the amount of asbestos in the drinking waters studied would be likely to yield an increased risk too small to detect.

The U.S. Consumer Product Safety Commission, in carrying out its responsibility for protecting consumers, sought guidance from a Chronic Hazard Advisory Panel on Asbestos. The latter body concluded that "asbestos at all levels of exposure ...[should be regarded] ... as a potential human carcinogen." Furthermore, the panel wrote, "It is prudent to behave as if asbestos fibers may be carcinogenic at low exposure levels and at small particle sizes" (U.S. Consumer Product Safety Commission, 1983). There has also been concern about asbestos in schools, as evidenced by reports from the U.S. Environmental Protection Agency (1980) and the U.S. General Accounting Office (1982).

In a more general approach to the issue, broadening it beyond asbestos, the Environmental Protection Agency asked the National Academy of Sciences:

> to evaluate the human health risks associated with nonoccupational exposure to asbestiform fibers, with emphasis on inhalation of outdoor and indoor air, and
>
> to determine the extent to which the physical-chemical properties of the fibers may be associated with the development of various human diseases and the extent to which such information may be incorporated into assessing health risks resulting from exposure to the fibers.

To conduct that study, the National Research Council established the Committee on Nonoccupational Health Risks of Asbestiform Fibers in August 1982. This is the report of that committee.

I personally would like to thank the committee members, who worked extremely hard and persistently to bring the project to fruition. I could not imagine a more thoughtful, energetic, and cooperative group for approaching this complex problem. On behalf of the committee, I would also like to thank the many persons from various groups and agencies who provided the committee with unpublished draft documents, or who took the time to answer questions and offer suggestions. They are too numerous to mention individually. However, Dr. Dennis Kotchmar, EPA project officer, deserves special mention, as do Mr. Colin Church, Dr. Robert Clifton, Dr. Jon Konzen, Dr. James Leineweber, Dr. Marvin Schneiderman, and Mr. Paul White.

The committee is also grateful to the capable and devoted NRC project staff, including Dr. Barbara Mandula, Ms. Pamela Smith, Ms. Dena Banks, Ms. Frances Peter, and the many others who assisted them at various times, especially Ms. Shirley Ash, Ms. Leslye Giese, Ms. Jacqueline Prince, Ms. Mary Ellen Scheckenbach, and Ms. Bernidean Williams. Special thanks are also due Dr. Warren Muir, who was a consultant to the committee. Finally, I wish to thank Dr. Robert Tardiff, who was executive director of BOTEHH when the project began; Dr. Devra Davis, present executive director of BOTEHH, who energetically shepherded the project through its final stages; and Drs. Frederick Robbins and Alvin Lazen of the Commission on Life Sciences for their continued interest and support.

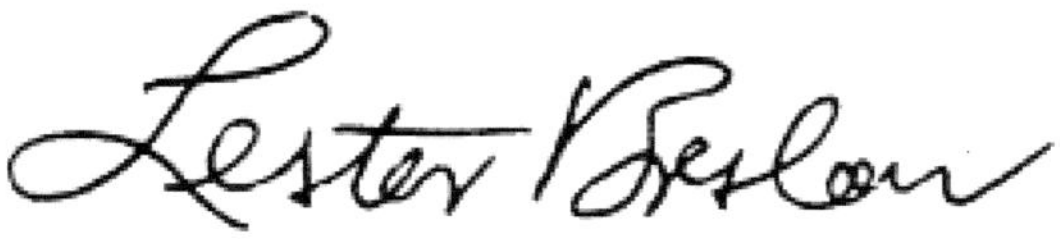

LESTER BRESLOW

CHAIRMAN

COMMITTEE ON NONOCCUPATIONAL HEALTH RISKS OF ASBESTIFORM FIBERS

References

National Research Council. 1983. Drinking Water and Health. Vol. 5. A report of the Safe Drinking Water Committee, Commission on Life Sciences. National Academy Press, Washington, D.C.

U.S. Consumer Product Safety Commission. 1983. Chronic Hazard Advisory Panel on Asbestos. Consumer Product Safety Commission, Washington, D.C.

U.S. Environmental Protection Agency. 1980. Asbestos-Containing Materials in Schools. Health Effects and Magnitude of Exposure. Support document for proposed rule 6 on friable asbestos-Containing materials in school buildings. Environmental Protection Agency, Washington, D.C.

U.S. General Accounting Office. 1982. Asbestos in Schools: A Dilemma. General Accounting Office, Washington, D.C.

Contents

Executive Summary

ORIGIN OF THE STUDY

Nonoccupational health risks associated with exposure to airborne asbestiform[1] fibers have aroused concern because the adverse effects from occupational exposure to some types of these fibers have been well documented and because asbestos as well as other mineral and synthetic particles with similar properties are widespread in the environment. Moreover, an excess occurrence of asbestos-related disease has been found among people who were not themselves occupationally exposed but who lived either near industrial facilities where asbestos was used or in households with asbestos workers. In this report, the Committee on Nonoccupational Health Risks of Asbestiform Fibers considers the health risks posed by nonoccupational airborne exposures to asbestos and other natural or synthetic asbestiform fibers. The issue is important because many people may be exposed to these materials, although at relatively low levels.

To reach a better understanding of the relationship between characteristics of asbestiform fibers and possible adverse health effects from nonoccupational exposures, the U.S. Environmental Protection Agency asked the National Academy of Sciences to undertake a study with two goals:

- to evaluate the human health risks associated with nonoccupational exposure to asbestiform fibers, with emphasis on inhalation of outdoor and indoor air, and
- to determine the extent to which the physical-chemical properties of the fibers may be associated with the development of various human diseases and the extent to which such information may be incorporated into assessing health risks resulting from exposure to the fibers.

The committee found that much more information is available about asbestos than about the other materials of concern. Wherever possible, the committee compared data on the nonasbestos fibers with data on asbestos. This comparison required assessment of information on asbestos as well as on other materials.

[1] The term "asbestiform" in this report refers to fibers that share some specific physical properties with asbestos. These are described later in this summary and in Chapter 2. The term is a mineralogical one that has been used for more than a century.

MAJOR FINDINGS AND RECOMMENDATIONS

Evaluation of Risk

Nonoccupational exposure to asbestiform fibers in air presents a risk to human health. The extent of this risk is highly uncertain, depending on the nature and amount of exposure and other factors. Evidence for the existence of the risk includes the following:

- Large excesses of lung cancer, mesothelioma, pulmonary fibrosis, and other pleural abnormalities have been found among workers occupationally exposed to asbestos. Presumably, nonoccupational exposures would result in qualitatively similar effects.
- Both a statistically excessive number of cases of mesothelioma and an excess frequency of pleural abnormalities have been observed among household contacts of asbestos workers.
- Asbestiform fibers are distributed extensively outside the workplace, although usually in minute quantities.
- The major pathological effects associated with human exposure to airborne asbestos have been duplicated experimentally in animals.
- Increases in cell replication and other abnormalities have been seen in cultures of tracheal lining cells from humans and animals after the cells were exposed to synthetic or natural asbestiform materials.

Estimating the extent of health risks from nonoccupational exposure to asbestiform fibers is fraught with uncertainty. Factors contributing to that uncertainty include the following:

- A great variety of asbestiform fibers has been found in the nonoccupational environment. These fibers occur in a range of sizes and vary in physicochemical characteristics, such as flexibility and durability.
- It is difficult to standardize methods for measuring amounts and characteristics of asbestiform fibers.
- A long time is required for health effects in humans to become detectable after exposure begins (often 20 to 40 years).
- There is inadequate knowledge of the mechanisms by which asbestiform fibers lead to cancer and other health effects.
- There are uncertainties in determining dose-response relationships from the occupational environment and then extrapolating them to the nonoccupational environment, where both exposure and population characteristics are usually very different and doses are typically much lower.

The committee made estimates of comparative risk of adverse health effects that might result from exposures to various asbestiform substances. It concluded that population risks from exposure to the other materials considered would generally be lower than the risks from exposure to chrysotile asbestos because the opportunities for airborne exposure to particles of respirable size were generally less for the other substances than for chrysotile. The nonasbestos materials considered were attapulgite (the trade name for the mineral palygorskite, which exists in asbestiform and nonasbestiform varieties); several man-made mineral fibers, such as fibrous glass, mineral wool, and ceramic fibers; carbon fibers; and fibrous erionite. These were selected because they seemed likely to have, or are known to have, at least some of the properties of asbestiform fibers.

The committee made a quantitative estimate of the risk of excess lung cancer and mesothelioma that might occur in persons breathing low levels of asbestos in the air. A concentration of 0.0004 fibers/cm^3 was deemed reasonable to use in such calculations because a variety of measurements of indoor and outdoor air indicated that 0.0004 fibers/cm^3 is the approximate average level that may be encountered. If a person inhaled air containing asbestos at that level throughout a 73-year lifetime, the committee's best judgment is that the lifetime risk of mesothelioma would be approximately nine in a million (range 0 to 350 per million, depending on assumptions regarding the relationship of dose to risk). Others have produced different estimates that are discussed in this report. Risks for continuous lifetime exposures to higher or lower levels would be proportionately higher or lower. Epidemiological data and the estimates derived from them indicate that the corresponding lifetime risk for lung cancer would be about 64 in a million for male smokers (range 0 to 290), 23 in a million for female smokers (0 to 110), and 6 and 3 in a million, respectively, for male and female nonsmokers. The risk to nonsmokers appears greater for mesothelioma than for lung cancer.

Because of the great reliance on assumptions and on clearly deficient exposure and effects data, the committee views these risk estimates as guides to the qualitative assessment of nonoccupational health risks from asbestos and asbestiform fibers—not as definitive estimates of the amount of disease to be anticipated. These estimates and other considerations lead to the following five conclusions about risk:

- Some deaths from mesothelioma and lung cancer will probably result from current and past levels of exposure to asbestos in ambient air.
- Excess deaths from other diseases, such as asbestosis, and from exposures to other asbestiform fibers are also possible but are not likely to be as numerous as those from asbestos-induced mesotheliomas or lung cancer.
- The numbers of annual or cumulative deaths expected to result from such exposures are very uncertain, but they are virtually certain to be lower, and probably much lower, than those resulting from past, heavier occupational exposures to asbestos.

- Deaths from past occupational exposures to asbestos can reasonably be estimated to total several thousand per year in the United States during the next few years. Among these, more deaths from lung cancer than from mesothelioma can be expected.
- The greatest risks of continuous lifetime exposure to asbestos would be to smokers, who would be most at risk of lung cancer. However, the risks to nonsmokers might well be greater for mesothelioma than for lung cancer, because of the strong dependence of mesothelioma rates on time from first exposure. The time dependence factor also implies that restricting exposures of children to asbestos would be even more effective than a corresponding restriction for adults in reducing the lifetime risk of mesothelioma.

Physicochemical Properties and Health Effects

Some of the physical properties of asbestiform fibers appear to be important in causing adverse health effects, but the specific properties that are necessary and sufficient are not known. One clearly important characteristic is respirability. In addition, longer, thinner fibers appear to be more pathogenic than shorter, thicker fibers, but there is not a minimum size below which no effects would be expected. However, nonfibrous particles generally do not induce mesotheliomas in animals. Number, rather than mass, and durability of fibers also seem to be significant factors in pathogenicity of asbestiform fibers.

All major commercial types of asbestos fibers used in the United States have been associated with lung cancer, mesothelioma, and asbestosis in humans. It is not known whether the physicochemical fiber properties responsible for fibrosis are similar to those involved in carcinogenesis.

Recommendations

The committee's findings and analysis led to the following recommendations:

1. Systematic monitoring and characterization of asbestiform fibers with standardized methods should be undertaken in nonoccupational environments, including urban, rural, indoor, and outdoor locations where exposure may be of special concern.
2. A program of systematic surveillance should be undertaken to determine the extent to which the occurrence of mesothelioma and lung cancer is associated with exposure to asbestiform fibers.
3. Cessation of cigarette smoking should be encouraged in view of the multiplicative effect of smoking and asbestos exposure in increasing the risk for lung cancer.
4. Steps should be taken to educate both the medical profession and the general public concerning possible exposures to asbestiform fibers and the resulting health effects.

The committee also made several recommendations concerning future research to resolve the many questions about the health risks of nonoccupational exposure to asbestiform fibers.

1. A standardized terminology for asbestiform fibers should be adopted. The terminology should be based on mineralogical analysis and should distinguish these fibers from other types of particles.
2. The various characteristics of asbestiform fibers or other particles used in experiments should be described as completely as possible.
3. Standardized methods for measuring and characterizing asbestiform fibers should be improved.
4. In vivo and in vitro laboratory studies with asbestiform fibers and nonfibrous substances should be conducted to investigate the physico-chemical properties that are responsible for the biological effects.
5. Clinical studies of lung cancer, mesothelioma, and fibrosis should be continued with emphasis on the possible role of asbestiform fibers.
6. Epidemiological studies are needed to clarify further the relationships between exposure to fibers and adverse health effects. These studies should include case-control studies for mesothelioma and lung cancer and prospective cohort studies among persons occupationally exposed to materials such as asbestos, attapulgite, and man-made mineral fibers.
7. To improve risk assessments, studies should be conducted to elucidate the relationships between amount of exposure and time factors and the development of adverse health effects.

SUMMARY OF THE STUDY

Background

Asbestos has been detected in both outdoor and indoor air, although almost always at concentrations far below the standard established by the Occupational Safety and Health Administration (OSHA) for the workplace. Since 1976 the workplace standard has been 2 fibers/cm^3 for fibers longer than 5 μm seen in a phase contrast light microscope under specified conditions. The general population is also exposed to other fibrous materials with some of the same physical properties as asbestos but whose effects on health are not well known. These materials include man-made mineral fibers such as fibrous glass and mineral wool, which are sometimes used as substitutes for asbestos, as well as certain natural asbestiform varieties of minerals not marketed as asbestos.

Sources of exposure to asbestiform fibers may be roughly divided into three broad categories:

- naturally occurring asbestiform fibers used commercially, such as asbestos;
- commercially used synthetic fibers with some properties similar to those of asbestos; and
- naturally occurring types of asbestiform fibers that are not used commercially.

There is a substantial amount of data on exposures in the workplace, but very little information on nonoccupational exposures. In the occupational setting, four diseases have been clearly associated with exposures to asbestos. These are (1) lung cancer; (2) mesothelioma, a rare but almost invariably fatal cancer of the tissues that line the chest cavity (pleural mesothelioma) or the abdominal cavity (peritoneal mesothelioma); (3) asbestosis, a nonmalignant, progressive fibrosis of the lung that may result in severe disability and death; and (4) nonmalignant pleural disease, including diffuse pleural thickening and effusions and the formation of fibrous and calcified plaques. The occurrence of these four diseases in various occupational settings and the presence of asbestiform fibers in the general environment led to current concern about potential health effects from nonoccupational exposures.

During the course of its study, the committee was confronted with several difficulties:

- Fibers in the general outdoor environment seem to differ in size and other physicochemical properties from those in the workplace; however, it is not easy to characterize these materials. Different types and samples of fibrous materials vary greatly in their physical properties, even when they are composed of the same mineral. Therefore, it is difficult to develop a consistent methodology for determining and expressing the characteristics and concentrations of fibers found in different environments or used in laboratory studies.
- Because most health effects data are based on workplace exposures, it is necessary to extrapolate results from relatively high occupational concentrations to the much lower concentrations of fibers typically found outside the workplace. Although the health consequences are presumably similar among workers and nonworkers, incidence rates would be expected to be lower and the nonmalignant changes less severe among persons nonoccupationally exposed to lower levels of asbestos. Thus, the effects would be more difficult to detect.
- Other factors associated with the diseases must be considered. For example, cigarette smoking multiplies the effect of asbestos in causing lung cancer.
- The mechanisms by which the fibers produce disease are not well understood, nor is it clear how the fibers reach various parts of the body.

- The length of time from initial exposure to the expression of certain health consequences is often several decades. Thus, current disease is the result of past exposures, whereas present exposures will produce disease only many years in the future. Exposure in childhood may increase the possibility of ultimate damage to health, because disease can occur long after external exposure has ceased and more years of life remain for children.

Thus, great uncertainty is likely to attend any conclusions drawn about the relevant fiber characteristics and the health risks that may accompany exposure.

The committee agreed that the major potential for future fiber-associated health problems is probably presented by inhalation exposures to airborne fibers rather than by the ingestion of these materials, for example, in water. Most of the committee's attention was therefore devoted to airborne fibers of respirable size, that is, to fibers less than approximately 3 μm in diameter.

The committee made quantitative risk assessments for lung cancer and mesothelioma from inhaled asbestos, but it did not attempt quantitative risk assessments for other cancers, from inhalation of other asbestiform fibers, or from ingestion of asbestiform fibers in water or food.

Materials of Concern

For purposes of this report, the term "asbestiform fibers" is used broadly to include both naturally occurring and certain synthetic inorganic and carbon fibers that share some specific physical properties with asbestos.

Asbestos, the prime example of an asbestiform material, consists of the commercially marketed asbestiform varieties of several silicate minerals. They are primarily chrysotile, crocidolite, and the asbestiform variety of some amphibole minerals marketed as "amosite." Chrysotile accounts for approximately 95% of the asbestos currently sold in the United States. Because of its great strength, flexibility, and heat resistance, asbestos came into extensive use during the 20th century for textiles, thermal and electrical insulation, and high strength reinforcement in such products as vinyl-asbestos flooring and asbestos-cement sheet and pipe. In 1982, the United States used approximately 6% of the world production of asbestos.

Five basic physical properties distinguish asbestiform fibers from other materials. The presence of these properties generally depends on the physical and chemical conditions under which the fibers grow. Compared with a nonasbestiform variety of the same mineral, the properties are:

- microscopic, fiberlike dimensions and morphology, i.e., the fibers are much longer than wide;
- enhanced strength and flexibility;
- inverse relationship between diameter and strength, i.e., the smaller the diameter, the greater the strength per unit cross-sectional area;
- enhanced physical and chemical durability; and
- high quality, relatively defect-free surface structure.

"High quality" fibers have all these properties to a great extent; "low quality" fibers possess them to a lesser extent. The presence of these properties does not necessarily indicate that a material is either carcinogenic or fibrogenic. Because these properties are interdependent and variable, naturally occurring asbestiform fibers, even those composed of the same mineral, have a range of physical characteristics. In contrast to fibers in the workplace, it is not currently possible to determine the sources of most fibers in the ambient environment or the extent to which these fibers have the above properties.

Mineralogical terms pertaining to asbestiform fibers have sometimes been used inaccurately in scientific reports, including the literature on biological effects. As a result, it may be impossible to discern the composition of materials studied and extremely difficult to draw conclusions about their physical properties and biological effects.

Relationship of Fiber Characteristics to Health Effects

Various physical properties of asbestiform fibers appear to play a role in causing adverse health effects; however, the specific properties that are necessary and sufficient to produce such effects have not been postively identified. Furthermore, it is not known whether the properties associated with a given effect, for example, lung cancer, are the same or different from those associated with other effects, such as fibrosis or mesothelioma. Some characteristics that appear to be important are discussed below, in approximately descending order of the strength of the positive evidence.

Respirability. For significant health effects to result from inhalation of asbestiform fibers, the fibers must reach the lower portions of the respiratory tract where they cause the most damage. Although the limiting upper diameter appears to be about 3 μm, fibers that are much longer than wide can penetrate deeply in the respiratory tract.

Length, Diameter, and Aspect Ratio (i.e., Ratio of Length to Diameter). Experiments inducing mesothelioma in rodents by injections of test material have indicated that long, thin fibers yield more tumors than do short, thick fibers. Samples with an overwhelming majority of fibers shorter than 5 μm yielded mesotheliomas in rats when injected intraperitoneally, but the pathogenic role of short fibers, especially those shorter than 3 μm, is unclear. Fibers longer than approximately 10 μm cannot be completely engulfed and inactivated by macrophages, and they have tended to produce more disease in animal tests than have the shorter fibers.

Other Properties. The number of fibers, which is also correlated with surface area, generally appears to be a more relevant measure than mass in determining pathogenicity. Durability also appears to be a factor. The more durable fibers appear to be more pathogenic in some studies than fibers that are less durable. The relevance of fiber surface charge to effects on human health remains to be demonstrated. Some experimental studies have indicated that surface charge appears to be involved in cytotoxicity. Although chemical composition is related to physical properties of asbestiform fibers, a direct role for chemical composition per se in biological activity has not been demonstrated.

Measurement and Extent of Exposure

Measurement. Information about asbestiform fibers in the ambient environment, although scanty, indicates that they differ from those in the workplace. Different techniques for measuring the concentrations in the two environments have been used. The phase contrast light microscope has been adequate for counting fibers in the workplace. However, that technique has been less useful for the ambient environment, where fiber identity and character are usually unknown; almost all fibers are too small to be seen by light microscopy; and concentrations, expressed as mass, are usually hundreds or thousands of times lower than those in the workplace.

Data on workplace fiber concentrations are generally given as numbers of fibers longer than 5 μm, whereas data on ambient concentrations obtained with transmission electron microscope techniques have usually been expressed as mass per unit volume. Substantial uncertainty may be introduced in calculations that assume that ambient and workplace exposures differ only in fiber concentration. Furthermore, it is not usually possible to convert mass measurements to fiber concentrations accurately because the various conversion factors that are used assume particular fiber dimensions, and these vary greatly with different environments and sampling techniques. During the early 1970s, mass measurements of asbestos made in various U.S. cities ranged from 1 to 100 ng/m^3. If we assume that 30 $\mu g/m^3$ is equivalent to 1 $fiber/cm^3$ (counting fibers longer than 5 μm through a light microscope), the mass measurements in those cities would lead to an expected concentration of 0.00003 to 0.003 asbestos fibers per cubic centimeter.

Extent of Exposure. In assessing the likelihood that individuals would be exposed to various asbestiform fibers, the committee considered patterns of use; production or consumption levels; fiber dimensions, i.e., whether the fibers are of respirable size; and potential for population exposure. In many situations, the fibers are tightly bound in a matrix during product manufacture and, therefore, might be expected to produce little subsequent exposure.

In the United States, the annual use of asbestos peaked in 1973 at almost 800,000 metric tons, but decreased to approximately 250,000 metric tons, or about 6% of world production, in 1982. However, much of the more than 30 million metric tons of asbestos used in the United States since 1900 is still present in its original application and provides a potential for exposure.

Attapulgite (palygorskite) is the only natural asbestiform material used in the United States in amounts greater than those of asbestos. Of the more than 700,000 metric tons used annually, most appears to be classifiable as asbestiform. Most attapulgite fibers are less than 5 µm long and have diameters of approximately 0.03 µm. Some uses of this material could result in the release of fibers, but the committee found no reported measurements of attapulgite in ambient air.

Synthetic fibers with some physical properties similar to those of asbestos include man-made mineral fibers, of which more than 1 million metric tons are produced annually in the United States. Typical diameters of most of these fibers exceed the respirable size range, although diameters of fine grades of fibrous glass and some rock wool and slag wool are mostly below 3 µm.

Some fibrous erionite found in deposits in the western United States falls into the respirable size range. Mining and natural weathering of this material could lead to significant local air concentrations, but the committee did not find any measurements of such concentrations. Moreover, the population exposed is probably small.

Current U.S. consumption figures and use patterns indicate that future exposure of the general population to attapulgite and fibrous glass is likely to be somewhat greater than exposure to chrysotile, whereas exposure to mineral wool, ceramic fibers, other asbestos fibers, and carbon fibers would be less. However, material already in place would also contribute to total exposure.

Health Effects Methodology

To develop an understanding of the health risks associated with exposure to environmental agents such as asbestiform fibers, investigators usually evaluate data from clinical, epidemiological, and laboratory studies. Clinical observations often provide the first suggestion that exposure to a particular substance may cause an adverse health effect. Epidemiological studies are then undertaken to attempt to confirm the hypothesized association and to quantify it. Laboratory studies of the response in animals (in vivo) and in cells growing outside the body (in vitro) can provide further information. If a substance administered to animals produces pathological effects similar to those found in humans, the case for its being a causative agent in humans is strengthened. For asbestos, the major diseases observed in humans have been produced in animals by exposure to asbestos.

In vitro and in vivo studies do not necessarily adequately reflect the amounts or routes of exposures experienced by humans, nor do they take into account individual susceptibilities or other substances to which people might be exposed. Thus, such studies should be extrapolated to humans only with great caution. Except for smoking, however, no environmental or genetic factors have been unequivocally shown to influence the chance that a person will develop an asbestos-induced disease.

Health Effects of Asbestos

Appendix A of this report contains a chronological list of the major findings associating adverse health effects with exposure to asbestos. The first disease to be associated with asbestos exposure was asbestosis, which was first noted in the early 1900s. From 1938 to 1949, numerous autopsy reports indicated that a high proportion of persons dying of asbestosis also had lung cancer. In the 1950s, when the sharp increase in lung cancer attributable to smoking was occurring in the United States and other industrial nations, epidemiologists found that occupational exposure to asbestos also increased the risk of lung cancer, especially among cigarette smokers. In the early 1960s, the association with mesothelioma was established among asbestos miners in South Africa.

Lung Cancer. Exposure to asbestos appears to increase a worker's underlying risk of getting lung cancer as much as fivefold. Since a smoker's risk of getting lung cancer is approximately 10 times greater than that of a nonsmoker, an asbestos worker who smokes has up to a 50-fold greater chance of dying from lung cancer than does a nonsmoker who does not work with asbestos. An increase in exposure, expressed as concentration of asbestos and duration of exposure, appears to increase the lung cancer risk. Epidemiological data suggest that this relationship is linear; the data do not indicate the presence of an exposure threshold below which there is no increased risk.

Mesothelioma Approximately 1,600 cases of mesothelioma occurred in the United States during 1980, according to projections from cases reported in the 10% of the U.S. population monitored by the National Cancer Institute's Surveillance, Epidemiology, and End Results (SEER) program. Although exposure to asbestos has been strongly associated with most mesothelioma cases studied, some cases may occur without apparent asbestos exposure. The evidence does not exclude the possibility that ambient exposure to asbestiform fibers was associated with mesotheliomas for which exposure could not be documented. The percentage of workers with mesothelioma has ranged from 0 to 2% among chrysotile miners and chrysotile textile workers, but has been as high as 10% among workers who manufactured crocidolite-containing gas masks. The disease seems to be independent of smoking but related to dose and to time from first exposure.

Asbestosis. All types of asbestos appear to be implicated in the development of asbestosis. Data indicate that the incidence rate increases and the disease becomes more severe with increasing dust exposure, which is expressed as concentration of dust and duration of exposure. It is not clear whether an exposure threshold exists. Persons in the early stages of this condition may be free of symptoms, but beyond a certain stage the disease seems able to progress even in the absence of further exposure.

Pleural Thickening. Another nonmalignant pathological effect of asbestos exposure is the formation of fibrous and sometimes calcified plaques and diffuse thickening of the pleural lining of the chest cavity. Effusion of fluid into the pleural cavity may also occur. Such pleural thickening is suggestive of asbestos exposure but is rarely a cause of significant, direct respiratory impairment.

Gastrointestinal Cancer. Excess gastrointestinal (GI) cancers have been found among some cohorts of asbestos workers, but the excesses were usually substantially less than for lung cancer. Dose-response data are not available. Recent animal feeding studies have failed to demonstrate asbestos induction of GI cancers. Moreover, because of inherent limitations in the epidemiological studies, including the limited sizes of the exposed populations and the lack of individual exposure data, it has not been possible to determine from these studies the extent to which there may be an association between GI cancers in humans and the presence of asbestiform fibers in drinking water.

Health Effects of Nonasbestos Asbestiform Fibers

Some natural asbestiform substances other than asbestos seem to have biological effects similar to those of asbestos. For example, erionite, a fibrous zeolite, readily induces mesothelioma in animal tests, and populations living in central Turkey, where it is present in volcanic tuff, are reported to have an excess incidence of lung cancer, mesothelioma, and pulmonary fibrosis. As another example, epidemiological studies are being conducted on workers exposed to attapulgite, but as yet there are essentially no data on humans indicating whether it is toxic when inhaled.

Exposure to man-made mineral fibers is relatively recent, and the occupational exposure levels apparently have not been as high as those for asbestos. Some epidemiological data do suggest, however, that diseases of the respiratory tract, such as pulmonary fibrosis and lung cancer, may result from long-term occupational exposure to these fibers.

Evidence Associating Fiber Properties with Adverse Health Effects

Asbestos and other asbestiform fibers appear to react with cells in a variety of ways, They may alter normal cell function, they may cause cell death, or they may directly or indirectly alter the genetic information and the way cells replicate, Studies of cells lining the respiratory passages suggest that asbestos may act as a promoter (in the initiator/promoter model of carcinogenesis). The in vitro evidence that asbestos can damage DNA directly or be mutagenic to genes or chromosomes is weak and inconclusive.

Laboratory studies have not identified one type of asbestos as being more potent than others. In animal inhalation experiments, however, asbestos generally appears to be more pathogenic than most other asbestiform fibers that have been tested. At present, none of the available in vitro models can be used to quantify the relative fibrogenic or carcinogenic potential of asbestiform fibers either in animals or in humans. Interpretation of results is hindered by the failure of most reported studies to define the test materials precisely, by the paucity of experiments showing dose-response information, and by the differences in response among species and cell types.

Results of studies of various groups of workers indicate that it is extremely difficult to assess the role of fiber type (e.g., chrysotile or crocidolite) in determining the risk for developing either lung cancer or mesothelioma. Analysis of the epidemiological studies is complicated because of variations in type of industry, the diverse fiber characteristics within an industry, and the usual inadequacy of exposure data. Some of the apparent discrepancies may be explained by differences in physical properties of the fibers, their concentrations, and their characteristics in the different environments. These possibilities need further testing.

Risk Assessments

In general, three steps are necessary before one can assess health risk from environmental exposures: determination that a material is toxic and identification of adverse effects; determination of dose-response relationships; and determination of the extent of exposure. At least some types of asbestiform fibers are toxic and have identifiable adverse health effects. However, few occupational studies have demonstrated dose-response relationships, and there is great variability among those few studies. Estimates of exposure outside the workplace are particularly difficult to obtain, and it is the risk from such exposure that is the focus of this report.

Other factors that introduce uncertainty into risk assessments for nonoccupational exposures include assumptions about the magnitude of effects at low doses; differences in the characteristics of fibers in the occupational and nonoccupational environments, especially regarding size and composition; and differences in the populations exposed, age at onset of exposure, and duration of exposure.

In this report, risk assessments are limited primarily to mesothelioma and lung cancer as end points and to inhalation as the route of exposure. For asbestos, sufficient information was available for the committee to make quantitative estimates—albeit with great uncertainty—of the risk for lung cancer or mesothelioma after inhalation exposure. These risk assessments were conducted for a "generalized" asbestos exposure, rather than for exposure to a specific type of asbestos. However, the committee assumed that the risk estimates would also apply if chrysotile were the primary agent of exposure. For the other types of fibers considered, the committee made comparative, i.e., qualitative, risk assessments that were subject to yet greater uncertainty.

For the quantitative risk assessment, the committee concluded that the epidemiological data supported the use of a linear, no-threshold model. Dose-response data from workplace studies were used in developing the equations. To estimate nonoccupational exposures, measurements of the mass of asbestos in the ambient environment were converted to the number of fibers longer than 5 μm that would have been found in the workplace at a similar mass concentration.

These measured concentrations indicated to the committee that 0.0004 fibers/cm^3 was a reasonable level to use in the risk assessment. However, there could be specific circumstances, such as schoolrooms with flaking asbestos, where persons are exposed to higher levels for limited periods. If a person were to inhale air containing asbestos at an average of 0.0004 fibers/cm^3 throughout a 73-year lifetime, the committee's best estimate is that the lifetime risk of mesothelioma would be approximately nine in a million (range 0 to 350 per million, depending on assumptions regarding the relationship of dose to risk). The corresponding lifetime risk for lung cancer would be about 64 in a million for male smokers (range 0 to 290), 23 in a million for female smokers (range 0 to 110), and 6 and 3 in a million for male and female nonsmokers, respectively.

The risk for mesothelioma is greater than that for lung cancer among nonsmokers because of the strong dependence of mesothelioma risk on time since first exposure. Occupational studies indicate that mesothelioma usually first appears about 20 years after onset of workplace exposures and that the incidence increases rapidly thereafter. The calculations suggest that a given exposure to asbestos in childhood markedly increases the lifetime risk of mesothelioma compared with an equivalent dose later.

The risk estimates remain uncertain, especially because they are based on the assumption that the data on occupational exposures are transferable to the nonoccupational situation. Smaller fiber size in the ambient environment would probably tend to lead to lower risk.

The comparative or qualitative risk assessments for the other asbestiform fibers were based on chrysotile and lung cancer as the baseline case. Population risk for particular fibers was compared with the population risk for lung cancer from chrysotile. In making comparative risk assessments, the committee considered such factors as respirability, biodisposition, and intrinsic toxicity as they are related to population exposures and to individual risk. The materials considered were crocidolite, other asbestos fibers as a group, attapulgite, fibrous glass, mineral wool, ceramic fibers, and carbon fibers. (Appendix H of this report presents the qualitative assessments for each substance.)

The risks for developing lung cancer or mesothelioma as a result of exposure to the other materials considered by the committee were usually much lower than those for chrysotile, principally because of a lower potential for airborne exposure or because the fibers are less respirable—not because their intrinsic toxicity is necessarily less. For example, both ceramic and carbon fibers can be found in respirable size ranges and may have some biological properties similar to those of asbestos, but production and opportunities for exposure are low, although increasing. The materials with potentially greatest impact are fibrous glass and attapulgite because of their current large production volume and extensive use.

1

Introduction

Asbestos-associated diseases generally have been related to occupational exposures, such as those experienced by some miners, insulators, and factory workers (Doll, 1955; Gloyne, 1935, 1951; Merewether, 1930; Selikoff, 1979; Selikoff et al., 1964; Wagner et al., 1960). Recently, however, there has been concern that exposures to asbestos and related fibers may present a health hazard to the general public. Asbestos has been widely used in the United States for building materials and in other applications. Consequently, there is exposure co asbestos from many possible sources—in some schools and other public and private buildings, in ambient air,[1] and in drinking water (National Research Council, 1983; Sebastien et al., 1982; U.S. Environmental Protection Agency, 1980).

Because asbestos and other asbestiform fibers[2] appear to be ubiquitous, virtually everybody is exposed co some extent. During autopsy, asbestos fibers have been detected in the lungs of most urban residents studied (Churg and Warnock, 1977; Langer et al., 1971; Pooley et al., 1970; Wagner et al., 1982). However, reported concentrations of asbestos in urban air are usually considerably below the current U.S. occupational standard of 2 fibers/cm^3.

Exposure of the public is particularly worrisome because the populations involved are large and include unhealthy persons. Moreover, exposure may begin in childhood, leaving a longer time for development of adverse effects. Furthermore, asbestos may enhance the carcinogenic effects of other materials. mere is little information about the health effects of most nonoccupational exposures to these fibers.

Despite many epidemiological studies of workers and experimental studies on animals, questions remain about which properties of asbestos are responsible for the adverse health effects and which conditions of

[1] Ambient air is outside air to which the public is exposed (U.S. Environmental Protection Agency, 1982b).

[2] These include asbestos and other fibers with some of the same physical properties as asbestos.

exposure are most likely to lead to such effects. Certain other natural mineral fibers, as well as man-made mineral fibers sometimes used as substitutes for asbestos and for other purposes, might have similar deleterious effects (Artvinli and Baris, 1983; Stanton, 1974; World Health Organization, 1983).

The term "asbestos" refers to the fibrous form of several specific silicate minerals that have been used commercially. Because of its high tensile strength, flexibility, and resistance to heat and chemical attack, asbestos is used in many products, including asbestos-cement pipes, insulation, friction materials, and flooring and roofing tiles (Suta and Levine, 1979).

The consumption of asbestos in the United States has greatly increased during this century (Selikoff and Lee, 1978). Annual U.S. consumption peaked at about 800,000 metric tons in 1973 and 1974, but in 1982 it dropped to 250,000 metric tons, or about 6% of world production (U.S. Bureau of Mines, 1978, 1983). Figure 1-1 shows U.S. asbestos consumption by year since 1890 and cumulative consumption since 1905. The millions of tons of asbestos already in place provide an ongoing potential hazard to workers and the public.

The most serious health effects associated with exposure to asbestos are lung cancer, mesothelioma (an almost invariably fatal form of cancer), and asbestosis (a noncancerous but debilitating and sometimes fatal disease). In addition, other nonmalignant lung changes have been documented. Appendix A describes the chronology of the major observations documenting the relationship between asbestos exposure and disease.

Persons exposed to asbestos nonoccupationally can be at increased risk of contracting these asbestos-associated diseases. In one of the first studies linking asbestos exposure and mesothelioma, the disease was found among residents of a mining area in South Africa. These subjects had presumably inhaled the material in the surrounding air (Wagner et al., 1960). In another study, persons living in households with asbestos factory workers in New Jersey were reported to be at increased risk of asbestos-associated disease (Anderson et al., 1979).

The diseases usually become evident clinically 20 to 40 years after initial exposure, and may occur even in the absence of continued exposure. Thus, many current cases of diseases associated with asbestos exposure are primarily the result of occupational exposures that the individuals experienced many years ago. It has been estimated that up to several hundred thousand excess deaths could result over the next few decades from such exposures already experienced (Hogan and Hoel, 1981; Nicholson et al., 1982; Walker et al., 1983). Results of current exposures would be manifested as disease in the future.

Because of the long latent period, it is difficult to reconstruct exposure histories. Moreover, variations in particle size and in other

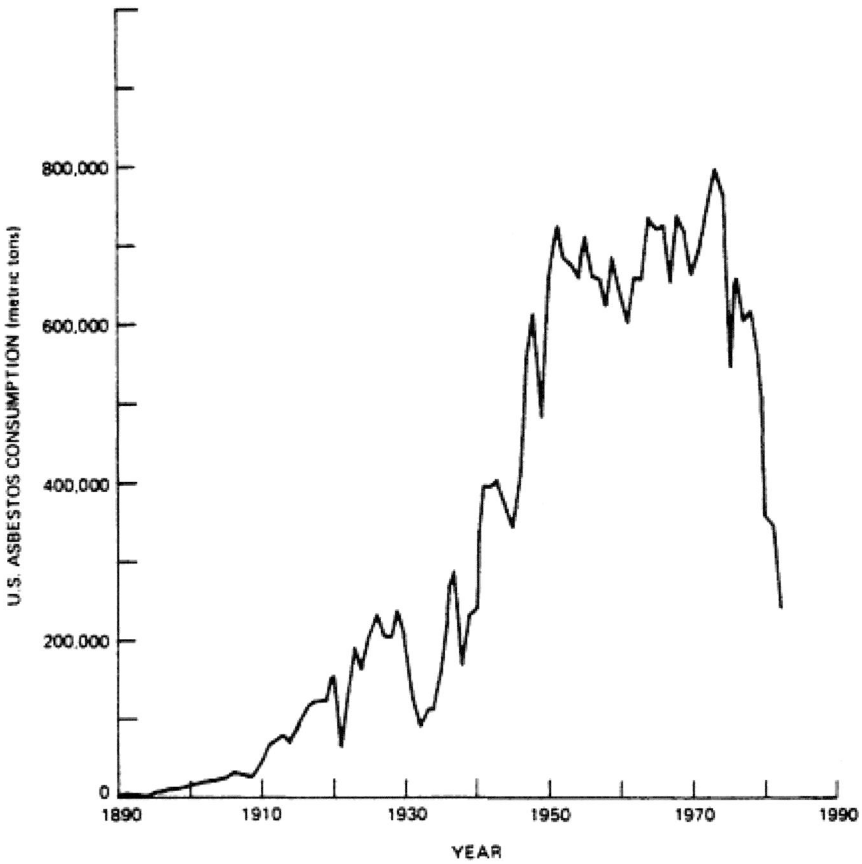

Figure 1-1A.
Annual U.S. consumption of asbestos from 1890 to 1982.

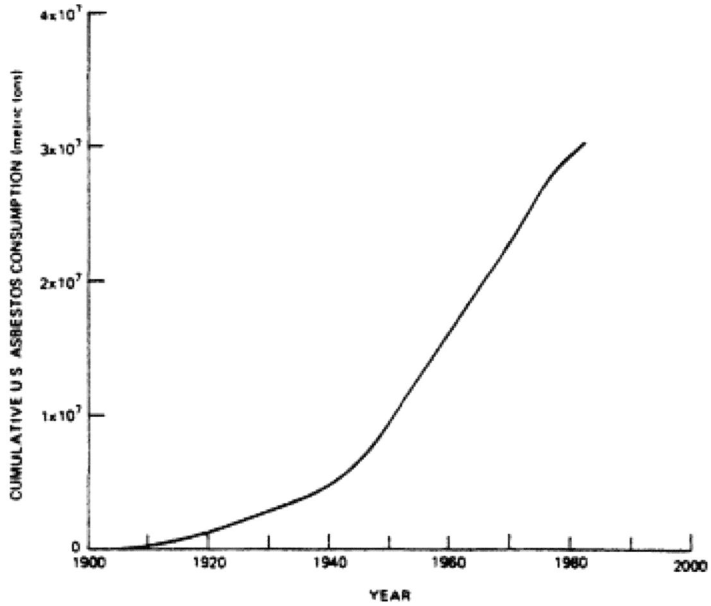

Figure 1-1B.
Cumulative U.S. consumption of asbestos from 1905 to 1982. Based on data from U.S. Bureau of Mines, 1973, 1978, 1983.

properties of asbestiform fibers may lead to different degrees of health risk from apparently similar exposure. The effects of exposure to the fibers may also be modified by other factors, such as smoking.

CONCURRENT NATIONAL RESEARCH COUNCIL AND GOVERNMENT ACTIVITIES RELATED TO ASBESTOS

While this committee carried out its task, numerous other efforts were under way to coordinate government activities and to summarize and interpret findings concerning the health effects of asbestos. The U.S. Environmental Protection Agency (1982a, 1983) issued reporting requirements related to asbestos in schools and reaffirmed its interest in limiting the amount of asbestos used in certain applications. In 1983 the EPA, the Occupational Safety and Health Association (OSHA), and the Consumer Product Safety Commission (CPSC) formed an interagency task force on asbestos to coordinate information-gathering and regulatory efforts concerning asbestos among the three agencies. For example, OSHA has for several years considered revising the permissible exposure limit for asbestos in the workplace. In 1976 the standard became 2 fibers/cm^3. An asbestos fiber for counting purposes means a particulate that has a physical dimension longer than 5 μm and a length-to-diameter ratio of 3:1 or greater (U.S. National Institute for Occupational Safety and Health, 1977, 1980). In early November 1983, OSHA issued an emergency temporary standard lowering the permissible exposure limit to 0.5 fibers/cm^3 (U.S. Occupational Safety and Health Administration, 1983), but a stay on the temporary standard was granted later in the month.

Asbestos as a health hazard was considered by the Chronic Hazard Advisory Panel (CHAP) on Asbestos, which was formed in January 1983 by the CPSC (Consumer Product Safety Act, 1981; U.S. Consumer Product Safety Commission, 1982, 1983). The panel was composed of persons nominated by the National Academy of Sciences. Its major purpose was to provide advice to CPSC on the risks of cancer associated with exposure to asbestos. The National Research Council (NRC) has also engaged in several activities related to asbestos. One was an analysis of data related to asbestos in drinking water, which was part of a study conducted by the NRC Safe Drinking Water Committee (National Research Council, 1983). The Committee on Nonoccupational Health Risks of Asbestiform Fibers was able to draw upon the findings of the CHAP and NRC reports and on other draft documents.

Another NRC activity is an ongoing study to identify and solve problems related to asbestos exposure in federal buildings. This report is being prepared by the Federal Construction Council Consulting Committee on Asbestos under the NRC Advisory Board on the Built Environment (National Research Council, in press).

THE COMMITTEE'S APPROACH

To study the health effects of nonoccupational exposure to asbestiform fibers, this committee took as its overview a "chain of events" depicted in Figure 1-2. This figure shows that fibers may occur naturally or be synthesized and that exposure of humans may result from either commercial or environmental "flows." These human exposures may then lead to biological reactions and adverse health effects.

While recognizing the difficulties involved in interpreting data related to health effects of asbestiform fibers, the committee considered the following questions:

1. What are the major sources of nonoccupational exposure to asbestiform fibers, and how great are such exposures?
2. Which properties of the fibers Seem to be most closely associated with adverse health outcomes? These properties may include length, diameter, chemistry, strength, durability, mass, and surface characteristics.
3. Is it possible to distinguish different levels of carcinogenic and fibrogenic risks among the different types of asbestos fibers? The question is difficult to address by either epidemiological or laboratory studies, because virtually all samples of fibers contain a range of fiber sizes and other fiber characteristics may differ among the various studies. Thus, it is difficult to relate observed effects to specific types of particles.
4. To what extent can the data on occupational exposures be used to develop risk estimates for the general public?

In order to respond to its charge from EPA, the committee considered various routes of exposure, but placed emphasis on the inhalation route. To elucidate the relevant properties of the fibers responsible for the adverse health effects, it evaluated physical, epidemiological, and toxicological data related to asbestiform fibers. It also estimated the health risk for certain populations under various assumptions of exposure. Although many of the data reviewed in this study concern asbestos, the committee has drawn conclusions that encompass other fibrous materials as well.

The committee has not carried out an exhaustive review of the literature, but has concentrated instead on those data that are most relevant to the charge. It found many excellent reviews and collections of articles related to asbestos and other fibrous materials that have appeared in recent years. Among the documents that were most useful during the course of this study were those prepared by Selikoff and Lee (1978), Washer (1980), Craighead and Hossman (1982), Walton (1982), and papers from a conference on biological effects of man-made mineral

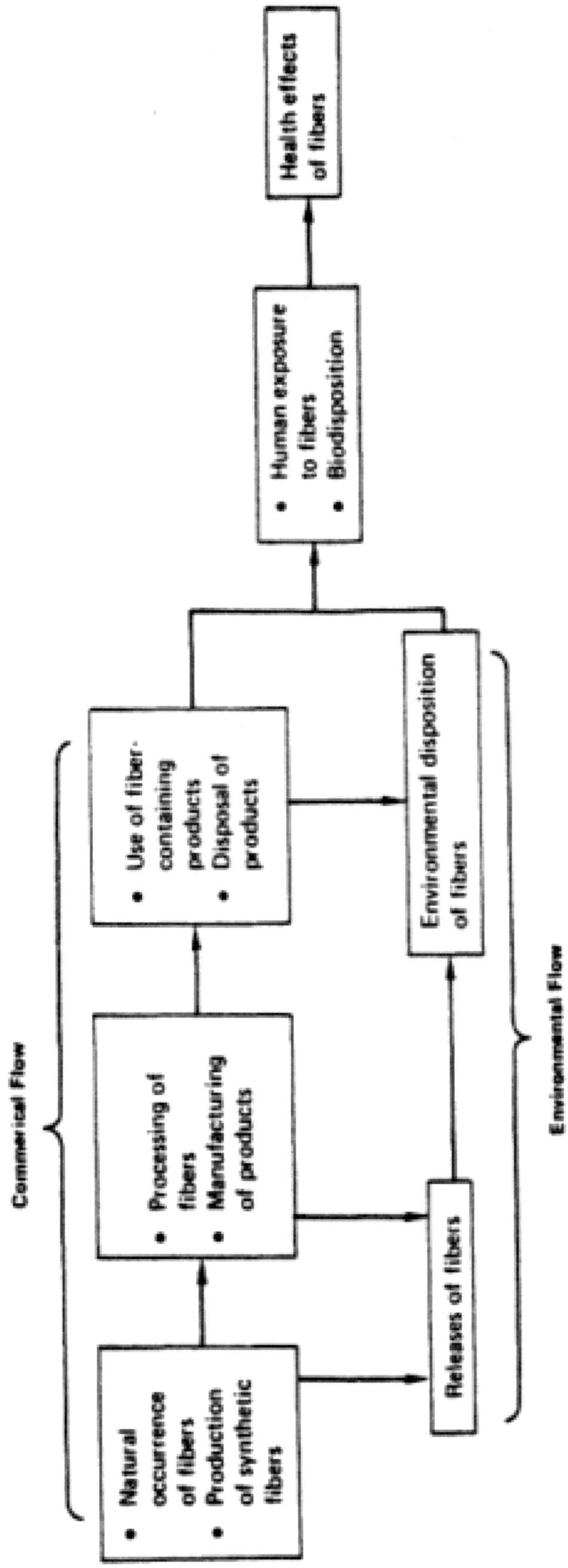

Figure 1-2.
The chain of phenomena leading to the health effects of asbestiform fibers. The three boxes on the upper line represent commercial flow, whereas the lower boxes show environments! flow. Either flow, if not controlled, may lead to human exposure and adverse health effects.

fibers, which was held in Copenhagen in April 1982. The proceedings of that conference have been summarized by the World Health Organization (1983).

The succession of chapters in this report reflects a logical sequence for pursuing this study. First, the committee defined the kinds of materials it was considering and described some of their properties. It then assessed exposure to these materials. Its next step was to consider the various ways of determining the amounts of fibers both in the workplace and in the ambient environment and to evaluate epidemiological and laboratory data. Finally, it integrated data from exposure, epidemiological and laboratory studies in order to make quantitative and comparative risk assessments.

REFERENCES

Anderson, H. A., R. Lilis, S. M. Daum, and I. J. Selikoff. 1979. Asbestosis among household contacts of asbestos factory workers. Ann. N.Y. Acad. Sci. 330:387-399.

Artvinli, M., and Y. I. Baris. 1982. Environmental fiber-induced pleuro-pulmonary diseases in an Anatolian village: An epidemiologic study. Arch. Environ. Health 37:177-181.

Churg, A., and M. L. Warnock. 1977. Correlation of quantitative asbestos body counts and occupation in urban patients. Arch. Pathol. Lab. Med. 101:629-634.

Consumer Product Safety Act. 1981. Section 1206 of the Omnibus Budget Reconciliation Act of 1981 (P.L. 97-35; 15 U.S.C. 2077, as amended).

Craighead, J. E., and B. T. Mossman. 1982. The pathogenesis of asbestos-associated diseases. N. Engl. J. Med. 306:1446-1455.

Doll, R. 1955. Mortality from lung cancer in asbestos workers. Br. J. Ind. Med. 12:81-86.

Gloyne, S. R. 1935. Two cases of squamous carcinoma of the lung occurring in asbestosis. Tubercle 14:445-451.

Gloyne, S. R. 1951. Pneumoconiosis. A historical survey of necropsy material in 1205 cases. Lancet 1:810-814.

Hogan, M.D., and D. G. Hoel. 1981. Estimated cancer risk associated with occupational asbestos exposure. Risk Analysis 1: 67-79.

Langer, A. M., V. Baden, E. C. Hammond, and I. J. Selikoff. 1971. Inorganic fibers including chrysotile in lungs at autopsy: Preliminary report. Pp. 683-694 in W. H. Walton, ed. Inhaled Particles III. The Gresham Press , Surrey.

Levine, R. J., ed. 1978. Asbestos: An Information Resource. U.S. Department of Health, Education, and Welfare, Public Health Service, National Institutes of Health.

Merewether, E. R. A. 1930. The occurrence of pulmonary fibrosis and other pulmonary affections in asbestos workers. J. Ind. Hyg. 12:198-222, 239-257.

National Research Council. 1983. Drinking Water and Health. Vol. 5. A report of the Safe Drinking Water Committee, Commission on Life Sciences. National Academy Press, Washington, D.C.

National Research Council. In press. Identifying and solving asbestos problems in existing federal buildings. Draft report of the Federal Construction Council Consulting Committee on Asbestos. National Academy Press, Washington, D.C.

Nicholson, W. J., G. Perkel, and I. J. Selikoff. 1982. Occupational exposure to asbestos: Population at risk and projected mortality—1980-2030. Am. J. Ind. Med. 3:259-311.

Pooley, F. D., P. D. Oldham, U. Chang-Hyun, and J. C. Wagner. 1970. The detection of asbestos in tissues. Pp. 108-116 in H. A. Shapiro, ed. Pneumoconiosis. Proceedings of the International Conference in Johannesburg. Oxford University Press, Cape Town.

Sebastien, P., J. Bignon, and M. Martin. 1982. Indoor airborne asbestos pollution: From the ceiling and the floor. Science 216: 1410-1413.

Selikoff, I. J. 1979. Mortality experience of insulation workers in the United States and Canada, 1943-1976. Ann. N.Y. Acad. Sci. 330: 91-116.

Selikoff, I. J., and D. K. Lee. 1978. Asbestos and Disease. Academic Press, New York. 549 pp.

Selikoff, I. J., J. Churg, and E. C. Hammond. 1964. Asbestos exposure and neoplasia. J. Am. Med. Assoc. 188:22-26.

Stanton, M. F. 1974. Fiber carcinogenesis: Is asbestos the only hazard? J. Natl. Cancer Inst. 52:633-634.

Suta, B. E., and R. J. Levine. 1979. Nonoccupational asbestos emissions and exposures. Pp. 171-205 in L. Michaels and S. S. Chissick, eds. Asbestos. Properties, Applications, and Hazards. Vol. 1. John Wiley & Sons, New York.

U.S. Bureau of Mines. 1973. Minerals Yearbook 1972. Bureau of Mines, Department of the Interior, Washington, D.C.

U.S. Bureau of Mines. 1978. Asbestos. Minerals Yearbook 1977. Bureau of Mines, Department of Interior, Washington, D.C.

U.S. Bureau of Mines. 1983. Asbestos. Preprint from the 1982 Minerals Yearbook. Bureau of Mines, Department of the Interior, Washington, D.C.

U.S. Consumer Product Safety Commission. 1982. Chronic hazard advisory panel on asbestos; invitation to submit suggestions for scientists to serve as members. Fed. Regist. 47:17323-17324.

U.S. Consumer Product Safety Commission. 1983. Report by the Chronic Hazard Advisory Panel on Asbestos. Consumer Product Safety Commission, Washington, D.C.

U.S. Environmental Protection Agency. 1980. Asbestos-Containing Materials in Schools. Health Effects and Magnitude of Exposure. Support document for proposed rule 6 on friable asbestos-containing materials in school buildings. Office of Pesticides and Toxic Substances, Environmental Protection Agency, Washington, D.C.

U.S. Environmental Protection Agency. 1982a. Asbestos; friable asbestos-containing materials in schools; identification and notification. Fed. Regist. 47:23360-23389.

U.S. Environmental Protection Agency. 1982b. National primary and secondary ambient air quality standards. Definitions. Code of Federal Regulations, Title 21, Part 50.1.

U.S. Environmental Protection Agency. 1983. Rules restricting the commercial and industrial use of asbestos fibers. Fed. Regist. 48:47880.

U.S. National Institute for Occupational Safety and Health. 1977. Asbestos Fibers in Air. NIOSH Manual of Analytical Methods. Second Edition. Vol. 1. National Institute for Occupational Safety and Health, Cincinnati.

U.S. National Institute for Occupational Safety and Health. 1980. Workplace Exposure to Asbestos. NIOSH-OSHA Asbestos Work Group. NIOSH Pub. No. 81-103. National Institute for Occupational Safety and Health, Cincinnati.

U.S. Occupational Safety and Health Administration, 1983. Occupational exposure to asbestos: Emergency temporary standard. Fed. Regist. 48:51086-51140.

Wagner, J. C., ed. 1980. Biological Effects of Mineral Fibres. Vols. 1 and 2. IARC Scientific Pub. No. 30. International Agency for Research on Cancer, Lyon. 1001 pp.

Wagner, J. C., C. A. Sleggs, and P. Marchand. 1960. Diffuse pleural mesothelioma and asbestos exposure in the North Western Cape Province. Br. J. Ind. Med. 17:260-271.

Wagner, J. C., G. Berry, and F. D. Pooley. 1982. Mesothelioma and asbestos type in asbestos textile workers: A study of lung contents. Br. Med. J. 285:603-606.

Walker, A. M., J. E. Loughlin, E. R. Friedlander, K. J. Rothman, and N. A. Dreyer. 1983. Projections of asbestos-related disease 1980-2009. J. Occup. Med. 25:409-425.

Walton, W. H. 1982. The nature, hazards and assessment of occupational exposure to airborne asbestos dust: A review. Ann. Occup. Hyg. 25:117-247.

World Health Organization. 1983. Biological Effects of Man-Made Mineral Fibers. Report on a WHO/IARC Meeting, Copenhagen, April 20-22, 1982. EURO Reports and Studies No. 81. World Health Organization, Copenhagen.

2

Asbestiform Fibers: Historical Background, Terminology, and Physicochemical Properties

Unlike many environmental substances that are discrete entities definable by a fixed chemical structure, asbestiform fibers comprise a group of materials that are less easily defined. They have a broad range of chemical compositions and crystal structures, sizes, shapes, and properties, and have been described with diverse terminology. These factors have led to some difficulties in studying and classifying the effects of these materials over the years. This chapter provides a brief historical overview of asbestos use, defines some of the mineralogical terms related to asbestos and other asbestiform fibers, describes the physical properties that characterize these fibers, and then discusses the biological relevance of the various physicochemical properties.

As used in this report, the term asbestiform fibers includes fibers that possess great strength and flexibility, durability, a surface structure relatively free of defects, and several other properties described later. Commercial quality asbestos is an example of an asbestiform fiber.

ASBESTOS IN HISTORY

In some ways asbestos resembles organic material, such as hair or cotton, more than it resembles minerals. Some ancient philosophers apparently had difficulty deciding whether asbestos should be considered a plant or a stone. Plinius (77 A.D.) compromised and referred to asbestos as "linum vivum" (durable linen). He postulated that it was originally a plant that adopted partial mineralogical properties to survive at high temperatures.

Asbestos has been used at least from the beginning of recorded history. The Egyptians used asbestos as embalming cloth; the Romans used it for cremation wrappings and for everlasting wicks in the lamps of the Vestal Virgins. Charlemagne is supposed to have had an asbestos tablecloth that he cleaned after feasts by tossing it into the flames of a fireplace. Marco Polo reported that asbestos clothing was used in China. In 1647, de Boot gave a recipe for a "miraculous asbestos ointment" to cure various infectious skin diseases (Figure 2-1).

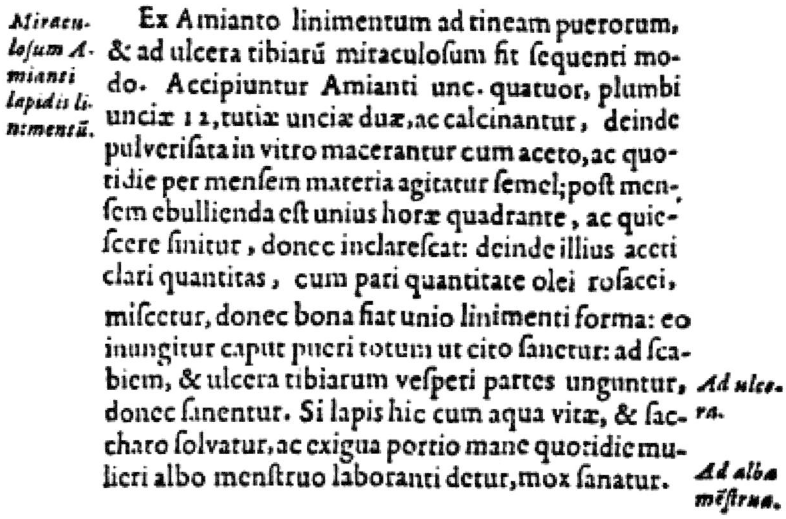
Miraculoſum Amianti lapidis linimentũ.
Ex Amianto linimentum ad tineam puerorum, & ad ulcera tibiarũ miraculoſum fit ſequenti modo. Accipiuntur Amianti unc. quatuor, plumbi unciæ 12, tutiæ unciæ duæ, ac calcinantur, deinde pulveriſata in vitro macerantur cum aceto, ac quotidie per menſem materia agitatur ſemel; poſt menſem ebullienda eſt unius horæ quadrante, ac quieſcere ſinitur, donec inclareſcat: deinde illius aceti clari quantitas, cum pari quantitate olei roſacei, miſcetur, donec bona fiat unio linimenti forma: eo inungitur caput pueri totum ut cito ſanetur: ad ſcabiem, & ulcera tibiarum veſperi partes unguntur, donec ſanentur. Si lapis hic cum aqua vitæ, & ſaccharo ſolvatur, ac exigua portio mane quotidie mulieri albo menſtruo laboranti detur, mox ſanatur.
Ad ulcera.
Ad alba mẽſtrua.

Figure 2-1.
de Boot's recipe from 1647 for an asbestos ointment. Roughly translated, it states: Multiple application, miraculous asbestos ointment for juvenile "tinea" (head-fungus?) and shinbone (skin?) ulcer. Take 4 oz asbestos, 12 oz lead (oxide?), 2 oz zinc oxide, and calcinate. Thereupon pulverize into glass while adding vinegar, and agitate it daily for a month. After a month, boil it for a quarter hour and let it cure until it becomes clear. Thereafter, add some vinegar, mix it with rose-petal oil until it becomes a homogeneous ointment.... From Zoltai, 1978.

Most of these and other early applications of asbestos were relatively isolated examples. Asbestos was not available in large enough amounts for widespread use until the extensive Canadian deposits were discovered lace in the 19th century. Subsequently, asbestos came into wide use for insulation, reinforcement of tiles and cements, and as an absorbent, thickener, and filler.

MINERALOGICAL TERMINOLOGY

Before discussing the properties associated with asbestiform fibers, a few definitions are provided. A MINERAL is usually defined as a naturally occurring inorganic and crystalline substance having a definite chemical composition and crystal structure. A mineral name usually ends in "-ite."

VARIETIES of minerals are distinguished when the physical appearance or properties of a mineral are modified by minor changes in chemical composition, crystal structure, and conditions of crystallization.

The term ASBESTOS is a commercial-industrial term rather than a mineralogical term. It refers to well-developed and hairlike long-fibered varieties of certain minerals that satisfy particular industrial needs. Table 2-1 lists the names and chemical formulas of the minerals included in the term asbestos. Other minerals used in industry, such as

TABLE 2-1. Mineralogy of Commercial Asbestos

Commercial Name	Mineral Name	Mineral Group	Chemical Formula
Chrysotile	Chrysotile	Serpentine	$(Mg, Fe)_6(OH)_8Si_4O_{10}$
Crocidolite	Riebeckite	Amphibole	$Na_2(Fe_{3+2}(Fe_{2+})_3(OH)_2Si_{822}$
Anthophyllite	Anthophyllite	Amphibole	$(Mg, Fe)_7(OH)_2Si_8O_{22}$
Amosite	Cummingtonitegrunerite[a]	Amphibole	$Mg_7(OH)_2Si_8O_{22}$ $Fe_7(OH)_2Si_8O_{22}$
	Actinolitetremolite[b]	Amphibole	$Ca_2Fe_5(OH)_2Si_8O_{22}$ $Ca_2Mg_5(OH)_2Si_8O_{22}$

[a] Hyphenated mineral names, such as cummingtonite-grunerite, represent MINERAL SERIES. The minerals in the series are structurally identical but can contain variable proportions of two or more different cations in the same structural site. Thus, these mineral series may be regarded as solid solution series. The variable cations in the cummingtonite-grunerite series are magnesium and iron; most minerals in this series have both elements, totalling seven atoms per chemical formula. The end members are identified by the hyphenated names, e.g., cummingtonite, which contains seven atoms of magnesium per chemical formula, and grunerite, which contains seven atoms of iron.
[b] Although asbestiform tremolite and actinolite occur in nature, large commercially mined deposits are rare. However, actinolite asbestos is found as a contaminant of amosite from South Africa, and tremolite asbestos is found as a contaminant of some talc and chrysotile deposits.

palygorskite,[1] may also crystallize as well-developed, thin hairlike fibers (i.e., in the asbestiform habit), but they are not called asbestos.

The different kinds of asbestos belong to two groups of minerals: serpentine and amphibole. The most common asbestos, chrysotile, is a member of the serpentine group. Because of their layered silicate structure, serpentine minerals usually crystallize as thin platy crystals; however, some of them, e.g., chrysotile, occasionally crystallize as thin hairlike fibers. In chrysotile, the structural layers are curled up to form scrolls or tubes (see Figure 2-2).

All the other kinds of asbestos belong to the amphibole group. Their crystal structure is characterized by parallel chains of silica tetrahedra. Because of the strength of these chains, amphibole crystals are either prismatic or acicular (needlelike). The asbestiform varieties of amphiboles have essentially the same crystal structure as the nonasbestiform varieties. Figure 2-3 shows schematically the structure of amphibole crystals looking down the silica chains.

Historically, mineralogists have had difficulty recognizing that "asbestos minerals" are actually varieties of several other minerals. Thus, Werner's recognition in the 18th century that amphibole asbestos is a variety of amphibole mineral was an important contribution to mineralogy (Freiesleben, 1817). Chrysotile was not identified as a variety of serpentine until 1853. Amosite was not recognized as a mixture of asbestiform actinolite and grunerite until 1948, and the term "amosite" is still used as a trade name for some asbestos.

CRYSTAL refers to a solid with a highly ordered, periodic arrangement of atoms. The arrangement of atoms is called the CRYSTAL STRUCTURE. CRYSTALLIZATION HABIT refers to the distinct nature and shapes of individual crystals or aggregations of several crystals. The crystallization habit of a mineral is usually identified by terms describing its appearance, such as equant (equidimensional), filiform (hairlike), etc., according to the dominant geometric shape. The basic properties of minerals usually do not vary with different crystallization habits, but a noteworthy exception is the asbestiform habit.

ASBESTIFORM HABIT refers to the unusual crystallization habit of a mineral when the crystals are thin, hairlike fibers. Historically, the definition of the asbestiform habit was based primarily on appearance, and the properties were only implied. At present, the definition of asbestiform habit is often augmented to include a statement on the

[1] The term "attapulgite" is a commercial designation for materials that consist of asbestiform and platy palygorskite. Although the latter term is more precise mineralogically, in this report the committee generally uses "attapulgite" for consistency. Not all palygorskite (attapulgite) is asbestiform.

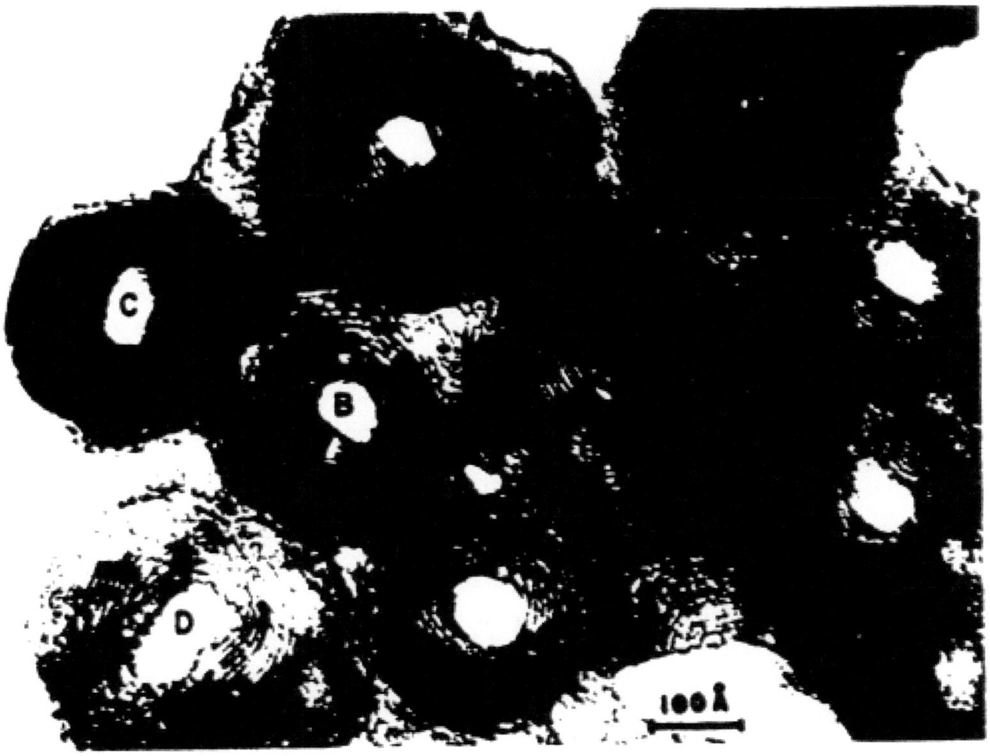

Figure 2-2.
Electron microphotograph of a cross section of chrysotile fibers displaying the scroll-like and tubular growth of the layered serpentine structure. From Yada, 1967.

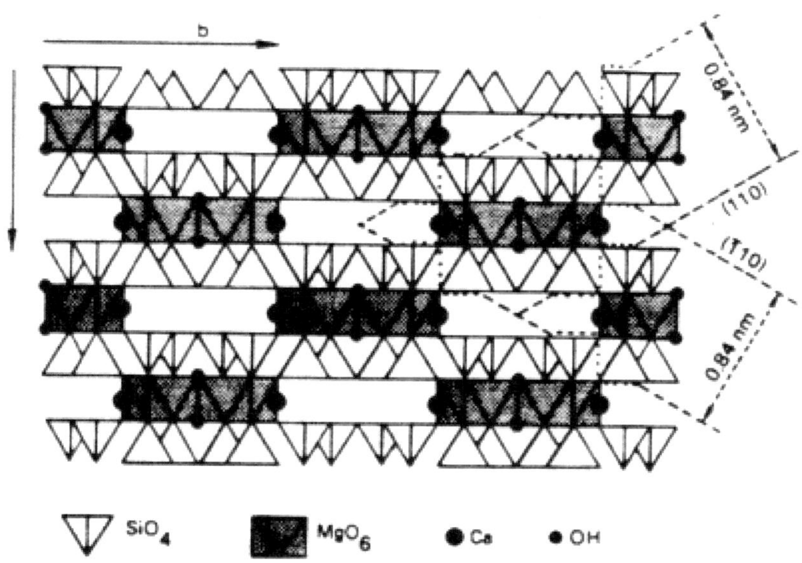

Figure 2-3.
Diagram of the structure and cleavage of amphibole crystals. Because of structural weakness, the crystal preferentially breaks along the (110) and (110) planes, parallel with the c-axis, yielding acicular fragments. From Zoltai, 1979.

properties of asbestiform fibers, i.e., shape; enhanced strength, flexibility, and durability; diameter-dependent strength; and unique surfaces. The fibers of asbestos are good examples of the asbestiform habit.

Asbestiform describes a special type of fibrosity. Fibrous is a broad term that includes, for example, asbestos as well as pseudomorphic fibrous quartz. Asbestos is composed of distinct fibers with unique properties, whereas most fibrous quartz breaks into odd shaped fragments unrelated to its apparent fibrous appearance. The proper use of mineralogical nomenclature for fibrous materials, particularly asbestos, and problems that have arisen from improper usage have been discussed in several reports (Campbell et al., 1977; Langer et al., 1979; Zoltai, 1978). Thus, the term asbestiform has been used in a variety of ways in the past, sometimes applying only to asbestos or to fibers that look like asbestos. This committee has developed and used a definition that is more circumspect mineralogically.

ACICULAR crystals are crystals that are extremely long and thin and have a small diameter. (An acicular crystal is a special type of PRISMATIC crystal. A prismatic crystal has one elongated dimension and two other dimensions that are approximately equal.) As defined by the American Geological Institute (1980), a mineral fragment must be at least three times as long as it is wide to be called acicular. Acicular crystals or fragments are not expected to have the strength, flexibility, or other properties of asbestiform fibers.

However, small diameter acicular crystals with a high aspect ratio may be ASBESTIFORM if they are strong and flexible. Larger diameter crystals, even if stronger and more flexible than the parent mineral, are usually described as FILIFORM or HAIRLIKE. The limiting upper diameter of whiskers (see definition below) is usually considered to be 15 μm; the same diameter may be used for the definition of asbestiform fibers.

FIBROUS refers to (1) single crystals that resemble organic fibers such as hair or cotton and (2) large crystals or crystalline aggregates that look like they are composed of fibers (i.e., long, thin, needlelike elements) (Dana and Ford, 1932). The apparent fibers do not need to be separable. If the fibers are separable and are strong and flexible, they are ASBESTIFORM. If they have the normal strength and brittleness of the mineral, they are ACICULAR. If the apparent fibers are not separable, the specimen may be a single crystal or a multiple (polycrystalline) aggregate displaying a fibrous pattern (resulting, for example, from striation or pseudomorphic replacement of an initially fibrous mineral).

The term MINERAL FIBERS has traditionally referred to crystals whose appearance and properties resembled organic fibers, such as hair and cotton. In some recent literature, however, the term sometimes refers only to the appearance of the material, and there can be confusion about whether particular properties are also implied.

CLEAVAGE refers to the preferential breakage of crystals along certain planes of structural weakness. Such planes of weakness are called cleavage planes. A mineral with two distinct cleavage planes will preferentially fracture along these planes and will produce ACICULAR fragments (Figure 2-3). Minerals with one cleavage plane produce PLATY fragments, and those with three or more cleavage planes yield POLYHEDRAL fragments. Minerals without cleavage planes fracture into IRREGULAR, nongeometric fragments. The strength and flexibility of cleavage fragments are approximately the same as those of single crystals. Cleavage cannot produce the high strength and flexibility of asbestiform fibers.

COMMINUTION is the breaking down of material into smaller (more minute) particles.

WHISKERS refer to synthetic crystals that share the properties of asbestiform fibers.

For more extensive definitions, see Campbell et al. (1977), Zoltai and Wylie (1979), and Walton (1982).

SOURCES OF MINERAL PARTICLES

Many types of mineral fragments are formed as the result of the constant weathering of rocks, as well as from various human activities. In general, the mineral composition of these particles approximately reflects the relative abundance of the minerals in the earth's crust. These particles are transported by water and air before being eventually deposited in unconsolidated sedimentary rocks, and the very small particles may remain in the environment (i.e., air and water) for extended periods.

A substantial proportion of these suspended particles have the apparent morphology of asbestiform fibers. However, most of these fiber-shaped particles are not asbestiform. For example, the suspended particles include elongated cleavage fragments of chain silicate and other minerals, such as the most common mineral, feldspar.

PHYSICAL PROPERTIES OF ASBESTIFORM FIBERS

A complete listing of the physical properties of asbestiform fibers would be very extensive. However, their common properties, as compared with nonasbestiform crystals of the same minerals, comprise a relatively short list:

- fiberlike morphology and dimensions
- enhanced strength and flexibility
- diameter-dependent strength
- increased physical and chemical durability
- improved surface structure (i.e., relatively free of defects)

In addition, the presence and the quality of these properties depends on the conditions present during fiber growth.

A continuum of these properties is possible. For example, "high quality" commercial asbestos has all these properties to a great extent, whereas other, more brittle fibers may have these properties to a lesser extent. Most whiskers and some amorphous materials, such as fibrous glass, may also have many of these properties, including fiber morphology, flexibility, and diameter-dependent strength. Therefore, in this report, some of the properties of asbestiform fibers are also assumed to apply to these other materials.

Many natural minerals, such as palysorskite (attapulgite), and some synthetic fibers have properties of asbestiform fibers to some extent. Appendix B lists many of these materials accompanied, in some instances, by brief comments related to human exposure or to health effects.

The properties listed above are discussed in the following section, primarily as they apply to asbestos.

Fiberlike Morphology

The shape of these fibers is characterized by small crystal diameter, by extreme length to width ratio (aspect ratio), and by smooth and parallel longitudinal faces. The longitudinal faces may be:

- rational crystallographic faces (indexable by lattice parameters) that are similar or identical to the prismatic faces of other crystals of the same materials;
- crystallographically irrational planes (not indexable by lattice parameters—one of the most unusual characteristics of high-quality amphibole asbestos fibers); or
- curved, scroll-like or tubular structures, as in chrysotile and carbon whiskers.

Although acicular crystals and acicular fragments may also display a high aspect ratio, that ratio is almost always small compared to that of asbestos, since nonasbestiform crystals are more brittle and break more readily across the longitudinal axis. Comminution of asbestos, especially the amphibole varieties, may also produce some fragments with length-to-width ratios very similar to those observed for acicular crystals and fragments, but these are usually only a small proportion of the total mineral mass and would still be expected to possess the properties of asbestiform fibers. At present, to determine whether a sample of particles seen in a microscope contains asbestiform fibers, it is senerally necessary to know the origin of the sample. However, on average, acicular fragments are shorter than asbestiform fibers (Campbell et al., 1979).

Enhanced Strength and Flexibility

Asbestos, whiskers, and fibrous glass with sufficiently small diameters have great strength and flexibility. The tensile strength of commercial quality asbestos fibers is 20 to 50 times greater than that of the nonasbestiform crystals of the same minerals. For example, the strength of grunerite crystals is approximately 1,000 kg/cm^2, whereas the strength of asbestiform grunerite (also called amosite) may reach 40,000 kg/cm^2. Whiskers and fine fibers of glass also possess extreme strength.

Although the usual crystals of most minerals are brittle and cannot be bent more than a few degrees, asbestiform fibers are highly flexible and may also be somewhat elastic. In general, measurement of the bending strength of fibers is an acceptable approximation of tensile strength.

Diameter-Dependent Strength

One of the properties shared by high quality fibers of asbestos, whiskers, and glass is their diameter-dependent strength. That is, the strength of the fibers per unit of cross-section area increases as the diameter decreases. Thus, the smaller the diameter of the fiber, the greater its strength.

The diameter-dependent variation in the strength of fine wires was first observed by van Müsschenbroeck (1729). In the ensuing centuries, similar observations were made by later investigators (e.g., Karmarsch, 1824; Gerstner, 1831), including famous bridge builders in the early 19th century (Dufour, 1823; Seguin, 1824; Telford, 1814).

An apparent strength-diameter effect was also observed in glass fibers by Threlfall (1890) and confirmed and quantitatively analyzed by Griffith (1921). The diameter-dependent strength of asbestos fibers was first studied by Nadgornyi et al. (1965). Later, the effect was observed in asbestiform varieties of other minerals by Maleev et al. (1972). Figure 2-4 illustrates the strength-diameter effect in fibrous glass and asbestos. Appendix C provides further discussion of the effect.

Increased Physical and Chemical Durability

Asbestos fibers are more resistant to physical stress than are nonasbestos varieties of the same mineral. For example, asbestiform fibers are much more difficult to grind to a powder in a mortar than are the corresponding nonasbestiform crystals. Furthermore, high quality amphibole asbestos does not possess prismatic cleavage planes.

Similarly, fibers of asbestos are more resistant to dissolution by acids than are other crystals of the same minerals. Thus, Walker (1981) noted that dissolution of grunerite cleavage fragments was initiated on all surfaces, whereas dissolution of the asbestiform grunerite fibers required stronger acid and began at the ends of the fibers—a process that resulted in the development of inverted cones at the end of the fibers. This observation suggests that the external structure of asbestiform fibers is more resistant to acids than is the internal structure. In many cases, the solid fibers became partially hollow cylinders before the surface dissolved. Glass and rock wool fibers also dissolve from the ends (Wojnárovits-Hrapka, 1977, 1978, 1979). (See Figure 2-5.)

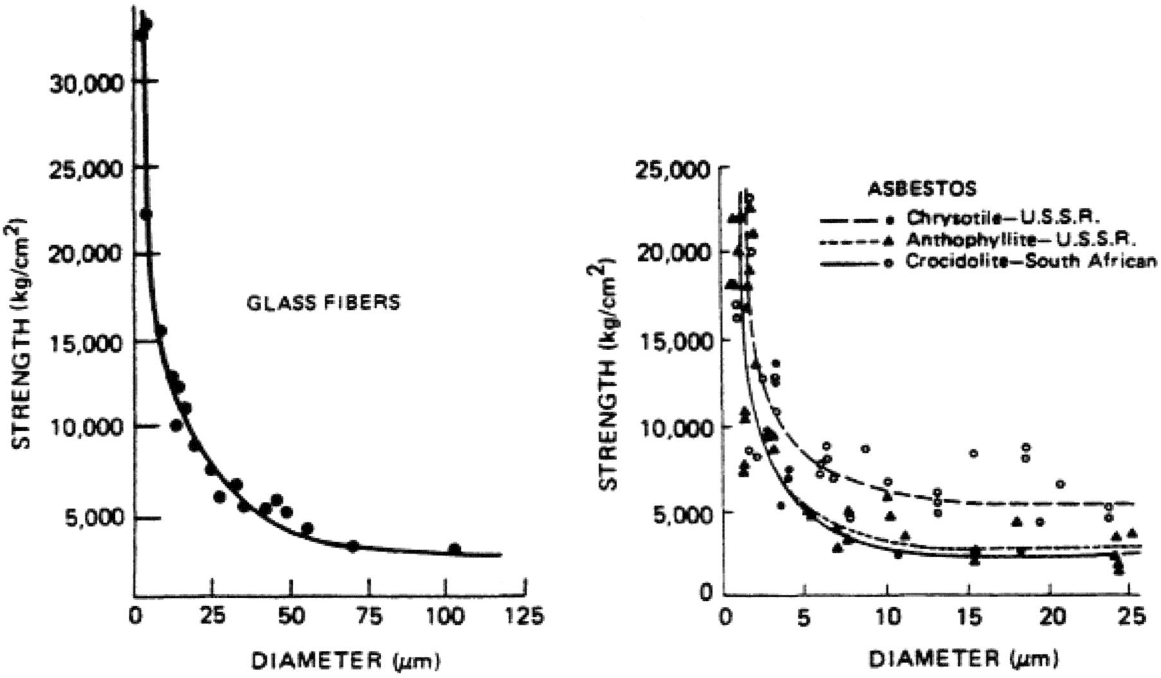

Figure 2-4.
Illustration of the strength-diameter effect. Data from Griffith, 1921 (glass fibers) and Nadgornyi et al., 1965 (asbestos).

Defect-Free Surface Structure

Many asbestos fibers have the shiny luster and high reflectivity indicative of a surface structure that is relatively free of defects. Investigators have noted the low density or the absence of surface defects in whiskers (Bokshtein et al., 1968; Brenner, 1956; Jones and Duncan, 1971; Mehan and Herzog, 1970; Webb et al., 1966) and in glass fibers (Bartenev and Izmailova, 1962; Griffith, 1921; Moorthy et al., 1956).

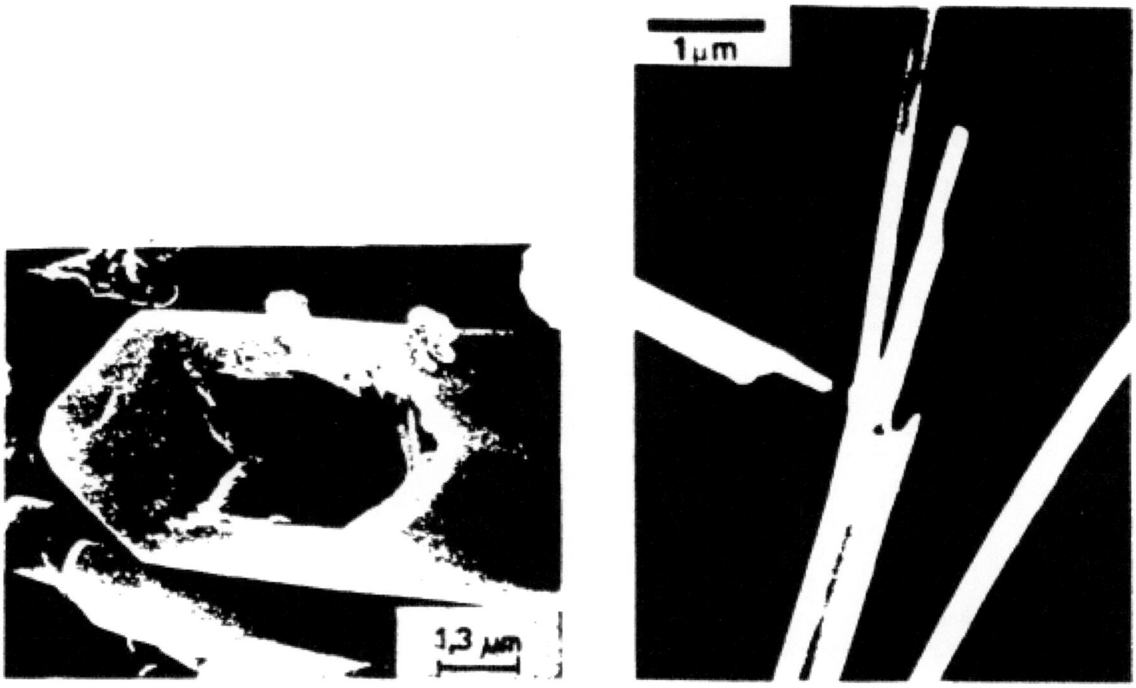

Figure 2-5.
The dissolution pattern of a glass fiber (from wojnárovits-Hrapka, 1977) and amosite fibers (from Walker, 1981).

The lack of surface defects may be partly responsible for the high strength of the surface layer of asbestiform fibers, The strength may also be enhanced by the differences in bonding between the internal and surface structures of these fibers (Gerstner, 1831; Griffith, 1921; Joffé et al., 1924; Orowan, 1933; Sella and Voigt, 1893; Weibull, 1939).

Growth-Dependent Fiber Quality

Although the conditions prevailing during crystallization can affect the physical and chemical properties of crystals, the effect is usually minor. However, the conditions of growth greatly influence the properties of asbestos, whisker, and glass fibers. A strong surface structure with relatively few defects can develop only when the crystal grows in only one direction. Such unidirectional growth can be achieved if, for example, there is unidirectional tension or sudden release of stress. In major asbestos deposits, therefore, the fibers usually crystallize parallel with tension and perpendicular to the wall of the fracture veins. In laboratories, whiskers are grown experimentally by creating various types of physical and chemical conditions that promote unidirectional growth (Wagner, 1970). Because the physical quality of the fibers depends on the growth conditions, fiber properties will vary as the growth conditions vary.

BIOLOGICALLY RELEVANT PHYSICOCHEMICAL PROPERTIES

The various pathological effects associated with asbestiform fibers are discussed in detail in Chapters 5 and 6. However, the properties of the fibers that may be relevant to those effects are introduced here, along with some of the evidence for their importance.

Respirability

Only fibers with mean aerodynamic diameters less than approximately 3 um enter the small airways. This feature is discussed in greater detail in the section on biodisposition in Chapter 5. See also Leineweber (1980), Timbrell (1965), and Walton (1982).

Size and Aspect Ratio (Length:Diameter)

Dimensional characteristics of fibers determine not only where they will deposit in the respiratory tract but also how a cell will respond to them. In animals, shorter fibers and particles may be engulfed by scavenger cells and thereby may be substantially prevented from interaction with other cell types. Thus, after being inhaled, these fibers may be present for extended periods in the cytoplasm of airway epithelial cells, in membrane-bound vesicles, or in macrophages (Mossman et al., 1977; Suzuki and Churg, 1969). Longer fibers, which are incapable of undergoing phagocytosis (i.e., being engulfed by cells), are associated with marked cytotoxic alterations in vitro in animals, but toxicity is reduced substantially when larger fibers are milled to smaller sizes (Brown et al., 1978; Kaw et al., 1982; Lipkin, 1980). Unfortunately, the reduction in toxicity cannot be attributed solely to the reduction in size, since milling also alters to some degree the crystallinity and surface features of the fibers, and these properties may also exert some effect (Langer et al., 1978). The greater toxicity of the longer fibers might be due to the inability of cells such as macrophages to engulf the fibers and/or inactivate the various sites on longer fibers.

In animals, a direct relationship between dimension and development of mesothelioma has been suggested by results of studies in which intrapleural, intrathoracic, and intraperitoneal injections have been administered. However, the appropriateness of extrapolating these data to humans is questionable in view of the massive dosages, species-specific variability, and different pathological findings, e.g., sarcomas and histiocytomas, in these animal studies. Moreover, although most mesotheliomas in humans seem to be associated with exposure to asbestiform fibers, spontaneous mesotheliomas appear in the mouse (Shapiro and Warren, 1949), rat (Hueper and Payne, 1962), and hamster (Fortner, 1961). These observations suggest that different mechanisms of disease induction may occur in various species.

Although data reported by most investigators show an increased risk of mesothelioma after exposure to long, thin fibers, in comparison to short, thick fibers, there does not appear to be a critical length below which fibers have no carcinogenic potential. For example, studies by Port and colleagues (1974) show that fiber preparations containing an overwhelming majority of fibers shorter than 5 um still possess measurable biological activity. Moreover, mesotheliomas have been induced by administering glass powder and other particulates, although the tumors occurred with less frequency than with long fibers (Wagner et al., 1973).

Bertrand and Pezerat (1980) used a new statistical approach to analyze the information generated by Stanton and colleagues (1977) from experiments using fibrous glass of various sizes. Bertrand and Pezerat suggested that carcinogenesis is a continuous increasing function of aspect ratio, but concluded that it is not possible to separate the effects of the two variables, length and diameter.

Durability

Many asbestiform fibers survive in biological systems for long periods. However, the physicochemical properties of asbestos and other fibers may undergo alteration after inhalation (Spurny et al., 1983). For example, the surface characteristics of fibers are modified after adsorption of surfactant and mucin; this coating reduces the cytotoxic properties of fibers (Desai and Richards, 1978; Harington et al., 1975; Jaurand et al., 1979; Morgan, 1974). In addition, fibers in general appear to undergo comminution or breakdown in the lung. The number of fibers per unit mass of asbestos also increases. Asbestos fibers tend to fragment longitudinally into thinner fibrils (Cook et al., 1982; Suzuki and Churg, 1969), whereas glass fibers cannot do so (Klingholz, 1977).

Chrysotile also is modified structurally after deposition in the lung, since magnesium ions (Mg^{++}), which contribute to both the structural integrity and positive surface charge of the fiber, are leached from the fiber (Jaurand et el., 1979; Langer et al., 1972). This leaching process apparently causes fragmentation of chrysotile and its faster disappearance from the lung in comparison to amphibole types of asbestos (Morris et al., 1967). Depletion of Mg^{++} decreases the cytotoxicity of chrysotile (Morgan et al., 1977) and the ability of this type of asbestos to cause mesothelioma in animals (Monchaux et al., 1981). The leaching of magnesium ions may alter the composition of chrysotile, but it does not tend to dissolve In tissues as glass does (Leineweber, in press).

Asbestos-related diseases, especially cancers, generally occur many years after first exposure. Autopsies and biopsies show that fibers are still present in the lungs and other tissues and often appear to be essentially intact years after the last known exposure. It is possible, therefore, that the exceptional physicochemical durability of asbestiform fibers is one of the basic requirements for their biological effects.

Flexibility and Tensile Strength

The relatively high flexibility of the asbestiform fibers enables them to bend without breaking and may facilitate their passage through the respiratory tract. Like asbestos fibers, fine-diameter glass fibers do not tend to break across their axes and are often as strong as asbestos. However, relatively large-diameter glass fibers tend to break perpendicularly to the fiber axis into "blocky" fragments. The flexibility of fibers is directly related to tensile strength.

Chemical Composition

The possible significance of certain elements contained in the chemical formulas of fibers in relation to disease is under study. In initial investigations of the health effects of asbestos, the chemical composition of the fibers was expected to be important. The most obvious candidate for the common chemical component was silicon, since all commercial forms of asbestos are silicates. The likelihood that silicon plays a role in carcinogenesis is minimized, however, by the exceptionally strong and almost indestructable bonding of silicon to oxygen in a tetrahedral structure. Furthermore, neither other silicates nor pure silica particles have carcinogenic properties similar to those of the asbestiform fibers (Churg, 1982).

Magnesium was next considered, since it is present in most asbestos and on the chrysotile surface. However, it was soon recognized that one of the major types of asbestos (asbestiform grunerite) contained relatively little magnesium and that another type (crocidolite) did not necessarily contain any magnesium in its chemical formula.

Although it has not been shown that chemical composition has a direct role in the pathogenic properties of asbestiform fibers, the chemical composition and structure obviously underlie many of the other properties of the fibers. Thus, chemical composition may play an important indirect role in determining which fibers exert pathological effects and what these effects are.

Some asbestiform fibers carry some foreign material on their surfaces and, in the case of chrysotile, in the centers of their fibrils. Zeolites also have large channels that may contain a variety of elements and compounds. These foreign materials could be carcinogenic, even if the host crystal is not.

Surface Area

The surface area of asbestiform fibers per unit volume is very large because of the small diameter of the fibers. Most commercial asbestos occurs in bundles that are broken open as the size of the unit mass is reduced. An increase in surface area and particle number then occurs. Several biological effects studied in the laboratory are related directly to an increase in fiber surface area. These include hemolysis by chrysotile (Schnitzer and Pundsack, 1970) and by amphiboles (Morgan et al., 1977; Schnitzer and Pundsack, 1970); cytotoxicity of chrysotile-when it is tested on alveolar macrophages from rabbits or humans (Yaeger et al., 1983); and general sorption of serum components (Desai et al., 1975). Presumably, an increase in surface area allows more cellular interaction, although the concomitant decrease in diameter may also play a role.

Surface Charge

Asbestos-induced cell damage appears to be initiated by a reaction of the plasma membrane that results either in cell lysis or in phagocytosis of the material (Mossman et al., 1983). The degree of cytolytic reactivity, as measured by a variety of techniques in vitro, including hemolysis and decrease in cell viability, is apparently dependent initially on the surface charge of the fiber (Light and Wei, 1977a,b; Reiss et al., 1980).

Red blood cells lyse after exposure to asbestos, and the release of hemoglobin can be quantified. The surface charge on fibers, as measured by the zeta potential, is related directly to the fibers' hemolytic activity (Light and Wei, 1977a,b). When chrysotile fibers are treated with acid, both the zeta potential and the hemolytic activity decrease. By contrast, the hemolytic potential for crocidolite increases as the fibers become more negatively charged. Schiller and colleagues (1980) have shown regional differences in surface charge on amphibole fibers. The charge characteristics of fibers also vary according to their size.

Standardized Asbestos Samples[2]

Samples of asbestos that come from different sources or have undergone modifications vary in many of the characteristics discussed.

[2] Much of this information was taken from an unpublished draft paper prepared by Paul W. Weiblen, University of Minnesota, 1983.

To facilitate comparisons of experiments and measurements among researchers throughout the world, five UICC standard reference samples for asbestos were prepared and partially characterized (Rendall, 1970, 1980; Timbrell, 1970; Timbrell and Rendall, 1972), The five half-ton samples and the mines they came from are: amosite (Penge, South Africa); anthophyllite (Paakkila, Finland); crocidolite (Koegas, NW Cape, South Africa); chrysotile A (Shabani, Rhodesia); chrysotile B (various Canadian mines). The samples were prepared by a specific blending and milling procedure. As tested by elutriator and cyclone, 67% to 87% of the fibers (by weight) have been reported as respirable (Rendall, 1970). For the four samples other than crocidolite, 8% to 15% of the fibers counted by electron microscope were reported to be longer than 10 μm; for crocidolite, 3% of fibers were found to exceed 10 μm in length (Timbrell, 1970). These samples do not completely satisfy all the current requirements for comparing biological and health effects of different asbestos samples, and it would be useful if a new set of standards were prepared taking into consideration all the fiber characterization criteria now considered important.

The U.S. Bureau of Nines has prepared and characterized samples of approximately one-half ton each of amosite, chrysotile, crocidolite, and nonfibrous tremolite for use in oral ingestion studies carried out by the National Institute of Environmental Health Sciences (Campbell et al., 1980).

SUMMARY

Asbestos is a generic name for the asbestiform variety of certain minerals that are used commercially. The term commercial asbestos encompasses five minerals: chrysotile, anthophyllite, riebeckite, cummingtonite-grunerite, and actinolite-tremolite. Many other minerals occasionally crystallize in the asbestiform habit and therefore may have the characteristic properties of asbestos.

Asbestiform fibers, including asbestos fibers, are mineral fibers that are characterized by a specific set of interdependent physical properties, including fiberlike shape, enhanced strength and flexibility, increased durability, strong and defect-free surface structure, and the dependence of these properties on conditions of growth.

The fiber properties that have been considered for possible association with deleterious health effects are respirability (i.e., fibers <3 μm diameter), size and aspect ratio, durability, flexibility and tensile strength, chemical composition, surface area, and surface charge.

Figure 2-6 and Table 2-2 illustrate some of the characteristics described above for fibers with progressively smaller diameters.

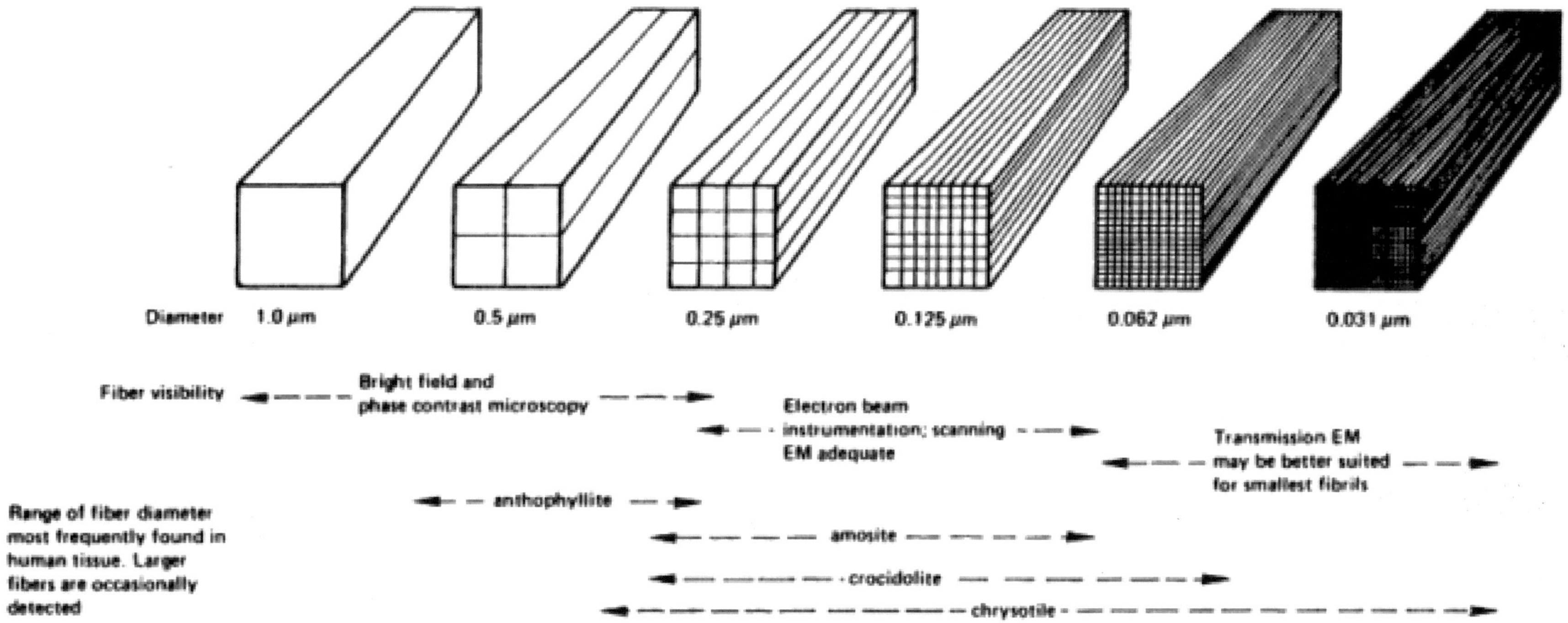

Figure 2-6.
Asbestiform fibers in different stages of comminution—the process whereby fibers are reduced to minute particles. A 1.0 × 1.0 × 8.0 μm fiber is the starting material. Each diameter is halved as the comminution process is carried through five cycles. Reduction down to 0.031 μm or 310 Å, as shown, is a reasonable size for a chrysotile fibril. EM = electron microscopy. Adapted from A. Langer, personal communication, 1983.

TABLE 2-2. The Effects of Comminution on Properties of Polyfilamentous Asbestiform Fibersa

Fiber Diameter (μm)	Fiber Number/mg[b]	Relative Time of Fall ($1/d^2$)[c]	Aspect Ratio (length/diameter)	Relative Surface Area[d]
1.000	4×10^7	1	8	4
0.500	1.6×10^8	4	16	6
0.250	6.4×10^8	16	32	10
0.125	2.56×10^9	64	64	18
0.062	1.024×10^{10}	256	128	34
0.031	4.096×10^{10}	1,024	256	66

[a] Adapted from A. Langer, personal communication, 1983.

[b] If mineral density is assumed to be about 2.80 g/cm^3, 1 mg of dust would contain approximately the number of fibers shown in this column for the diameter shown. The increase in particle number is about three orders of magnitude when length is constant and the diameter of individual particles is decreased to about 3% of initial value.

[c] Falling speed of a fiber is approximately inversely proportional to the square of the fiber diameter (l/d^2). A chrysotile fiber with a 0.03 μm diameter takes approximately 1,000 times longer to settle (neglecting other factors) out of an aerosol as compared to a 1-μm diameter fiber.

[d] Change in surface area with comminution. Units are relative. Ends of fiber not considered in these calculations. Relative surface area = 2N-2.

RECOMMENDATIONS

1. To facilitate communication among persons studying fibrous materials, mineralogical terminology should be used appropriately in all discussions and reports concerning fibrous materials. In particular, a distinction should be made between asbestiform fibers and elongated mineral particles that are not fibrous. When such a distinction cannot be made, it should be so stated.
2. Methods should be developed for both macroscopic and microscopic quantitative determination of the physical properties of fibers, such as their tensile strength.
3. In carrying out research to correlate the physical and chemical properties of fibers responsible for their pathological effects, the fibers should be characterized as completely as possible. Where studies are conducted to determine the effects of natural fibers, characterization should include such parameters as surface and internal fiber strength (discussed in Appendix C), surface charge, and density of surface defects.

REFERENCES

American Geological Institute. 1980. Glossary of Geology. R. L. Bates and J. A. Jackson, eds. American Geological Institute, Washington, D.C.

Bartenev, G. M., and L. K. Izmailova. 1962. Defect-free glass fibers. Dokl. Nauk. SSSR. Chem. Techn. Sect. 146:196-198.

Bertrand, R., and H. Pezerat. 1980. Fibrous glass: Carcinogenicity and dimensional characteristics. Pp. 901-911 in J. C. Wagner, ed. Biological Effects of Mineral Fibers, Vol. 2. IARC Scientific Pub. No. 30. International Agency for Research on Cancer, Lyon.

Bokshtein, S. Z., S. T. Kishkin, M. P. Nazarrova, and I. I. Svetlov. 1968. Size effect and anisotropy in the strength of sapphire whiskers at room temperature. Sov. Phys. Solid State 9:1488-1494.

Brenner, S. S. 1956. Tensile strength of whiskers. J. Appl. Phys. 27:1481-1491.

Brown, R. C., M. Chamberlain, D. M. Griffiths, and V. Timbrell. 1978. The effect of fibre size on the in vitro biological activity of three types of amphibole asbestos. Int. J. Cancer 22:711-727.

Campbell, W. J., R. L. Blake, L. L. Brown, E. E. Cather, and J. J. Sjoberg. 1977. Selected Silicate Minerals and their Asbestiform Varieties; Mineralogical Definition and Identification-Characterization. U.S. Bureau of Mines, Information Circular No. 8751. U.S. Bureau of Mines, Washington, D.C.

Campbell, W. J., E. B. Steel, R. L. Virta, and M. H. Eisner. 1979. Relationship of Mineral Habit to Size Characteristics for Tremolite Cleavage Fragments and Fibers. Report of Investigations No. 8367. U.S. Bureau of Mines, Washington, D.C.

Campbell, W. J., C. W. Huggins, and A. G. Wylie. 1980. Chemical and Physical Characterization of Amosite, Chrysotile, Crocidolite, and Nonfibrous Tremolite for Oral Ingestion Studies by the National Institute of Environmental Health Sciences. U.S. Bureau of Mines Report of Investigations No. 8452. U.S. Bureau of Mines, Washington, D.C.

Churg, A. 1982. Reaction of the lung to silica, silicates, and asbestos. Pp. 201-228 in Environmental Pathology: An Evolving Field. A. R. Liss, Inc., New York.

Cook, P. M., L. D. Palekar, and D. L. Coffin. 1982. Interpretation of the carcinogenicity of amosite asbestos and ferroactinolite on the basis of retained fiber dose and characteristics in vivo. Toxicol. Lett. 13:151-158.

Dana, S. D., and W. E. Ford. 1932. A Textbook of Mineralogy. J. Wiley and Sons, New York.

de Boot, A. B. 1647. Gemmarum et Lapidum Historia. Lugdunid Bataborum, Amsterdam. 550 pp.

Desai, R., and R. J. Richards. 1978. The adsorption of biological macromolecules by mineral dusts. Environ. Res. 16:449-464.

Desai, R., P. Hext, and R. Richards. 1975. The prevention of asbestos-induced hemolysis. Life Sci. 16:1931-1938.

Dufour, G. H. 1823. Description du pont suspendu en fil de fer construit à Genève. Bibl. Universelle 24:280-299.

Fortner, J. C. 1961. The influence of castration on spontaneous tumorigenesis in the Syrian (golden) hamster. Cancer Res. 21:1491-1498.

Freiesleben, J. C. 1817. A. G. Werner's Letztes Mineral-System. Craz and Gerold, Freiburg and Vienna.

Gerstner, F. G. P. yon. 1831. Handbuch der Mechanik. Vol. 1. J. Spurny, Prague.

Griffith, A. A. 1921. The phenomena of rupture and flow In solids. Philos. Trans. R. Soc. London, Set. A 221:163-198.

Harington, J. S., A. C. Allison, and D.V. Badami. 1975. Mineral fibers: Chemical, physicochemical, and biologic properties. Adv. Pharm. Chemother. 12: 291-402.

Hueper, W. C., and W. W. Payne. 1962. Experimental studies in metal carcinogenesis: Chromium, nickel, iron, arsenic. Arch. Environ. Health 5:445-462.

Jaurand, M. C., J. Bignon, P. Sebastien, and J. Goni. 1979. Leaching of chrysotile asbestos in human lungs. Correlation with in vitro studies using rabbit alveolar macrophages. Environ. Res. 14:245-254.

Joffé, A., M. W. Kirpitschewa, and M. A. Lewitzky. 1924. Deformation und Festigkeit der Kristalle. Z. Phys. 22:286-302.

Jones, B. F., and R. G. Duncan. 1971. The effect of fiber diameter on the mechanical properties of graphite fibers manufactured from polyacrylonitrile and rayon. J. Mater. Sci. 6:1225-1227.

Karmarsch, L. 1824. Versuche über die Festigkeit der zu Draht gezogenen Metalle. Jhrb. Polytech. Inst. Vienna 18:54-115.

Kaw, J. L., F. Tilkes, and E. G. Beck. 1982. Reaction of cells cultured in vitro to different asbestos dusts of equal surface area but different fibre length. Br. J. Exp. Pathol. 63:109-115.

Klingholz, R. 1977. Technology and production of man-made mineral fibres. Ann. Occup. Hyg. 20:153-159.

Langer, A. M., J. B. Rubin, I. J. Selikoff, and F. D. Pooley. 1972. Chemical characterization of uncoated asbestos fibers from the lungs of asbestos workers by electron microprobe analysis. J. Histochem. Cytochem. 20:735-740.

Langer, A. M., M. S. Wolff, A. N. Rohl, and I. J. Selikoff. 1978. Variation of properties of chrysotile asbestos subject to milling. J. Toxicol. Environ. Health 4:173-178.

Langer, A. M., A. N. Rohl, M. Wolff, and I. J. Selikoff. 1979. Asbestos, fibrous minerals and acicular cleavage fragments: Nomenclature and biological properties. Pp. 1-22 in R. Lemen and J. M. Dement, eds. Dusts and Disease. Pathotox Publishers, Park Forest South, Ill.

Leineweber, J. P. 1980. Dust chemistry and physics: Mineral wool and vitreous fibers. Pp. 881-900 in J. C. Wagner, ed. Biological Effects of Mineral Fibres, Vol. 2. IARC Scientific Pub. No. 30. International Agency for Research on Cancer, Lyon.

Leineweber, J. P. In press. Solubility of fibers in vitro and in vivo. Presented at the Biological Effects of Man-Made Mineral Fibers, Occupational Health Conference, Copenhagen, April 20, 1982. World Health Organization.

Light, W. G., and E. T. Wei. 1977a. Surface charge and hemolytic activity of asbestos. Environ. Res. 13:135-145.

Light, W. G., and B. T. Wei. 1977b. Surface charge and asbestos toxicity. Nature 265:537-539.
Lipkin, L. E. 1980. Cellular effects of asbestos and other fibers: Correlations with in vivo induction of pleural sarcoma. Environ. Health Perspect. 34:91-102.
Maleev, M. N., A. P. Krusilina, and V. N. Rosanckij. 1972. Ultimate strength of naturally fibrous rutile, antimony and jamesonite crystals. fin Russian] C. R. Acad. Bulg. Sci. 25:1085-1088.
Mehan, R. L., and J. A. Herzog. 1970. Mechanical properties of whiskers. Chapter 6 in A. P. Levitt, ed. Whisker Technology. Wiley Interscience, New York.
Monchaux, G., J. Bignon, M. C. Jaurand, J. Lafuma, P. Sebastien, R. Masse, A. Hirsch, and J. Gone. 1981. Mesotheliomas in rats following inoculation with acid-leached chrysotile asbestos and other mineral fibers. Carcinogenesis 2:229-236.
Moorthy, V. K., F. V. Tooley, and G. F. Stockdale. 1956. influence of water immersion treatment on tensile strength of glass: Effect of temperature. J. Am. Ceram. Soc. 39:395-398.
Morgan, A. 1974. Absorption of human serum albumin by asbestiform minerals and its application to the measurement of surface areas of dispersed samples of chrysotile. Environ. Res. 7:330-341.
Morgan, A., P. Davies, J. C. Wagner, G. Berry, and A. Holmes. 1977. The biological effects of magnesium-leached chrysotile asbestos. Br. J. Exp. Pathol. 58:465-473.
Morris, T. G., W. H. Roberts, Re E. Silverton, J. W. Skidmore, J. C. Wagner, and G. W. Cook. 1967. Comparison of dust retention in specific pathogen free and standard rats. Pp. 205-213 in C. N. Davies, ed. Inhaled Particles and Vapours, Vol. II. Pergamon Press, London.
Mossman, B. T., B. Ley, J. B. Kessler, and J. E. Craighead. 1977. Interaction of crocidolite asbestos with hamster respiratory mucosa in organ culture. Lab. Invest. 36:131-139.
Mossman, B., W. Light, and E. Wei. 1983. Asbestos: Mechanisms of toxicity and carcinogenicity in the respiratory tract. Ann. Rev. Pharmacol. Toxicol. 23: 595-615.
Müsschenbroeck, P. van. 1729. Physicae experimentales et geometriae. L. Batavorum and S. Lichtmans, Leiden.
Nadgornyi, E. M., L. F. Grigoreva, and A. P. Ivanov. 1965. The mechanical properties of synthetic fibrous fluoramphiboles and certain forms of natural asbestos. [In Russian] Izv. Akad. Nauk SSSR, Neoerg. Mater. 1:1117-1123.
Orowan, E. 1933. Die erhöhte Festigkeit dunner Faden, der Joffe-Effekt und verwandte Erscheinungen yon Standpunkt der Griffitachen-Bruchtheorie. Z. Phys. 86:195-213.
Plinius, Secundus, C. 77 A.D. Historia Naturalis. 27 books.
Pott, F., F. Huth, and K. Friedrichs. 1974. Tumorigenic effects of fibrous dusts in experimental animals. Environ. Health Perspect. 9:313-315.
Rendall, R. E. G. 1970. The data sheets on the chemical and physical propeties of the UICC standard reference samples. Pp. 23-27 in H. A. Shapiro, ed. Pneumoconiosis. Proceedings of the International Conference in Johannesburg. Oxford University Press, Cape Town.

Rendall, R. E. C. 1980. Physical and chemical characteristics of UICC reference samples. Pp. 87-96 in J. C. Wagner, ed. Biological Effects of Mineral Fibres, Vol. 2. IARC Scientific Pub. No. 30. International Agency for Research on Cancer, Lyon.

Reiss, B., S. Solomon, J. Weisburger, and C. M. Williams. 1980. Comparative toxicities of different forms of asbestos in a cell culture assay. Environ. Res. 22: 109-129.

Schiller, J. E., S. L. Payne, and S. E. Khalafalla. 1980. Surface charge heterogeneity in amphibole cleavage fragments and amphibole asbestos fibers. Science 209:1530-1532.

Schnitzer, R. J., and F. L. Pundsack. 1970. Asbestos hemolysis. Environ. Res. 3:1-13.

Seguin, M. 1824. D'Annonay: Sur la ténacité de fer. Ann. Chim. Phys. 25:109-111.

Sella, A., and W. Voigt. 1893. Beobachtungen über die Zerreissungsfestikeit yon Steinsalz. (Wied.) Ann. Phys. Chem. 48:636-656.

Shapiro, D. M., and S. Warren. 1949. Cancer innervation. Cancer Res. 9:707-711.

Spurny, K. R., F. Pott, W. Stober, H. Opiela, J. Schörmann, and G. Weiss. 1983. On the chemical changes of asbestos fibers and MMMFs in biologic residence and in the environment: Part 1. Am. Ind. Hyg. Assoc. J. 44:833-845.

Stanton, M. F., M. Layard, A. Tegaris, E. Miller, M. May, and E. Kent. 1977. Carcingenicity of fibrous glass: Pleural response in the rat in relation to fiber dimension. J. Natl. Cancer Inst. 58:587-603.

Suzuki, M. D., and J. Churg. 1969. Structure and development of the asbestos body. Am. J. Pathol. 55:79-107.

Telford, T. 1814. Experiments on the direct and transverse resistance of iron wire of different lengths and dimensions. Pp. 243-254 in Appendix to P. Barlow Essay on the Strength and Stress of Timber. Second Edition.

Threlfall, R. 1890. The elastic constants of quartz threads. Phil. Mag. and J. of Sci. Fifth Set. 30:99-116.

Timbrell, V. 1965. The inhalation of fibrous dusts. Ann. N.Y. Acad. Sci. 133:255-273.

Timbrell, V. 1970. Characteristics of the International Union Against Cancer standard reference samples. In H. A. Shapiro, ed. Pneumoconiosis. Proceedings of the International Conference in Johannesburg. Oxford University Press, Cape Town.

Timbrell, V., and R. E. G. Rendall. 1972. Preparation of the UICC standard reference samples of asbestos. Powder Technol. 5:279-287.

Wagner, J. C. 1970. VLS mechanism of crystal growth. Chapter 3 in A. P. Levitt, ed. Whisker Technology, Wiley Interscience Publications, New York.

Wagner, J. C., G. Berry, and V. Timbrell. 1973. Mesothelioma in rats after inoculation with asbestos and other materials. Br. J. Cancer 28:173-185.

Walker, J. S. 1981. Asbestos and the asbestiform habit of minerals. M.S. Thesis, University of Minnesota, Minneapolis.

Walton, W. H. 1982. The nature, hazards and assessment of occupational exposure to airborne asbestos dust: A review. Ann. Occup. Hyg. 25:117-247.

Webb, W. W., H. D. Bartha, and T. B. Shaffer. 1966. Strength characteristics of whisker crystals, microcrystals and macrocrystals. Chapter 14 in J. J. Burke, N. L. Reed, and V. Weiss, eds. Strengthening Mechanism. Syracuse University Press.

Weibull, W. 1939. A statistical theory of the strength of materials. The Phenomenon of Rupture of Solids. Proc. No. 151 and 153. Ing. Vetensk. Akad., Stockholm.

Wojnárovits-Hrapka, I. 1977. Structural examination of inorganic fibrous materials. Part I. [In Hungarian] Epitoanyag 29:498-503.

Wojnárovits-Hrapka, I. 1978. Structural examination of inorganic fibrous materials. Part II. [In Hungarian] Epitoanyag 30:13-18.

Wojnárovits-Hrapka, I. 1979. Crystallization of synthetic inorganic fibers used for thermal insulation. Epitoanyag 31:281-286, 361-366, 422-429.

Yada, K. 1967. Study of chrysotile asbestos by a high resolution electron microscope. Acta Crystallogr. 23:704-707.

Yaeger, H., Jr., D. A. Russo, M. Yanez, D. Gerardi, R. P. Nolan, E. Kagan, and A. M. Langer. 1983. Cytotoxicity of a shore-fiber chrysotile asbestos for human alveolar macrophages: Preliminary observations. Environ. Res. 30:224-232.

Zoltai, T. 1978. History of asbestos-related mineralogical terminology. Pp. 1-18 in C. C. Gravatt, P. D. La Fleur, and K. F. J. Heinrich, eds. Proceedings of a Workshop on Asbestos: Definitions and Measurement Methods, July 18-20, 1977. NBS Spec. Pub. No. 506. National Bureau of Standards, Gaithersburg, Md.

Zoltai, T. 1979. Asbestiform and acicular mineral fragments. Ann. N.Y. Acad. Sci. 330:621-643.

Zoltai, T., and A. G. Wylie. 1979. Definitions of asbestos-related mineralogical terminology. Ann. N.Y. Acad. Sci. 330:101-109.

3

Assessing Nonoccupational Exposures to Asbestiform Fibers

Lack of information about exposure is often the major impediment to assessing health risks associated with environmental substances. In this chapter, the committee defines exposure and explores the sources of asbestiform fibers, both naturally occurring and man-made. It also describes the general movement of fibers in commerce and in the nonoccupational environment, notes the difficulties in determining amounts of fibers and in defining exposure, presents descriptive estimates of exposure levels and of the numbers of people exposed to various fiber types, and discusses the magnitude and significance of uncertainties about exposures to asbestiform fibers. In discussing the various types of fibers, asbestos is described first to provide perspective for the discussion of the other fibers.

DEFINITIONS OF EXPOSURE

To understand the extent of current and future health risks from exposures to substances of concern, it is necessary to characterize past, current, and projected future exposures. Information on past exposures serves as a guide for interpreting observed health impacts in epidemiological research and as a basis for estimating cumulative exposures. Information on current and projected future exposures provides information useful in making decisions about regulating exposure levels.

The goal of exposure assessment is to estimate the distribution of various levels of exposure over a population or subpopulation so that the information can be integrated with data on the substance's toxicity. Figure 3-1 provides one example of a distribution of asbestos exposure for some urban populations (Suta and Levine, 1979). In that example, exposure is expressed as units of mass per unit volume of air. Exposure information on asbestos is also often expressed by using the fiber concentration in air or water (fibers/cm^3 or fibers/liter, respectively) and the duration and pattern of exposure (e.g., 40 hours/week, 48 weeks/year, for 23 years).

Attempts at exposure assessment involve many assumptions, complications, and difficulties. To characterize exposures completely, one would like to know:

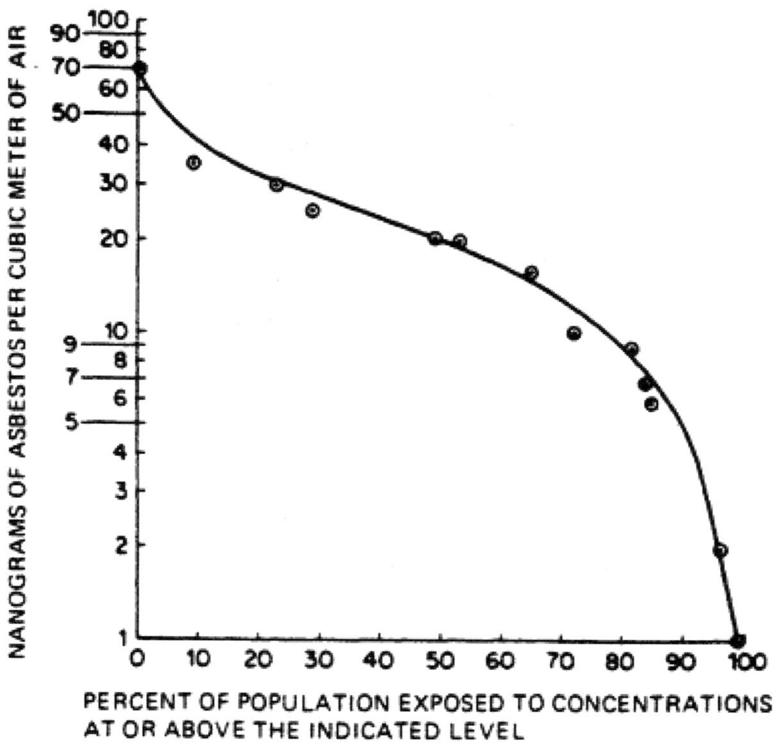

Figure 3-1.
Distribution of exposures to asbestos in ambient air of urban areas. From Suta and Levine, 1979.

- Who is exposed?
  - age
  - sex
  - race
  - health status
  - other exposures, e.g., tobacco smoke

- To which fibers are they exposed?
  - type of fiber
  - dimensions of fibers
  - other fiber characteristics

- How are they exposed?
  - occupational
  - community (near known sources of material of concern)
  - consumer use of manufactured products
  - general environmental

- By what routes?
  - respiratory
  - oral
  - other

- What pattern?
  - daily peak intake
  - annual fiber intake
  - cumulative fiber intake
  - cumulative exposure, e.g., fibers/cm^3 times number of years
  - concentration of exposure, e.g., fibers/cm^3 or fibers/liter

- How frequently, and how long?
  - continuously
  - regular, periodic, e.g., 8 hours/workday; once per month
  - irregular, but repeated
  - single incidents
  - age during exposure

- Through what chain of events?
  - natural weathering
  - mining and milling
  - manufacturing processes
  - transportation
  - storage
  - use
  - industrial discharges
  - waste disposal
  - environmental transport

- How many people are exposed by various routes and under various conditions?
  - single routes of exposure
  - multiple routes and types of exposure, e.g., oral and respiratory, occupational and consumer

In general, these questions are not easily answered, and fibrous materials such as asbestos pose some special difficulties. For example, fibers remain in the lungs after external exposure has ceased. In addition, there is no consensus on the best way to measure and express toxicologically significant doses, e.g., whether to use mass, fiber counts or fibers with particular characteristics. Measures of total mass are possibly not related to toxicity as reliably as appropriate fiber counts. Moreover, the various methods of collecting and counting fibers often do not correlate veil with one another. However, to compare dose-response relationships among studies and to predict health effects from exposure or dose measurements, data concerning exposure and dose must be expressed in the same units, even though there is uncertainty about the appropriate conversion factors (see Chapter 4).

Two major approaches are used for exposure assessment: one is based on measurements of exposure data and the other on calculations from more indirect indicators of exposure. In the first approach, exposure data are gathered as directly as possible. For example, a portable sampler worn by a person may provide good measurements of exposure. Host measurements are less direct, however, and the assessor must relate measured concentrations in air, water, or food to absorbed dose through some model of the exposure, absorption, and elimination processes. The amount of material present in the body of the exposed person provides an additional way of assessing exposure.

The measurement approach is founded on real exposure data rather than on a framework of assumptions; however, measurement procedures are expensive and many measurements are usually required if generalizations are to be made for a variety of situations.

By contrast, calculation-based approaches begin with less direct measurements of exposure, e.g., measurements of production volumes or chemical and physical properties. Then, ultimate distributions of exposures are estimated through a series of calculations or mathematical models that attempt to represent the behavior of the substance. Although this second approach obviates the need for multiple measurements of fiber concentrations, it must depend on a series of assumptions and mathematical respresentations that may be exceedingly poor descriptions of real phenomena but that must be kept relatively simple to avoid excessive computational costs. The validity of the input data—whether measured or simply estimated—may also be questionable.

A conceptual model for determining fiber exposures is discussed in Appendix D. This model is useful for making rough exposure estimates when few or no measurements exist. It incorporates a scheme representing commercial and environmental flows of fibers, including such factors as natural occurrence, imports and exports, disposal, ambient concentrations, and biodisposition.

The positive features of both approaches described above could be combined by calibrating the calculations against exposure measurements in known situations and then using the models to extrapolate or interpolate to unknown situations. Ideally, the actual amount of materials entering the human body would be measured for the most common conditions of exposure encountered by humans, taking into account differences in exposure both over time and by location.

ASBESTIFORM FIBERS AND THEIR SOURCES

The major properties of the asbestiform fibers of concern to this committee are described in Chapter 2. Figure 3-2 shows a simple classification system for fibers with those properties. This classification is based on commercial use rather than on other distinctions among the fibers. Thus, commercially used asbestos and natural nonasbestos fibrous materials such as attapulgite are shown in the figure, whereas fibrous erionite, which is not used in commerce, is not specifically noted. Rather, such fibers are included in the general category "noncommercial natural mineral fibers."

Asbestiform fibers probably account for the vast majority of the mass of most of these materials. Huggins et al. (1962) indicate that virtually all attapulgite consists of asbestiform fibers, even though the fibers are short. The committee was unable to determine whether or not the material commercially exploited as attapulgite is all fibrous. By contrast, the fibrous form of erionite is rarer (T. Zoltai, University of Minnesota, personal communication, 1983).

There are many sources of exposure to asbestiform fibers. In addition to exposures from natural sources, humans are exposed during such activities as mining, milling, manufacturing, use, and disposal of fiber-containing products. Because the committee was asked to study nonoccupational exposures, this report is focussed on environmental discharges or releases, rather than on exposures in the workplace.

Naturally occurring mineral fibers are a source of exposure through natural weathering or human disturbance of mineral deposits. Fibers measured in air far removed from known asbestos sources (Thompson and Morgan, 1971) or in drinking water are probably derived largely from such sources.

Similarly, mining and milling of asbestos are direct sources of fiber release into air and, occasionally, into water. Manufacturing of synthetic fibers may be considered a process that is parallel to the milling of asbestos. However, the fibers discharged during manufacturing probably represent a substantially smaller portion of the production output than would result from asbestos milling, because of differences in the processes and because cost considerations probably encourage greater efforts to minimize losses through discharge in the production of synthetic fibers.

Manufactured fiber products can be divided into two major classes: primary products and secondary products. Primary products are those made directly from asbestiform fibers (see Table 3-1). The different fibers and their respective primary uses are not completely interchangeable. Secondary products are made from primary products. For example, asbestos paper and cord (primary products) may be used for making electric and

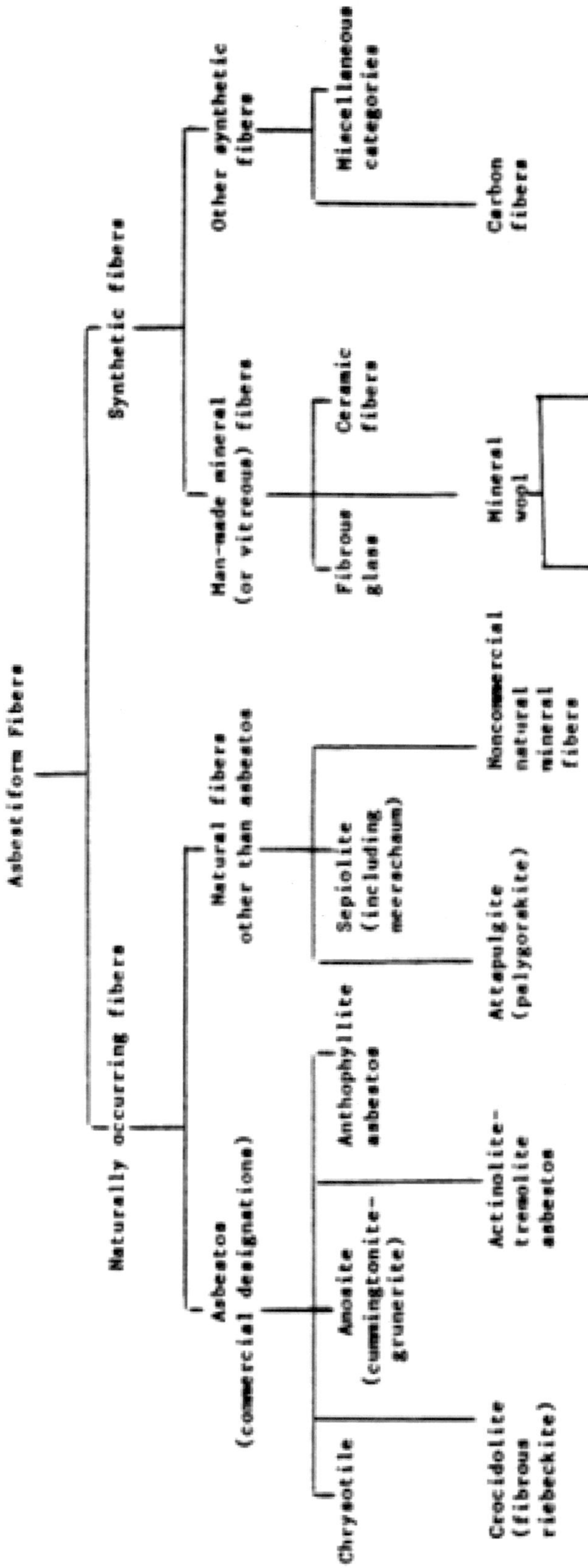

Figure 3-2.
Classification of asbestiform fibers.

TABLE 3-1. Primary Products of Different Fiber Types[a]

	Primary Product in Which Fibrous Material is Supplied						
Fibrous Material	Bulk Fibers	Paper	Cord	Textiles	Blanket	Friction Material	Asbestos-Cement
Chrysotile asbestos	X	X	X	X		X	X
Crocidolite and other asbestos	X (minor use)	X (minor use)					X
Attapulgite	X	X					
Other natural fibers	X						
Fibrous glass	X	X	X	X	X		
Rock wool	X				X		
Slag wool	X				X		
Ceramic fiber	X	X		X	X		
Carbon fiber	X				X		
Other man-made fibers	X				X		

[a] In this and subsequent presentations he materials are assumed to be largely asbestiform. However he committee does not know what proportion would be considered asbestiform particularly for attapulgite.

thermal insulation (secondary products). The major secondary uses of these fibers, based on total consumption, are shown in Tables 3-2 and 3-3.

The United States imports approximately 90% of the asbestos it uses, principally from Canada. On the other hand, it produces essentially all the attapulgite it uses and exports approximately 15% of its total production (U.S. Bureau of Mines, 1982).

The products that yield the greatest potential for exposure are not necessarily those produced in the greatest amounts. Conditions of use also influence exposure potential. For example, because the asbestos fibers in asbestos-cement pipe are relatively tightly bound in their cement matrix (as compared to other uses, such as in insulation), they may present less potential for exposure than some other uses. These different exposure potentials are discussed in the following sections for the various classes of fibers: asbestos, attapulgite and other natural fibers, man-made mineral fibers, and other synthetic fibers.

EXPOSURE POTENTIAL FOR ASBESTOS

Types of Exposure

Exposures to asbestos fall in the following four categories:

- occupational
- community (near known sources)
- consumer (use of manufactured products)
- general environmental

Occupational Exposure. Because the heaviest exposures to asbestos occur in the workplace, they have received the most attention. There has been particular interest in exposures associated with the following activities:

- asbestos mining and milling
- asbestos product manufacturing
- shipyard activities
- installation and removal of insulation in buildings
- brake lining manufacturing and replacement

However, these occupational exposures are not of concern in this study except as they provide reference points and influence total exposure in conjunction with nonoccupational exposures.

Community Exposures. Closely related to occupational exposures are community exposures, which encompass exposures of residents in communities where there are significant industrial sources of asbestos or other fibers. Such sources include mills, asbestos product manufacturing facilities, and brake manufacturing plants. These exposures can occur in

TABLE 3-2. U.S. Consumption of Asbestos Fibers in Secondary Products during 1982[a]

Secondary Product	Consumption (thousand of metric tons)	Chrysotile (%)
Asbestos-cement pipe	37.6	57
Asbestos-cement sheet	10.8	100
Flooring products	49.0	99+
Roofing products	7.0	100
Packing and gaskets	13.6	99
Thermal insulation	0.2	0
Electrical insulation	0.7	100
Friction products	52.9	100
Coatings and compounds	25.0	100
All other	49.7	99
Total	246.5	93

[a] Adapted from U.S. Bureau of Mines 1983.

TABLE 3-3. Estimated U.S. Consumption and Production of Selected Nonasbestos Fiber Products

Fiber and Use	1981 Consumption (thousands of metric tons)	References
Attapulgite		U.S. Bureau of Mines, 1982
Drilling mud	173.5	
Fertilizers	50.2	
Filtering (oil + grease)	18.7	
Oil and grease absorbents	178.2	
Pesticides and related products	106.5	
Pet waste absorbent	105.8	
Medical, pharmaceutical, cosmetic ingredient	0.06	
All other uses	79.5	
Total	712.46	
	1977 Production (thousands of metric tons)	
Fibrous glass		
Wool	1,100	Kirk-Othmer, 1980
Textile	340	Kirk-Othmer, 1980
Fine fiber	5	J. Leineweber, Manville Corp., personal communication, 1983
Total	1,445	
	Estimated Annual Production (thousands of metric tons)	
Mineral wool	200	J.D. Cornell, U.S. Gypsum Co., personal communication, 1983
Ceramic fiber ("current")		W.J. Breitsman, Carborundum Corp., personal communication, 1983
High temperature insulation	20	
All others	1	
Total	21	
Carbon fiber (including uses in aerospace structures, automotive structures, and sporting goods)	0.56	U.S. Bureau of Mines, 1982

a variety of rays. Fibers may be transported near the source via air and rarer or liberated from the clothes of a household member who works with the fibrous material. Community exposures are sometimes grouped with general environmental exposures.

Suta and Levine (1979) have identified eight types of facilities that lead to community exposures to asbestos:

- mines and mills
- friction product plants
- gasket, packing, or insulation plants
- asbestos-textile plants
- asbestos-cement plants
- asbestos vinyl flooring plants
- roofing products plants
- asbestos paper plants

Mines and mills are usually situated close to one another in rural communities. In the United States, all the mills are located within 100 km of the mine. According to the U.S. Bureau of Mines (1983), four active asbestos mining and milling operations existed in the United States in 1980, and there were three in 1982. The other facilities listed above can be located in either urban or rural settings. Those situated in or near urban areas have the greatest potential for exposing large numbers of people.

Consumer Exposures. These exposures result from the use of specific products outside the workplace. For example, the wear of vinyl asbestos floor tile can liberate detectable levels of asbestos into room air, as can disturbance of old installed asbestos insulation (Sebastien et al., 1982). Other sources have included hair dryers and other electrothermal appliances, which have been known to release asbestos in breathable form (Organization for Economic Cooperation and Development, 1982). Rice coated with talc has been reported to contain fibers that were apparently asbestos (Blejer and Arlon, 1973), presumably because the talc contained such fibers. Asbestos fibers have also been reported in beer and wine (Cunningham and Pontefract, 1973) as well as in drinking water as a result of migration from asbestos-cement pipe (American Water Works Association, 1974). Because both natural and waste asbestos can also reach drinking water through contamination of its source, drinking water is usually classified as an exposure from the general environment.

The Asbestos Information Association (1975) has reported more than 3,000 uses for asbestos. Many of these are probably hypothetical, many others entail very small quantities of asbestos and negligible potential for exposure, and yet other uses have disappeared over time. Nevertheless, there are scores and possibly hundreds of significant uses, most of which relate to the properties listed below:

- thermal insulation
- electrical insulation
- chemical inertness
- tensile strength
- ability to act as a filter

As shown in Table 3-2, the largest quantities of asbestos are used in the following products:

- asbestos-cement sheet and pipe
- flooring products, e.g., vinyl asbestos tile
- friction products, e.g., brake and clutch linings
- packing and gaskets
- coatings, e.g., patching compounds
- roofing products

These products accounted for almost 90% of U.S. consumption of asbestos in 1982. Some applications may have led to substantial earlier exposures through uses in filtration of parenteral drugs, filters for cigarettes, and insulation for home appliances such as hair dryers. Large amounts of asbestos were also formerly used in spray insulation for structural steel, especially in commercial and industrial buildings and in ships.

Nonoccupational exposures attributable to the use of manufactured products have often been assumed to be relatively low, because almost all these products contain asbestos in a binding matrix, such as cement, plastic, rubber, or resin. However, exposures can occur if fibers are liberated from these matrices through such occurrences as traffic on asbestos flooring, wear of brake linings,[1] and abrasion or leaching from pipe or paper. The Consumer Product Safety Commission is undertaking studies to determine the amounts of asbestos that might be released during typical consumer use of some products (P. White, Consumer Product Safety Commission, personal communication, 1983). In addition, fibers are often released during the disposal of asbestos products. For example, demolition and renovation of asbestos-insulated buildings may result in elevated transient concentrations of fibers if proper precautions are not taken.

Exposures to asbestos may also result from the use of products made from asbestos-contaminated substances. One example is talc, widely used as a pigment, extender, or processing aid in ceramic tile, paint, paper, plastics, and, in smaller quantities, as a component of cosmetic powders, foods, drugs, pesticides, and many other products. Although talcs can be virtually free of fibrous materials, they have also been reported to

[1] The material released from brake linings is in large part thermally altered (Harben, 1980).

contain asbestos fibers[2] in quantities sometimes constituting almost one-half the total product weight (Dement and Zumwalde, 1979). Talcum powders have also been reported to contain measurable amounts of asbestos (Rohl et al., 1976). Because more than 800 metric tons of talc are consumed annually in the United States (U.S. Bureau of Hines, 1982), exposures to asbestos may occur through these various uses. Another commercially important natural substance that could be contaminated with asbestos is vermiculite (Bank, 1980).

General Environmental Exposures. These exposures are usually attributable to fibers in ambient air and drinking water. To a lesser extent, they have resulted from ingestion of food and beverages. Asbestos fibers in air may result from human activities and from natural weathering of asbestos deposits. Drinking water may be contaminated by leaching from rocks, by deposition of airborne asbestos, or by runoff from dumps or ore deposits.

Unlike community exposures, exposures to asbestos in the general environment cannot be clearly identified with a causative human activity. However, general environmental concentrations may come from natural sources or from the transport of fibers from human sources many kilometers away.

The two principal routes of exposure to asbestos in the general environment are inhalation of ambient air and, in some areas, ingestion of drinking water. (After clearance from the lung, some of the inhaled asbestos is also swallowed with mucous secretions from the respiratory tract.) Exposures through the skin and possible ingestion of asbestos in foods are presumed to be much less important.

Only the finer fibers remain suspended in ambient air for long times. Therefore, general environmental exposures to asbestos entail a larger proportion of fine fibers than do occupational or community exposures. Such exposures also occur 24 hours per day throughout the year—a total of 8,760 hours per year—in contrast to about 1,800 hours per year for occupational exposures and short, intermittent exposures from product use.

The asbestos content of drinking water is heavily influenced by the character of the rocks and soils present in the water supply basin. Another source is asbestos-cement water pipe. The release of fibers from that source appears to be relatively slow under some conditions (Hallenbeck, 1978), but may be considerable if the water is aggressive to asbestos-cement pipe (Buelow et al., 1980; Millette et al., 1979a). Discharge of asbestos-containing wastes into water supplies could lead to

[2] Samples of talc mined in New York State contained tremolite and other particles with aspect ratios greater than 3:1. It is possible that most of these are not asbestiform fibers, as defined by this committee (T. Zoltai, University of Minnesota; R. Clifton, Bureau of Hines, personal communication, 1983).

high local concentrations, but such incidents have been infrequently reported. Croft (1982) has suggested that asbestos fibers in tap water may enter ambient air in residences as the water is sprayed or evaporates from the faucet.

Asbestos appears to degrade in the environment exceedingly slowly. However, mechanical forces may break the fibers into successively smaller particles. Attack by acidic waters in the environment is possible, and some thermal decomposition may take place. Decomposition is likely when asbestos-containing wastes are incinerated (Cogley et al., 1982). The deposition and eventual burial of fibers in soils and sediments are probably the major natural processes by which asbestos leaves the ambient environment.

Quantitative Exposure Estimates

It is difficult to make quantitative estimates of exposure to asbestos. A common unit of cumulative dose for occupational exposures is obtained by multiplying the average concentration of fibers in workplace air by the number of years that an individual worked there (full-time equivalent). The concentration of fibers in workplace air is expressed as fibers >5 μm long/cm^3, as counted by the light microscope (LM) under specified conditions (U.S. National Institute for Occupational Safety and Health, 1977). A convenient way of abbreviating this expression of exposure is (fibers/cm^3)yr. However, as discussed more extensively in Chapter 5, cumulative exposure measures do not take into account dose rate per unit time, duration of exposure, and ages at exposure. These three factors, particularly the third one, could be very important in determining effects on health.

Another measure of exposure that allows comparison of different exposure situations is expressed as "lifetime fibers." This quantity is derived by integrating over time the product of fiber concentrations in media such as air and water (which are the sources of exposure) and the intake rates of those sources. Some of the fibers inhaled are soon exhaled and, thus, are not available for retention in the body. Because the exhaled portion has not been specifically determined and because that portion is presumed to be reasonably uniform over all inhalation exposure situations, the committee did not apply any adjustment factors in calculating lifetime fibers. Similarly, the majority of fibers in ingested water probably pass through the digestive tract without penetrating its lining. The corresponding adjustment factor for determining lifetime fibers from this source also is not known, but would probably be different from that for inhalation. This difference should be remembered when interpreting the following calculations.

When interpreting health effects information obtained from occupational studies, it may be necessary to convert nonoccupational exposures to equivalent occupational dose expressed in (fibers/cm^3)yr. To do so, the number of lifetime fibers is divided by the volume of air inhaled at work in I year. If one were to assume an inhalation rate of approximately 10 m^3 air per 8-hour workday (International Commission on Radiological Protection, 1975) and 200 workdays per year, the amount of air inhaled each work year would be approximately 2,000 m^3, or 2 × 109 cm^3. Therefore, approximately 2 × 109 lifetime fibers would be inhaled during an occupational exposure of I fiber/cm^3 for I year. To extend this calculation, as many as 4 × 109 fibers would be inhaled annually by a worker exposed to air containing the U.S. Occupational Safety and Health Administration (OSHA) standard of two LM fibers/cm^3—a count based on fibers >5 μm long counted with a light microscope.[3] A working lifetime exposure to 2 fibers/cm^3 could conceivably result in inhalation of 2×10^{11} fibers; however, the number of people recently being exposed to such quantities is probably quite small—perhaps a few thousand. Occupational exposures of 10^{10} to 10^{11} lifetime fibers may accrue to a few hundred thousand people, and perhaps a million or so others may be exposed to 10^9 lifetime fibers through peripheral sources (Daley et al., 1976).

At the other end of the spectrum, Suta and Levine (1979), who summarized a great deal of data related to asbestos exposure have estimated that the rural U.S. population (60 million people) might be exposed Co concentrations ranging from 0.01 to 0.1 ng/m^3. They estimate further that the urban U.S. population—perhaps 170 million people—is exposed to asbestos concentrations higher than I ng/m^3 in ambient air. Spurny et al. (1979) also presented data showing fiber concentrations of approximately I ng/m^3. If we choose a nominal conversion of 30 LM fibers per nanogram,[4] an annual inhaled air volume of 7,300 m^3 (20 m^3/day × 365 days), and a 70-year lifespan, a lifetime exposure could reach 10^5 to 10^6 fibers for rural dwellers and 10^7 fibers for the less exposed urban dwellers. Virtually none of the population would experience lifetime exposures as high as 10^9 fibers.

Most community exposures might average about 10^8 LM lifetime fibers for perhaps 15 million people, a figure consistent with the distribution of ambient air exposures (Suta and Levine, 1979). For example, people living near metal mines that contain asbestos-contaminated ores might experience such levels (Bank, 1980; Kuryvial et al., 1975), whereas people living very near asbestos mines and mills would probably experience considerably higher levels.

Exposures in asbestos-insulated school buildings have caused considerable concern. Asbestos concentrations in schoolroom air have been estimated to range from approximately 10 to more than 1,000 ng/m^3

[3] In early November 1983, OSHA issued an emergency temporary standard (ETS) for workplace asbestos that lowered the permissible exposure to 0.5 fibers/cm^3 (U.S. Occupational Safety and Health Administration, 1983), but later in the month a stay was issued on the ETS.

[4] The committee used this conversion factor while recognizing its variability (Schneiderman et al., 1981).

(Nicholson et al., 1978; U.S. Environmental Protection Agency, 1980). Assuming that 1 ng/m^3 contains 30 LM fibers, that exposure occurs during 1,000 hours of school yearly for 12 years of school, and that the breaching rate is approximately 0.75 m^3/hr one would estimate the exposures to range from approximately 3×10^6 3×10^8 lifetime fibers for the 2 to 6 million students attending such schools. The 100,000 to 300,000 teachers in Chose schools could accrue higher lifetime doses from these concentrations (U.S. Environmental Protection Agency, 1980).

There are few measurements or calculations for estimating exposures from the use of manufactured products. In one study, Sebastien et al. (1982) reported concentrations of approximately 30 ng/m^3 in the indoor air of buildings with vinyl asbestos flooring. This concentration is converted to a lifetime exposure of approximately 5×10^7 fibers, assuming 2,000 hours of exposure annually over 40 years. In another report, Le Guen and Burdett (1981) recorded concentrations as high as 10 ng/m^3 in public buildings with asbestos insulation. Most ocher product exposures would be much less frequent or prolonged, although possibly of higher intensity. Thus, although some uses of manufactured products may result in people being exposed to relatively high fiber concentrations, use of manufactured products probably does not contribute greatly to the lifetime exposure of the average urban dweller.

Exposures to asbestos in drinking water may have an impact on human health. A committee of the National Research Council (1983) has summarized several studies on this subject. In Connecticut, exposures ranged from 10^4 to^5 $\times$ 10^5 electron-microscope fibers per liter, or approximately 170 to 12,000 LM fibers per liter. In San Francisco, concentrations as high as 3×10^6 LM fibers/liter have been reported, and in the Puget Sound area, levels ranging from about 10^5 to 3×10^6 LM fibers/liter were found. At an annual water consumption rate of 500 liters for 70 years, lifetime exposures could run from 6×10^6 to 10^{11} fibers.

Suta and Levine (1979) reported that asbestos mass concentrations in drinking water ranged from a high of about 100 µg/liter to less than 0.01 µg/liter. Some of the data from which this distribution was calculated are suspect. If taken at face value, however, these data suggest a lifetime ingestion of 4×10^7 to 4×10^{11} LM fibers, assuming 30 fibers/ng and an annual water consumption of about 500 liters. Approximately 10% of the population (23 million people) would receive lifetime exposures greater than 10^9 fibers, and not much more than 1% (2 million) would receive lifetime exposures greater than 10^{10} fibers. Nevertheless, these exposures—in terms of fibers ingested—are greater than the lifetime exposures from inhalation of ambient air. As noted in Chapters 5 and 6, however, it has been difficult to document adverse health effects of ingested asbestos.

Ingestion of asbestos in foods probably does not constitute a large portion of total exposure. For example, Cunningham and Pontefract (1973) found I to 10 million electron microscope fibers per liter of various beverages. This is approximately 0.02 to 0.2 million LM fibers/liter, a range similar to that for drinking water. However, some of the fibers found in beverages probably originated from filters used in processing.

Relative Contributions of Various Sources. Meylan et al. (1979) presented data suggesting that asbestos production, use, and disposal could result in annual emissions of 100 to 300 metric tons into the air and 50 to 100 metric tons to surface water. The upper figures reported by these investigators are based on the assumption. that the incineration of asbestos-containing wastes is a major source of emissions—an assumption that is probably not justified because some of the asbestos is likely to undergo thermal breakdown, which occurs as a function of temperature and type of fiber. Cogley et al. (1982) estimated that manufacturing processes discharge approximately 100 metric tons of asbestos into the air each year and about the same amount into water. They believe that emissions into air from disposal activities are minor. They also estimated that air emissions from mining and milling could reach 1,400 metric tons per year.

Although none of these estimates have been reported to be very accurate, they can be used to check the reasonableness of ambient measured concentrations. A l-km-thick layer of air over the 48 contiguous United States contains about 10^{16} m^3 of air, and all the rivers in the country discharge about 2×10^{15} liters of water per year (Brown et al., 1976). Assuming that the air mass moves across the United States in about 5 or 6 days (1.5% of a year), then about 1.5% of the annual asbestos discharges from manufacturing and use would yield concentrations in this air layer of about 0.2 to 0.5 ng/m^3 and mining and milling would yield up to 2 ng/m^3. Assuming that wet and dry deposition would remove most of the asbestos on the rest of its way around the world in approximately I month, the measured variation from 0.01 ng/m^3 to 1.0 ng/m^3 in air far from industrial sources could well be explained by the discharges estimated.

Discharges from manufacture and use primarily involve paper or friction products such as brake linings. Additional discharges would result from the natural weathering of deposits or incidental uses of asbestos such as in road surfacing (Serra and Connor, 1981). The discharges from mines and mills, which consist of fibers and bundles larger than those from other sources, are presumably deposited relatively close to their sources and do not contribute as much to general ambient concentrations.

If all discharges into water were confined to rivers, the average concentration would simply be the quotient of the discharge rate and the aggregate river flow rate, or approximately 0.02 to 0.05 µg/liter. The latter figure is close to the median value estimated by Suta and Levine

(1979). However, sedimentation as veil as discharges into lakes would reduce the average concentration, suggesting that natural sources of fibers such as serpentine deposits may be responsible for a significant amount of the waterborne asbestos. Of the sources attributable to human activity, asbestos paper manufacturing appears to account for the largest amount (Meylan et al., 1978). Asbestos-cement is also a large contributor (Cogley et al., 1982).

Accuracy, Uncertainty and Reliability of Estimates. The estimates of asbestos exposures discussed above are based on a series of data inputs, assumptions, models, and calculations that are individually and collectively rather tenuous. As noted in Chapter 4, many difficulties accompany attempts to measure levels of asbestos and to convert various measurements to comparable units. One analytical chemist (D. M. Coulson, personal communication, 1982) has stated that a given laboratory report is at best a ballpark estimate and that interlaboratory variations of several hundred percent are not unusual.

A particularly critical assumption is that dose measured in either fibers/cm^3 multiplied by years of exposure or in total lifetime fibers is the biologically significant exposure variable. Thus, the committee did not attempt to estimate details of the exposure pattern over time. In Chapter 7, it is shown that this assumption provides a reasonably good fit to the data when assessing lung cancer risks, but that age at first exposure and duration of exposure may be more important for mesothelioma risks.

The estimates are also based on the assumption that exposures are constant over periods as long as 20 to 70 years. Given the rise and fall of the asbestos industry, such an assumption is unlikely to be generally true. If most of the measurements were taken at times of high production and use rates, the lifetime exposure estimates could be grossly exaggerated.

The estimates of populations at risk are also crude. For example, no details of living, shopping, and working patterns were included in estimates of exposures to airborne concentrations and no firm relationships were established between the content of water supplies, the content of delivered tap water, and the actual populations consuming them.

The inevitable conclusion is that errors in estimating the lifetime fiber exposures for the various exposed populations could be very large. Differences between the least exposed and most exposed persons in a given population could easily be several orders of magnitude, and even the average exposure of the population could be considerably in error. Although the size of a specific population with known exposure conditions can be estimated with more certainty, it too can be substantially in error. The diversity of uncertainty factors and the lack of measurement of their variability make quantitative uncertainty estimates untenable, except in a very subjective way. Thus, the numbers cited in the previous sections can be used only to suggest where attention should be focussed, not to guide firm decisions. They are useful, however, in indicating the current best estimates of the relative levels of exposure in different situations. Note that the deficiencies in estimating past exposures lead to uncertainties regarding the dose-response relationships for health effects.

Trends. Little can be said about trends in exposures to asbestos. Occupational and related exposures increased rapidly after about 1940 and then decreased in the 1960s after risk factors associated with such exposures became known. Regulatory standards and a decline in the demand for asbestos products have led to lower occupational exposures and possibly to a reduction in community and general environmental exposures. (See Figure 1-1; U.S. Environmental Protection Agency, 1982.)

For manufactured products, the trends may be mixed. Spray asbestos insulation is no longer being installed, and many of the filtration and appliance insulation uses have diminished or stopped (Consumer Product Safety Commission, 1983). Some uses have continued, partly because of assumed low emission potentials or lack of adequate substitute materials, for example, in vinyl tiles, brake linings, and asbestos-cement water pipe.

After disposal of asbestos-containing products, especially old insulation and building materials, fibers formerly bound in a matrix may be liberated. This disposal-related exposure could continue to increase for many years if secure burial or decomposition techniques are not used. Overall, the distribution of lifetime exposures will probably shift toward lower levels, although the growth of the population will increase the number of people at risk for each class of exposure.

Population Exposures. Societal risk depends both on the levels of risk corresponding to the individual exposure levels and on the number of people so exposed. If risks are proportional to lifetime fiber exposures, as the linear dose-response models assume, then relative societal risk can be modeled by multiplying the various exposure levels by the number of exposed persons. The same result can be obtained by adding the logarithms of the two variables—a natural procedure for numbers that range over many orders of magnitude. If the exposure levels and population exposed to each level are plotted on log-log graph paper (as in Figure 3-3), then the diagonal lines are isopleths of equivalent total population exposure, measured as lifetime fibers for the particular population. The isopleths would also delimit regions of equivalent societal risk, with points near the vertical axis representing low exposures of large numbers of people and points near the horizontal axis indicating high exposures to few people. In general, the further away from the lower left-hand corner, the higher the societal risk. The horizontal axis indicates individual exposure.

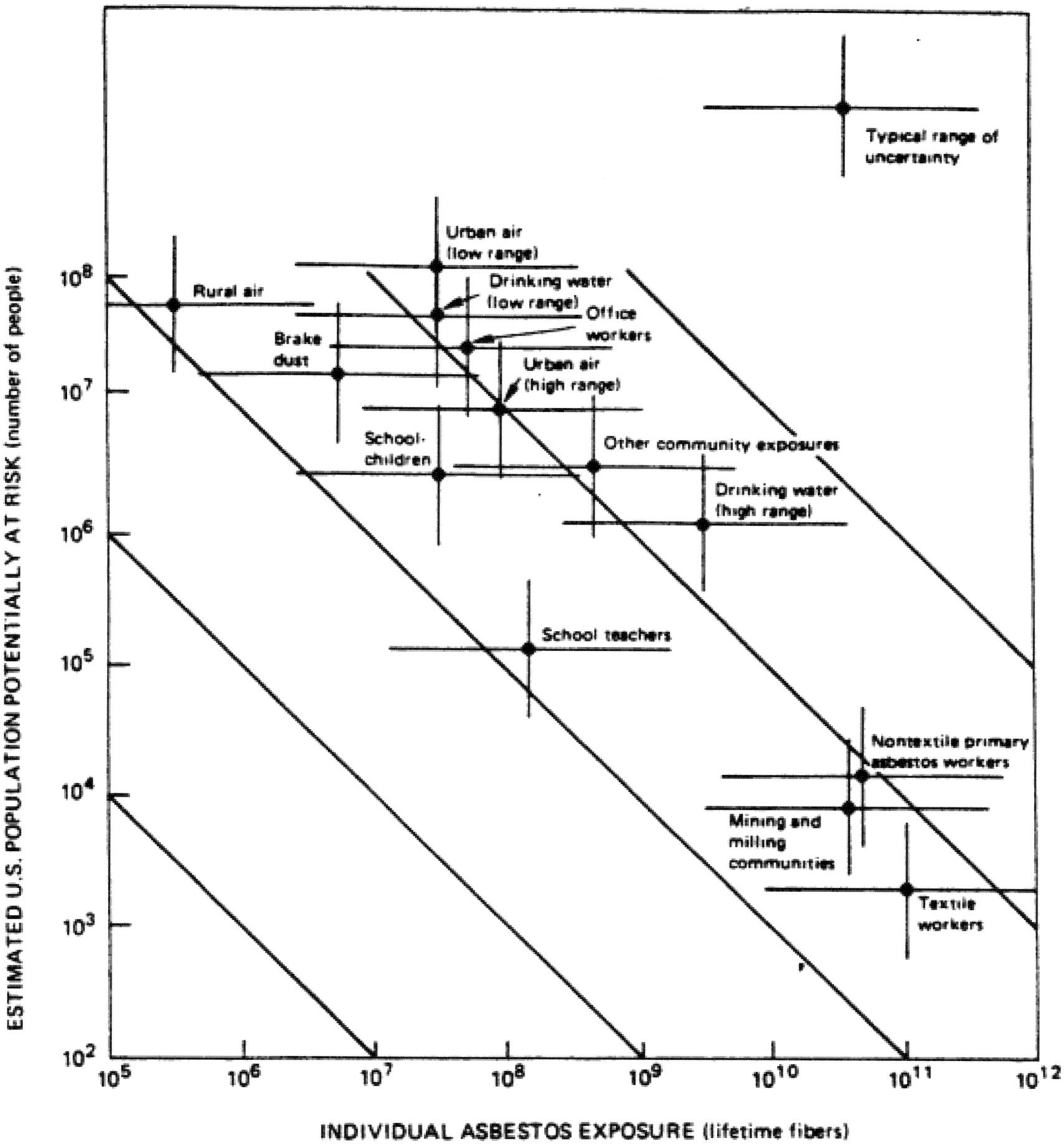

Figure 3-3.
Estimated lifetime exposures and numbers of people in various groups potentially exposed to asbestos. The points represent approximate estimates, and the lines indicate the ranges of uncertainty. As constructed, the uncertainty is about an order of magnitude for the population estimates and about two orders of magnitude for the exposure estimates. The committee was unable to make explicit estimates of the uncertainty limits, which would vary among the different populations. The points were derived from measurements or models for the groups represented; many of the points (e.g., the schoolchildren point) can be traced back to data provided in the section in this chapter entitled Quantitative Exposure Estimates.

Figure 3-3 also shows selected exposures[5] estimated by the committee as described in the section entitled "Quantitation Exposure Estimates." Each source is represented by a point, and the horizontal and vertical lines extending from those points indicate the uncertainties in the variables. The population estimates are generally more accurate than the exposure estimates. If one accepts the estimates, the following conclusion can be drawn from this chart: assuming total population exposures and risks are the criteria governing the level of concern, then some of the nonoccupational exposure classes may rival some occupational exposures in overall population risk. For most of the populations noted in the figure, however, it would be very difficult to detect health effects attributable to ambient concentrations of asbestos because of the small relative excesses expected (Marsh, 1983; National Research Council, 1983).

EXPOSURE TO OTHER NATURAL MINERAL FIBERS

Some natural fibrous materials other than asbestos have the properties of asbestiform materials described in Chapter 2, but the only asbestiform variety of mineral with commercial importance comparable to that of asbestos is attapulgite. Although the common acicular crystals of wollastonite resemble fibers, none is known to possess the properties of asbestiform fibers as defined by the committee in Chapter 2. Of the remaining mineral fibers listed in Appendix B as possibly asbestiform, only meerschaum, a block fibrous sepiolite, is of some commercial importance. A few metric tons of meerschaum are imported each year, and essentially all of it is carved into smoking pipes (U.S. Bureau of Mines, 1982). The committee did not consider meerschaum further because this material is used in such small amounts and because it remains intact in its natural form and does not readily release fibers.

The exposure of humans to other known natural asbestiform fibers is associated with natural weathering, the incidental use of fibrous materials in road-surfacing operations and in similar applications, or the occurrence of fibers as impurities in other minerals of commercial importance. For example, asbestos may be found in deposits of talc and a few other materials. Of the natural asbestiform minerals not commercially exploited, the committee reviewed only the fibrous zeolite called erionite, primarily because of its possible association with cancers in Turkish villages (Artvinli and Baris, 1982; Lilis, 1981). Figure 3-4 shows areas of the United States believed to be possible "incidental" sources of asbestiform fibers. These areas contain mineral deposits that could be, but are not necessarily, asbestiform (Kuryvial et al., 1974).

[5] Estimated number of people in a group are shown versus the estimated exposure per individual. Individual exposures within the group can easily span four or five orders of magnitude, and even the best representative value can be in error by an order of magnitude.

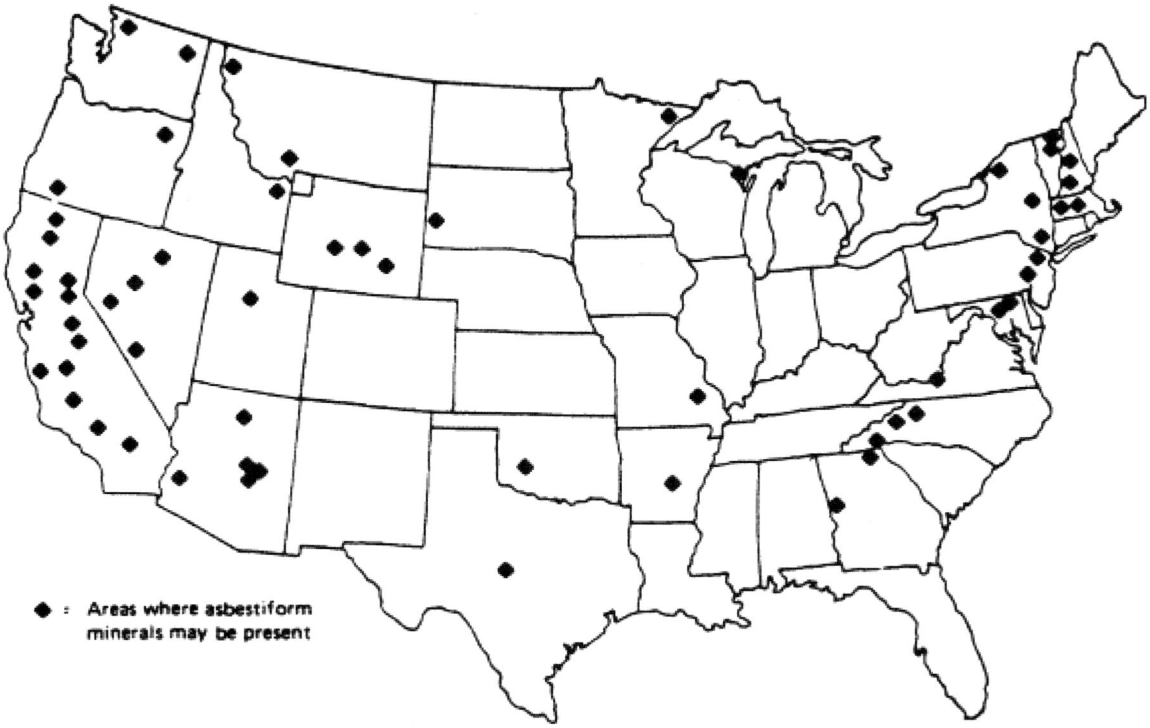

Figure 3-4.
Areas containing possible asbestiform phases of minerals. From Kuryvial et al., 1974.

Attapulgite

Attapulgite belongs to a group of commercially defined clays known as fuller's earths. It is a nonplastic clay, usually with a high magnesium content and with decolorizing and purifying properties. The United States is a leading producer of attapulgite, essentially all of which is mined in the vicinity of Attapulgus, Georgia, and Quincy, Florida. Domestic consumption is currently greater than 700 thousand metric tons—almost triple that of asbestos. An additional 100 thousand metric tons is exported (U.S. Bureau of Mines, 1982).

Attapulgite consists principally of short asbestiform fibers of the mineral palygorskite (Huggins et al., 1962; Zoltai and Stout, 1984). As with other minerals, some material will exhibit asbestiform properties to a greater degree than will other material. Of the uses listed in Table 3-3, some are more likely to involve higher quality fibers (S. Ampien, U.S. Bureau of Nines, personal communication, 1983). Material of lower quality, that is, having the characteristics of asbestiform fibers to a lesser extent, is acceptable for use in oil and grease absorbents, pesticide fillers, and pet waste absorbents. In France, attapulgite is used in drugs for the treatment of gastrointestinal diseases (Bignon et al., 1980); in the United States, it is a component of nonprescription antidiarrheal drugs (Physicians' Desk Reference, 1983). Bignon et al. (1980) reported that the French drugs contain fibers as long as 3.6 μ m (median length, approximately 1 μm) with typical diameters of approximately 0.03 μm. Lengths of 0.5 μm to 1 μm appear to be typical in attapulgite from the United States (Huggins et al., 1962).

The committee was unable to find data on airborne concentrations of attapulgite fibers. Because attapulgite is mined and processed in a region of relatively low population density, population exposures from these operations should be relatively low. Some uses, such as in pet waste absorbents, fertilizers, and pesticides, could release substantial amounts of attapulgite into the air. Attapulgite has also been found in water supplies (Millette et al., 1979b).

The levels of exposure to attapulgite and the numbers of people exposed could rival those for asbestos, even when measured as mass rather than as number of fibers. Because of the smaller size of attapulgite fibers, both in length and diameter, the numbers of fibers and their respirability would probably exceed those for asbestos. Clearance mechanisms, such as phagocytosis, would probably also be more effective. Bignon et al. (1980) reported two case studies in which attapulgite fibers were found in human lungs and urine.

Erionite

Unlike the population in parts of Turkey, no one in the United States is likely to live in dwellings constructed of erionite-containing materials. However, there are several deposits of zeolites in Arizona, California, Nevada, and Oregon, and some of them have been reported to contain fibrous erionite (Rom et al., 1983; Wright et al., 1983). Some of this material has been mined, possibly for use in ion-exchange processes, for retention of nitrogen in fertilizers, and for use in concrete aggregate or road surfacing. Some of these applications could lead to significant local air concentrations, as would natural weathering. The natural processes could also be sources of concentrations in drinking water. However, because ambient erionite concentrations have not been reported and because the population density in the intermountain western states is generally low, the committee believes there are few significant exposures to this substance.

Erionite fibers are similar to asbestos fibers, although they are probably, on average, shorter. Their maximum length is about 50 μm. Widths have been reported to range from 0.01 to 5.0 μm, averaging 0.1 μm in some samples (Suzuki, 1982) but most commonly ranging from 0.25 to 1.5 μm in others (Wright et al., 1983).

EXPOSURE TO MAN-MADE FIBERS

Man-Made Mineral Fibers

Man-made mineral fibers (MMMFs)—sometimes called man-made vitreous fibers—are glassy and amorphous rather than crystalline. The MMMFs include fibrous glass, mineral wool (i.e., rock wool and slag wool), and ceramic fibers. MMMFs compete with asbestos in some markets and have replaced it in others. Because they are amorphous, MMMFs do not split longitudinally; they do sometimes break transversely, yielding shorter, but not thinner, particles.

Fibrous Glass. Fibrous glass consists of monofilaments of silicate or borosilicate glass usually produced by melting amorphous silicates and forcing the melt through an orifice, followed by air, steam, or flame attenuation. The current processes allow production of relatively narrow ranges of fiber sizes, depending on the commercial need. The three main classes are textile fiber, wool fiber, and fine fiber, and there are many subclassifications within these broad classes. Textile fiber is the coarsest, typically 10 to 15 μm in diameter, 6 but may range from 6 to 20 μm (JRB Associates, Inc., 1981). Wool fiber usually ranges from about 3 to 10 μm in diameter (Konzen, 1982), but can be 1 to 25 μm (JRB Associates, Inc., 1981). Fine fiber is usually considered to be 1 μm nominal diameter or less.[6]

Fibrous glass accounts for approximately 80% of all MMMFs. At least 90% of the fibrous glass is produced as wool fibers, which are used primarily for thermal or acoustical insulation and for filtration. The largest category by far is thermal insulation, most of which is used to insulate buildings. These fibers are also used as duct linings, as insulation for pipes and appliances, and in ceiling tiles for acoustical insulation.[6]

Textile grades of fibers are used extensively in reinforcing resinous materials, e.g., in "fiber glass" automobile bodies or boat hulls (Watts, 1980). They are also used in various cloths (especially for draperies), papers, electrical insulation, and cording. Textile grades account for 5% to 10% of all fibrous glass.[6]

Approximately 0.5% by weight of fibrous glass produced falls within fine fiber size ranges. Because these fibers are expensive to produce, they are found only in specialized markets. Their two major uses are thermal insulation for aerospace vehicles and filtration, mostly to reduce the particulate content of air going to sensitive areas, such as the clean rooms of semiconductor plants.[6] The aerospace insulation is usually made as a fiber blanket sandwiched between metal or woven fiber cloth (Health and Safety Commission, 1979) and is installed between the inner and outer shells of the vehicle. The filter material is usually incorporated into a paperlike matrix with a small amount of binder.[6]

[6] J. Leineweber, Manville Corp., personal communication, 1983.

Less than 10% of all glass fibers are smaller than 3 μm in diameter. Fine fiber diameters are generally smaller than 3 μm (Konzen, 1982) and cluster around 1 μm, but may range from 0.2 μm to 5 μm, with typical airborne fiber lengths ranging from 5 to 20 μ (Esmen, 1982). Less than 2% of all other fibrous glass categories are smaller than 3 μm in diameter. Very fine or superfine grades of fibrous glass have diameters predominantly less than I μm. Thus the majority of the respirable fibers produced are probably in fine fiber grades; however, the uses for fine fibers do not appear to offer great opportunities for exposure. For example, the few measurements that have been made indicate that few fibers escape into the air during air filtration applications; otherwise, the utility of the filters would be compromised.[7]

Occupational exposures to fibrous glass have tended to be considerably lower than those to asbestos, mainly because of innate processing differences (JRB Associates, Inc., 1981) and the higher cost of producing fibrous glass. Typical levels in workplaces have been approximately 0.1 fiber/cm^3 as measured with a light microscope (Balzer, 1976; Corn, 1976; Esmen, 1982; Health and Safety Commission, 1979; Johnson et al., 1969; Shannon et al., 1982), although concentrations may exceed 10 fibers/cm^3 in areas where fine fibers predominate (JRB Associates, Inc., 1981). Concentrations were probably higher before the use of oils and binders to suppress dust (Hartung, 1982), which were used relatively early in the industry.

The fact that atmospheric concentrations of fibrous glass in the workplace are lower than those for asbestos by about an order of magnitude suggests that plant emissions might be lower by about the same factor on a pound-for-pound production basis. Although total production is currently greater for fibrous glass than for asbestos products, the portion of fibers in the respirable range is lower. Thus, total emissions of fine glass fibers are probably considerably lower than asbestos emissions. Balzer (1976) reported that ambient concentrations of fibrous glass in California air were approximately 0.002 fibers/cm^3 and that the average diameter of the fibers was 4 μm; 2/3 of the fibers were detectable by optical microscopy. Although the significance of this isolated report is uncertain, the reported concentration, which amounts to 2,000 fibers/m^3, is much higher than any reported for asbestos in ambient air, even in urban areas. If manufacturing emissions are lower for fibrous glass than for asbestos, as suggested earlier, some other explanation would be needed if the Balzer counts prove to be accurate and representative. For example, a point source might have been nearby. One possible nonmanufacturing source for glass fibers is in-place building insulation, which contains the fibrous material in relatively loose form (albeit with binders).

In addition to being exposed from outside air, a majority of the U.S. population is probably exposed to some extent by living or working in

[7] J. Leineweber, Manville Corp., personal communication, 1983.

buildings with fibrous glass insulation. The exposures would probably be highest shortly after installation or disturbance of the insulation. The committee was unable to locate reports of measured concentrations of glass fibers in buildings.

Many products contain fibrous glass. Smith (1976) has reported 35,000 individual product applications. Even if the vast majority of them are hypothetical or trivial, many possible sources of nonoccupational exposure still exist. However, fibrous glass production and its use in building insulation are likely to be the major sources.

Mineral Wool. Two types of fibers fall under the general rubric of mineral wool. Rock wool is the term for glass fibers made by melting natural igneous rocks and then drawing, blowing, or centrifuging the melt into fibers. Slag wool is made by similar processes, except that the feedstock is the already-melted slag from iron blast furnaces or other metal-slagging processes. Total mineral wool production in the United States is estimated to be approximately 200,000 metric tons.[8] Because of the generally less elaborate processes for manufacturing these two types of mineral wool, their diameter distribution tends to be broader than that of fibrous glass, and the product contains relatively large amounts of "shot" or residual unfiberized droplets of the molten material (Pundsack, 1976).

Rock wool and slag wool can serve many of the same purposes as fibrous glass. Host of it is used for either building insulation or specialty "technical" insulation for industrial processes. It is applied primarily as thermal insulation, but some is used for sound dampening.[8] Applications include power plants, chemical processes, and other heavy industrial manufacturing. Much smaller amounts are used in commercial buildings and even less in residences.[8] In current practice, binders are added to the mineral wool so that it can be supplied in the form of blankets or other shaped forms, rather than as loose fiber.

The reported measurements of slag and rock wool fiber concentrations in the workplace fall between those found for asbestos and those for fibrous glass, as one might expect from the processes involved and the relative costs of production.

Most of the reported fiber concentrations range from 0.2 to 0.5 fibers/cm^3, but concentrations as high as 2 fibers/cm^3 have been observed (Esmen, 1982; Health and Safety Commission, 1979; Ottery et al., 1982). Per pound of throughput, fiber emissions could be expected to be intermediate between fibrous glass and asbestos. Because the production is lower than that for fibrous glass and the uses are somewhat more likely to be industrial than residential, it is likely that population

[8] J. D. Cornell, U.S. Gypsum Corp., personal communication, 1983.

exposures to mineral wools are generally lower than those for fibrous glass, although the proportion of fine fibers my be greater.

The nominal diameter for mineral wools appears to be similar to that for glass wools—approximately 6 to 8 µm. However, there is a greater tendency for these wools to contain fine fibers. In the United States, as much as two-thirds of the fiber count may be less than 3 µm in diameter (Esmen, 1982). In some European rock wool plants, however, the portion of respirable fibers may be considerably lower (Ottery et al., 1982).

Ceramic Fiber. Ceramic fibers are produced by melting kaolin clay or a combination of alumina and silica to form aluminosilicate glasses and then blowing the melt to form the fibers. Host of these fibers are used for high temperature insulation. Some alumina and zirconia fibers are produced for even higher temperature applications; these are the fibers most often referred to as refractory (Health and Safety Commission, 1979). Total annual production is approximately 20,000 metric tons, but there is a capacity to manufacture at least double that figure.[9]

Ceramic fibers are used mostly for high temperature insulation. Smaller quantities are used for expansion joint stuffing. Approximately 85% of the fibers produced are sold in the form of blankets or modular building blocks. Bulk fiber, paper, and textile forms are also marketed. The principal industrial purchasers of ceramic fibers are manufacturers of steel and other metals, ceramics, petrochemicals, and catalytic converters for automotive vehicles. Typical uses include insulation for kilns, furnaces, ovens, ocher types of heaters, and, to a lesser extent, consumer appliances. Virtually all the fibers produced are encapsulated or incorporated into structures. The target range of diameters is 2 to 3.5 µm, but the diameters can range from less than I µm to 12 µm. Fiber lengths are often several centimeters, but many fibers a few micrometers in length are also produced (JRB Associates, Inc., 1981).[10]

In general, occupational exposures to ceramic fibers seem to fall within the same range as those for mineral wools, i.e., usually well under 1 fiber/cm^3, but they occasionally exceed that figure (Esmen et al., 1979; Fowler, 1980; Health and Safety Commission, 1979). Airborne fibers have a median diameter of about 1 µm and a median length of about 10 µm. Thus, many of the airborne fibers appear to be respirable (Esmen, 1978). Given the relatively low production volume, the moderate workplace concentrations, and the specialized applications, however, ceramic fibers are probably responsible for rather low general population exposures.

[9] W. J. Breitsman, Carborundum Corp., personal communication, 1983.

[10] Information also received from W. J. Breitsman, Carborundum Corp., personal communication, 1983.

Exposure to Other Man-Made Fibers

In comparison to the MMMFs, other fibers that might be considered asbestiform are produced in relatively small quantities. Among these are fibers of carbon, graphite, alumina, boron, potassium titanate, silicon carbide, and a variety of organic fibers such as Aramid or PTFE (polytetrafluoroethylene, or Teflon). The organic fibers usually enter the same general markets as the textile grade glass fibers and are correspondingly thick in diameter. Because these fibers are not of respirable size, exposures to them are not examined in this report. Even if they were respirable, it would be difficult to classify them as asbestiform under this committee's definition.

Most of the inorganic man-made fibers are marketed principally as reinforcement for various kinds of composite materials used in fabricating structures or equipment that must be strong but lightweight. For example, alumina fibers can be incorporated in an aluminum melt to produce fiber-reinforced metal (Chemical and Engineering News, 1980). Potassium titanate was marketed for reinforcing plastic friction materials in brakes, filters, and high temperature insulation, but was withdrawn from the market in the mid-1970s (C. F. Reinhardt, E. I. duPont, personal communication, 1978). Such fibers are also generally too large in diameter to be respirable, and they are presumed to have a very low exposure potential because they are sealed rather permanently in their matrix. Except for the carbon fibers, inorganic fibers are not discussed further in this report. At present, their production is limited, and their uses would not be expected to lead to substantial exposure.

In this document, the term carbon fiber is used to describe both the carbon and graphite fiber classes, although such fibers may be manufactured by different processes (Beardmore et al., 1980; Zumwalde and Harmison, 1980). These fibers are typically of the same general sizes as man-made wools, i.e., approximately 7 µm nominal diameter, and at least in normal use, they fall mostly within a quite narrow range of diameters (Johnson, 1982). They may exceed 2 or 3 mm in length. Less than 25% of them are shorter than 80 µm and have diameters less than 3 µm (Delmonte, 1981; Zumwalde and Harmison, 1980). There is some evidence of longitudinal cleavage after these fibers have been burned or worked (e.g., after sawing a composite that contains them) (Wagman et al., 1979).

Like the other mineral fibers mentioned in this section, most carbon fibers enter the reinforced materials market, e.g., in aerospace, automotive, and sports products such as golf club shafts. The matrices for the fibers are typically epoxy or polyimide resins (Kear and Thompson, 1980). The fibers are often treated first with another plastic product such as tetrafluoroethylene to make them less brittle (Harben, 1980). The U.S. Bureau of Mines (1982) reported that only about 250 metric tons of high-modulus (i.e., with the high-strength properties most like an asbestiform fiber) carbon fibers were produced in the United

States in 1980, but the rate of production growth is high, having doubled almost every year for the past 5 years (U.S. Bureau of Mines, 1982). One unusual new use of these fibers is in surgical implants that are reported to improve the healing of corn ligaments and tendons (Arehart-Treichel, 1982).

The committee found little information on exposures to carbon fibers. Both the small quantities produced and their applications primarily in composites suggest that little exposure occurs. The greatest opportunity for human exposure probably arises when the composite is accidentally or intentionally burned. Although the matrix is often decomposed under chose conditions, the fibers remain relatively intact (Wagman et al., 1979). In face, the first concerns about carbon fibers involved their potential effects on electronic systems after a fire had released them as conducting "wires" in semiconductor circuits.

Overall, nonoccupational exposures to carbon fibers are probably extremely low in comparison with Chose to most of the ocher asbestiform fibers discussed in previous sections. The potential for such exposures could change, however, if the use of carbon fibers continues to grow and diversify.

SUMMARY AND RECOMMENDATIONS

In assessing exposures to asbestiform fibers that could cause adverse health effects, the committee considered (1) synthetic and natural fibers that are used extensively in commerce and (2) natural fibers that are widely distributed by natural processes. As examples of commercial fibers, the committee assessed exposure to chrysotile, crocidolite, and ocher asbestos fibers; attapulgite; fibrous glass, mineral wool, and ceramic fibers; and carbon fibers. Fibrous erionite was chosen as an example of a noncommercial, naturally produced and distributed asbestiform fiber. Asbestos and attapulgite fibers are also released by natural processes, as are other natural fibers found in ambient air.

Many types of information would be helpful in assessing population exposures to various materials. However, because the most readily available information usually pertains co production or consumption levels, use patterns, fiber dimensions, and populations exposed, this type of information was used for the exposure assessment described in this chapter.

Current chrysotile consumption in the United States is approximately 230,000 metric tons per year. Attapulgite production is greater, and fibrous glass production apparently greater still. Mineral wool, crocidolite, ceramic fibers, ocher types of asbestos, and carbon fibers are produced or used in smaller quantities, approximately in Chat descending order.

All types of asbestos have fibers within the respirable range, i.e., less than approximately 3 μm in diameter, as do attapulgite and erionite. However, the nominal diameters of most of the synthetic fibers exceed the respirable range. Exceptions are some types of ceramic fibers, which are near the upper limit of the respirable range, and the fine grades of fibrous glass. With the possible exception of carbon fibers, most synthetic fiber products include some fibers of respirable size. Carbon fibers may split to finer, respirable fibers upon mechanical or thermal stress.

Asbestos fibers can be hundreds of micrometers long, although most of them detected in the ambient environment far from production sources are less than 3 μm long. Attapulgite fibers are generally less than 20 μm long. Target lengths for synthetic fibers are often measured in centimeters rather than in micrometers, but many shorter fibers are also produced.

Many of the commercial fibers are used only in binding matrices such as in reinforced plastics or paper products. Fibrous glass, mineral wool, attapulgite, and to some extent ceramic fibers are sometimes used unbound as relatively loose fibers. Because of their limited applications and present low production volumes, ceramic and carbon fibers probably have a relatively low exposure potential. Because of its limited natural occurrence, the same is true of fibrous erionite. Increased production and diversification of use is likely to be a significant factor for future exposures to carbon and ceramic fibers. The use of asbestos in the United States has declined in recent years.

As with most materials, lack of information on exposures to the various fibers limits the ability of investigators to identify the adverse health effects resulting from such exposure. Thus, there is a need to improve this information base and to establish correlations between exposures and health effects.

REFERENCES

American Water Works Association. 1974. A study of the problem of asbestos in water. J. Am. Water Works Assoc. 66:1-22.

Arehart-Treichel, J. 1982. A healing scaffold. Sci. News 122:219.

Artvinli, M., and Y. I. Baris. 1982. Environmental fiber-induced pleuro-pulmonary diseases in an Anatolian village: An epidemiologic study. Arch. Environ. Health 37:177-181.

Asbestos Information Association. 1975. Asbestos—General Information. Asbestos Information Association of North America, Washington, D.C.

Balzer, J. L. 1076. Environmental data; airborne concentrations found in various operations. Pp. 76-151 in Occupational Exposure to Fibrous Glass. Proceedings of a Symposium. Pub. No. 76-151. National Institute for Occupational Safety and Health, Cincinnati.

Bank, W. 1980. Asbestiform and/or Fibrous Minerals in Mines, Mills, and Quarries. Informational Report IR 1111. U.S. Mine Safety and Health Administration, Washington, D.C.

Beardmore, P., J. J. Harwood, K. R. Kinsman, and R. E. Robertson. 1980. Fiber-reinforced composites: Engineered structural materials. Science 206:833-840.

Bignon, J., P. Sebastien, A. Gaudichet, and M. C. Jaurand. 1980. Biological effects of attapulgite. Pp. 163-181 in J. C. Wagner, ed. Biological Effects of Mineral Fibres. Vol. 1. IARC Scientific Pub. No. 30. International Agency for Research on Cancer, Lyon.

Blejer, H. P., and R. Arlon. 1973. Talc: A possible occupational and environmental carcinogen. J. Occup. Med. 15:92-97.

Brown, S. L., B. R. Holt, and K. E. McCaleb. 1976. Systems for Rapid Ranking of Environmental Pollutants. CRESS Report No. 2. Stanford Research Institute, Menlo Park, Calif.

Buelow, R. W., J. R. Millette, E. F. McFarren, and J. M. Symons. 1980. The behavior of asbestos-cement pipe under various water quality conditions: A progress report. J. Am. Water Works Assoc. 72:91-102.

Chemical and Engineering News. 1980. Alumina fibers used to strengthen metals. Chem. Eng. News 58:24, June 30.

Cogley, D., N. Krusell, R. McInnes, P. Anderson, and R. Bell. 1982. Life Cycle of Asbestos in Commercial and Industrial Use Including Estimates of Releases to Air, Water, and Land. Final in house report. Report No. GCA-TR-79-73-G. GCA Corporation, Bedford, Mass. 265 pp.

Corn, M. 1976. Sampling strategy, air sampling methods, analysis, and airborne concentrations of fibrous glass in selected manufacturing plants. Pp. 91-96 in Occupational Exposure to Fibrous Glass. Proceedings of a Symposium. Pub. No. 76-151. National Institute for Occupational Safety and Health, Cincinnati.

Croft, W. 1982. Detection of high levels of asbestos fibers in the air of residential homes using asbestos-contaminated water. Proc. Am. Assoc. Can. Res. 23:72 (Abstract #281).

Delmonte, J. 1981. Technology of Carbon and Graphite Fiber Composites. Van Nostrand-Reinhold, New York.

Dement, J. M., and R. D. Zumwalde. 1979. Occupational exposures to talcs containing asbestiform minerals. Pp. 287-305 in R. Lemen and J. M. Dement, eds. Dusts and Disease. Proceedings of the Conference on Occupational Exposures to Fibrous and Particulate Dust and Their Extension into the Environment. Pathotox Publishers, Inc., Park Forest South, Ill.

Esmen, N. A. 1982. Short-term survey of airborne fibres in U.S. manufacturing plants. Presented at the Biological Effects of Man-Made Mineral Fibres, Occupational Health Conference, Copenhagen, April 20-22. World Health Organization.

Esmen, N. A., M. Corn, Y. Y. Hammad, D. Whittier, N. Kotsko, M. Haller, and R. A. Kahn. 1979. Exposure of employees to man-made mineral fibers: Ceramic fiber production. Environ. Res. 19:265-278.

Fowler, D. P. 1980. Industrial Hygiene Survey of Occupational Exposures to Mineral Wool. Contract No. 210-76-0120. National Institute for Occupational Safety and Health, Cincinnati.

Hallenbeck, W. H., E. H. Chen, C. E. Hesse, K. K. Patel-Mandlik, and A. H. Wolff. 1978. Is chrysotile asbestos released from asbestos-cement pipe into drinking water? J. Am. Water Works Assoc. 70:97-102.
Harben, P. 1980. What's new after asbestos? Ind. Miner.:51-57, September.
Hartung, W. J. A. 1982. Technical history of MMMF. Presented at the Biological Effects of Man-Made Mineral Fibres, Occupational Health Conference, Copenhagen, April 20-22. World Health Organization.
Health and Safety Commission. 1979. Man-Made Mineral Fibres: Report of a Working Party to the Advisory Committee on Toxic Substances. Her Majesty's Stationery Office, London. 36 pp.
Huggins, C. W., H. V. Denny, and H. R. Shell. 1962. Properties of Palygorskite, an Asbestiform Mineral. Report of Investigation 6071. U.S. Bureau of Mines, Department of the Interior, Washington, D.C.
International Commission on Radiological Protection. 1975. Report of the Task Group on Reference Man. Prepared by a Task Group of Committee 2 of the ICRP. ICRP Report No. 23. Pergamon Press, New York. 480 pp.
Johnson, D. J. 1982. Structure and physical properties of carbon fibers. Chem. Ind.:847-856, September 18.
Johnson, D. J., J. S. Healey, H. E. Ayer, and J. R. Lynch. 1969. Exposure to fibers in the manufacture of fibrous glass. Ind. Hyg. Assoc. J. 30: 545-550.
JRB Associates, Inc. 1981. Technical Support in the Classification of Toxic Substances—Fibrous Glass Industry. Vol. 1. Final report to U.S. Occupatioal Safety and Health Administration. JRB Associates, Inc., McLean, Va. 184 pp.
Kear, B. H., and E. R. Thompson. 1980. Aircraft gas turbine materials and processes. Science 208:847-856.
Kirk-Othmer. 1980. P. 877 in Encyclopedia of Chemical Technology. Vol. 11. Third Edition. John Wiley & Sons, New York.
Konzen, J. L. 1982. Production trends in fiber sizes of man-made mineral fiber (MMMF) insulation. Presented at the Biological Effects of Man-Made Mineral Fibres, Occupational Heath Conference, Copenhagen, April 20-22. World Health Organization.
Kuryvial, R. J., R. A. Wood, and R. E. Barrett. 1974. Identification and Assessment of Asbestos Emissions from Incidential Sources of Asbestos. EPA-650/2-74-087. Report prepared by Battelle Columbus Laboratories for the Office of Research and Development, Environmental Protection Agency, Washington, D.C.
Le Guen, J. M., and G. Burdett. 1981. Asbestos concentrations in public buildings—a preliminary report. Ann. Occup. Hyg. 24:185-189.
Lilis, R. 1981. Fibrous zeolites and endemic mesothelioma in Cappadocia, Turkey. J. Occup. Med. 23:548-550.
Marsh, G. M. 1983. Review of epidemiologic studies related to ingested asbestos. Environ. Health Perspect. 53:49-56.
Meylan, W. M., P. H. Howard, S. S. Lande, and A. Hanchett. 1978. Chemical Market Input/Output Analysis of Selected Chemical Substances to Assess Sources of Environmental Contamination: Task III. Asbestos. EPA 560 6-78-005. Environmental Protection Agency, Washington, D.C.

Millette, J. R., P. J. Clark, and H. F. Pansing. 1979a. Exposure to Asbestos from Drinking Water in the United States. ORD-EPA Environmental Health Effects Research Report EPA-600/1-79-028. Environmental Protection Agency, Washington, D.C.

Millette, J. R., J. D. Twyman, E. C. Hansen, P. J. Clark, and M. F. Pansing. 1979b. Chrysotile, palygorskite, and halloysite in drinking water. Scanning Electron. Microsc. 1:579-586.

National Research Council. 1983. Drinking Water and Health, Vol. 5. A report of the Safe Drinking Water Committee, Commission on Life Sciences. National Academy Press, Washington, D.C.

Nicholson, W. J. 1978. Control of Sprayed Asbestos Surfaces in School Buildings: A Feasibility Study. Final report. Contract 1-ES-2113.

National Institute of Environmental Health Sciences, Bethesda, Md. Organization for Economic Cooperation and Development. 1982. Control of Toxic Substances in the Atmosphere: Asbestos (Preliminary draft). Air Management Policy Group of the Environment Committee, Organization for Economic Cooperation and Development, Paris.

Ottery, J., J. Cherrie, J. Dodgson, and G. Harrison. 1982. A Summary Report on Environmental Conditions at 13 European Man Made Mineral Fibre Plants. Report No. TW/82/Draft. Institute for Occupational Medicine, Edinburgh.

Physicians' Desk Reference. 1983. Physicians' Desk Reference for Nonprescription Drugs, Fourth Edition. Medical Economics Co., Inc., Oradell, N. J. 804 pp.

Pundsack, F. L. 1976. Fibrous glass—manufacture, use, and physical properties. Pp. 11-18 in Occupational Exposure to Fibrous Glass. Proceedings of a Symposium. Pub. No. 76-151. National Institute for Occupational Safety and Health, Cincinnati.

Rohl, A. N., A. M. Langer, I. J. Selikoff, A. Tordini, and R. Klimentidis. 1976. Consumer talcums and powders: Mineral and chemical characterization. J. Toxicol. Environ. Health 2:255-284.

Rom, W. N., K. R. Casey, W. T. Parry, H. M. Corey, and F. Moatamed. 1983. Health implications of natural fibrous zeolites for the intermountain west. Environ. Res. 30:1-8.

Schneiderman, M. A., I. C. Nisbet, and S. M. Brett. 1981. Assessment of risks posed by exposure to low levels of asbestos in the general environment. Prepared for Institut für Wasser, Boden, und Lufthygiene des Bundesgesundheitsamtes. No. 4. Dietrich Reimer Verlag, Berlin.

Sebastien, P., J. Bignon, and M. Martin. 1982. Indoor airborne asbestos pollution: From the ceiling and the floor. Science 216:1410-1413.

Serra, R. K., and M. A. Connor, Jr. 1981. Assessment and Control of Chrysotile Asbestos Emissions from Unpaved Roads. EPA-450/3-81-006. Environmental Protection Agency, Washington, D.C.

Shannon, H. S., M. V. Hayes, J. A. Julian, and D. C. F. Muir. 1982. Mortality experience of glass-fibre workers. Presented at the Biological Effects of Man-Made Mineral Fibres, Occupational Health Conference, Copenhagen, April 20-22. World Health Organization.

Smith, H. V. 1976. History, processes, and operations in the manufacturing and uses of fibrous glass—one company's experience. Pp. 19-26 in Occupational Exposure to Fibrous Glass. Proceedings of a Symposium. Pub. No. 76-151. National Institute for Occupational Safety and Health, Cincinnati.

Spurny, K. R., W. Stoeber, H. Opiela, and G. Weiss. 1979. On the evaluation of fibrous particles in remote ambient air. Pp. 1-40 in The Science of the Total Environment. Elsevier, Amsterdam.
Suta, B. E., and R. J. Levine. 1979. Nonoccupational asbestos emissions and exposures. Pp. 171-205 in L. Michaels and S. S. Chissick, eds. Asbestos: Properties, Applications, and Hazards. John Wiley & Sons, New York.
Suzuki, Y. 1982. Carcinogenic and fibrogenic effects of zeolites: Preliminary observations. Environ. Res. 27:433-445.
Thompson, R. J. 1978. Ambient air monitoring for chrysotile in the United States. Pp. 355-363 in Proceedings of the Workshop on Asbestos: Definitions and Measurement Methods. Gaithersburg, July 18-20, 1977. NBS Spec. Pub. 506. National Bureau of Standards, Gaithersburg, Md.
Thompson, R. J., and G. B. Morgan. 1971. Determination of asbestos in ambient air. Pp. 154-157 in Proceedings of the Symposium on Identification and Measurement of Environmental Pollutants, June 14-17, Ottawa, Ontario, Canada.
U.S. Bureau of Mines. 1982. Minerals Yearbook 1981. Volume I. Department of the Interiors Washington, D.C.
U.S. Bureau of Mines. 1983. Asbestos. Preprint from the 1982 Minerals Yearbook. Department of the Interior, Washington, D.C.
U.S. Environmental Protection Agency. 1980. Asbestos-Containing Materials in Schools. Health Effects and Magnitude of Exposure. Support document for proposed rule on friable asbestos-containing materials in school buildings. Office of Pesticides and Toxic Substances, Environmental Protection Agency, Washington, D.C.
U.S. Environmental Protection Agency. 1982. National Emission Standards for Asbestos. Section B. Code of Federal Regulations. Title 40, Part 61.20-61.25.
U.S. Occupational Safety and Health Administration, 1983. Occupational exposure to asbestos: Emergency temporary standard. Fed. Regist. 48:51086-51140.
Wagman, J., H. R. Berger, J. L. Miller, and W. D. Conner. 1979. Dusts and Residues from Machining and Incinerating Graphite/Epoxy Composites: A Preliminary Study. Environmental Sciences Research Laboratory, Report No. EPA-600/2-79-196, Environmental Protection Agency, Research Triangle Park, N.C. 24 pp.
Watts, A. A., ed. 1980. Commercial Opportunities for Advanced Composites. ASTM Special Technical Publication 704. American Society for Testing and Materials, Philadelphia.
Wright, W. W., W. N. Rom, and F. Moatmed. 1983. Characterization of zeolite fiber sizes using scanning electron microscopy. Arch. Environ. Health 38:99-103.
Zoltai, T. 1979. Asbestiform and acicular mineral fragments. Ann. N.Y. Acad. Sci, 330:621-643.
Zoltai, T., and J. H. Stout. 1984. Mineralogy: Concepts and Principles. Burgess Publishers, Minneapolis.
Zumwalde, R. D., and L. T. Harmison. 1980. Carbon/Graphite Fibers: Environmental Exposures and Potential Health Implications. National Institute for Occupational Safety and Health, Cincinnati.

4

Measurement of Exposure to Asbestiform Fibers

For more than 50 years, asbestos-containing dust in the workplace has been measured to characterize occupational exposure to these particles. These measurements were needed to correlate specific health effects in workers with their exposure to the dust, to ensure the proper functioning of dust control equipment, and to evaluate compliance with the fiber and/or dust standards or guidelines in effect at that time. In developing these measurement methods, attempts were made to balance and maximize specificity, sensitivity, and biological relevance for the different dust components. As measurement technology and knowledge of agents and disease mechanisms advanced, new sampling and analytical methods were developed with the goal of obtaining measurements that would be useful in protecting workers. (See reviews by Ayer and Lynch, 1961; Holt, 1957; Walton, 1982.)

Attempts are now being made to determine the concentration of fibers in other environments, such as in buildings and in areas removed from known fiber sources. Techniques useful for the workplace are not always easily applied to other situations, where concentrations of materials are likely to be hundreds or thousands of times lower.

In this chapter, the committee describes the measurement methods used to determine the concentration of asbestos in a given environment. Although the discussions are focussed on the specific methods used to measure asbestos, many of these methods may also be used to measure other asbestiform fibers. The development of the techniques is presented within a historical perspective.

MEASUREMENT TECHNIQUES

Table 4-1 summarizes the principal methods used in the quantification and identification of asbestiform fibers (Burdett et al., 1980). The earliest methods measured mass. In the gross mass methods, airborne dust was collected by filtration, precipitation, or impaction, and the total dust was determined by simple weighing on conventional balances. X-ray diffraction techniques were used to identify mineral phases present in the dust; magnesium analysis was used as an index of chrysotile asbestos

TABLE 4-1. Asbestiform Fiber Measurement Methods[a]

Measurement	Collection	Quantification	Identification
Mass, gross	Filter	Gravimetric	Mineral identification by x-ray; chrysotile identification by magnesium analysis
	Electrostatic precipitator	Gravimetric (piezoelectric)	Not applicable
	Impaction	Beta-absorption	Not applicable
	Hi-vol/filter	Microscopic	Mineral identification by x-ray
Mass, respirable	Horizontal elutriator/filter	Gravimetric	Mineral identification by x-ray; chrysotile identification by magnesium analysis
	Cyclone/filter	Gravimetric	Mineral identification by x-ray; chrysotile identification by magnesium analysis
Count	Impingement	Light microscope	Identification by morphology
	Impaction	Light microscope	Identification by morphology
	Thermal precipitator	Light microscope	Identification by morphology
	Membrane filter	Light microscope phase contrast	Identification by morphology; mineral identification by dispersion staining
	Nuclepore filter	TEM,[b] SEM,[c] image recognition	Mineral identification by SAED;[d] chemical composition by EDXA[e]
	Nuclepore filter	Light scattering	Identification of fibers by magnetic alignment

[a] Adapted from Burdett et al., 1980.
[b] TEM-Transmission electron microscope.
[c] SEM-Scanning electron microscope.
[d] SAED-Selected area electron diffraction.
[e] EDXA-Energy-dispersive x-ray analysis.

content. When there was a need to collect and measure samples over short times, such as in the evaluation of controls or brief exposure episodes, the mass of the small amount of material could be measured by very sensitive piezoelectric or beta-absorption instruments.

Major drawbacks to these analytical methods were the insensitivity of the x-ray method in the detection of small particles, the nonspecificity in the resolution of chrysotile from the other serpentine minerals, and the similar nonspecificity of the magnesium assay. Because much of the mass measured by gross methods consisted of particles too large to penetrate into the lung, techniques were often used to remove the larger particles before assay. The horizontal, parallel plate elutriator was preferred in the United Kingdom, whereas industrial hygienists in the United States tended to use small cyclone devices.

All the mass methods yield results stated in terms of mass of dust per unit volume of air. In occupational environments, the units commonly used are milligrams of dust per cubic meter of air, whereas the much lower dust masses found in nonoccupational ambient environments are more conveniently expressed as nanograms of dust per cubic meter of air.

Counting methods are far more sensitive than mass determinations, since samples with too little mass to be weighed are usually adequate for counting.[1] Furthermore, since small particles far outnumber large particles, counting emphasizes the respirable dust. Lastly, fibers can be counted separately from other particles.[2]

Particles deposited directly on microscope slides by impaction or thermal precipitation can be counted by light microscopy. However, a more even dispersion can be obtained by impinging a jet of dust-ladened air on a surface submerged in a liquid. The liquid is then transferred from the impinger to a counting cell where the particles are allowed to settle so they can be seen and counted in the same focal plane. These methods have low and differing efficiency and resolving power. The membrane filter, however, is a very efficient dust collector. After being rendered transparent, thereby making the fibers visible, the filter can be examined by phase contrast microscopy. The best resolution is

[1] For example, 1 ng of chrysotile dust would yield 400 fibers 5 μm in length and 0.5 μm in diameter. A nanogram is about a thousand times lighter than most analytical balances can weigh with precision and accuracy.

[2] As noted in Chapter 2, shape alone does not determine whether a particle is asbestiform. In a workplace where asbestos fibers were the major dust present, the distinction was presumably not of major practical importance. For occupational environments, asbestos fibers are counted if they are more than 5 μm long and at least three times longer than they are wide (National Institute for Occupational Safety and Health, 1977).

obtained by the transmission electron microscope, which can resolve particles made up of only a few hundred atoms. Somewhat larger particles may be identified by techniques that reveal their chemistry (a probe technique) or crystallographic characteristics (by electron diffraction).

Results of impinger counts are usually expressed in millions of particles per cubic foot; dust concentrations measured by other methods are typically expressed as particles or fibers per cubic centimeter. In some electron microscope techniques, fibers or dispersed fibrils are counted, and the results are then converted to units of mass per volume.

MEASURING ASBESTOS DUST IN THE WORKPLACE

The Impinger Technique

Early investigators of workplace exposures to asbestos fibers in the United States used the impinger technique, then commonly used in mines. Dust was collected in an alcohol medium, usually over a short period (e.g., 20 to 30 minutes), and the suspension was examined by light microscopy at 100X total magnification. All particles in the dust were counted. Very few fibers were seen, partly because of the low resolving power of that optical system. The counting of large numbers of samples was tedious, and interobserver measurement differences led to systematic bias.

The first asbestos dust "standard" in the United States was based on measurements made with impingers by Dreessen et al. (1938). These investigators correlated observed health effects with measured dust exposures in the asbestos textile industry and tentatively concluded, with reservations, that limiting exposure to 5 million particles per cubic foot (5 mppcf) of air may be effective in preventing asbestosis. No correlation with cancer of any type was attempted. They recognized, as did later investigators, that counts of all particles provided a very indirect index of disease potential.

The Membrane Filter Technique

In the membrane filter technique, efficient, convenient collection media are used for assaying the work environment (Edwards and Lynch, 1968; Holmes, 1965; Leidel et al., 1979). A portion of the filter may be rendered transparent and then examined with a phase contrast light microscope. Fibers with an aspect ratio greater than 3 to 1 are counted on a prescribed, representative area of the filter[3] (National Institute for Occupational Safety and Health, 1977). This technique is sufficiently sensitive to allow fibers in workplaces to be counted with measurable precision and accuracy.

[3] See chapter 2 for a discussion of mineralogical definitions.

Prior to the 1960s, fibers of several lengths were counted separately and reported (Lynch, 1965). During the 1960s, the U.S. Public Health Service followed the counting strategy developed in the British textile industry, and counted only fibers >5 μm in length—a length that was later incorporated into the U.S. occupational asbestos standard (U.S. Occupational Safety and Health Administration, 1971). The longer asbestos fibers were believed to be the agents responsible for asbestosis (Beattie and Knox, 1961). In addition, when only the "longer" fibers were counted, greater precision was attained from repetitive fiber counts on the same specimen (Addingly, 1966).

MEASURING ASBESTOS DUST IN THE AMBIENT ENVIRONMENT

The number of fibers >5 μm in length counted on membrane filters by phase contrast light microscopy is used as an index for exposure in the industrial workplace. However, these fibers may constitute only a small portion of the total number of fibers present. When the fibers collected on membrane filters, which collect particles as small as 0.01 μm in diameter, are counted by transmission electron microscopy, up to 100 times more fibers may be detected than are visible by light microscopy. (See Lynch et al., 1970, for accounts of studies in the textile industry, and Rohl et al., 1976, for measurements in the brake repair industry.) The ratio of transmission electron microscope fibers to fibers visible in the light microscope may be a function of fiber type, industry, degree of manipulation, distance from emission source, and other factors. Fibers in the ambient environment far from point sources of asbestos emissions are generally much shorter than 5 urn, thinner than 0.5 μm, and, thus, predominantly smaller than the resolution capacity of the light microscope (Spurny and Strober, 1981).

In the ambient environment, electron beam instruments can be used to measure fiber concentration and to characterize single, isolated fibers (Langer and Pooley, 1973). Other mineral particulates may pose serious background problems. For example, in areas where rocks and minerals are crushed for processing, particles resembling asbestos may be emitted into the ambient environment (Langer et al., 1979).

Because chrysotile accounts for more than 90% of the asbestos used in the United States, the Environmental Protection Agency (EPA) has used it as an index of asbestos exposure. However, it was considered impractical to recover the fibers routinely without introducing artifacts or altering fiber size. Therefore, only the chrysotile mass, as determined with the electron microscope, has been monitored routinely (Thompson, 1978).

In the standard technique, large volumes of air are pulled through membrane filters. Portions of the filters are ashed in nascent oxygen at low temperatures to remove interfering organic matter. This ash is then dispersed in water by ultrasound, and the residue is filtered onto another membrane filter. Then, either this filter is "rubbed out" in a nitrocellulose medium and portions of the nitrocellulose film examined by electron beam instrumentation or it is directly transferred to an electron microscope grid for analysis. Both methods reduce the fibers to unit fibrils, thus enhancing homogenization of the specimen and reducing scan time, but information about the original nature of the fibers is lost.

RELATIONSHIPS AMONG VARIOUS EXPOSURE MEASUREMENT METHODS

Data on numbers of fibers in the workplace have been used in correlating exposure and health effects in various occupational studies (British Occupational Hygiene Society Committee on Asbestos, 1983; Dement et al., 1982; Liddell et al., 1982). In order to be able to compare diverse studies and to assess health risks from ambient exposures, it would be useful to establish a relationship among the various methods of determining exposure. Specifically, what are the relationships among the several methods used in estimating asbestos dust in the workplace and in the ambient environment?

Consistent relationships among these methods do not exist. They are subject to analytical error and subjective bias (Thompson, 1978). As examples, the electron microscope technique and its associated sampling and analytical techniques have an experimental error of approximately 15% to 30% of the measurement value. Relative standard deviations of 45% are not unusual in light microscope counts. In addition, measurements made in a particular environment at different times will vary because the actual concentrations vary.

The different techniques measure a variety of indices, which often do not remain in constant proportion to each other from sample to sample. For example, with the phase contrast light microscope, fibers longer than 5 μm are counted as a single species, whereas shorter fibers are not counted at all. Therefore, a given fiber count obtained by this technique would undoubtedly represent very different numbers of fibers and mass concentrations than the same fiber count obtained by electron microscopy. In some cases, reproducible conversion factors may be determined when large numbers of paired samples are analyzed by the various methods. However, these conversion factors usually cannot then be applied to samples obtained under a different set of conditions.

Table 4-2 summarizes some reported attempts to determine conversion factors among the various methods. The ratios in that table are based on direct, independent estimates, except for those in parentheses, which were calculated from other ratios. Although the accuracy of these estimates is not known, an order of magnitude either way would probably. embrace most situations. These ratios are equivalent only in the sense that they would be expected if side-by-side measurements were made in an environment similar to that in which the data were originally obtained.

TABLE 4-2. Relationships Among Methods of Measuring Exposure to Asbestos in the Workplace[a]

	Equivalent Values Expected from Various Measurement Methods			
Base Value[b]	Impinger (mppcf)	Phase Contrast Light Microscope (PCLM) (>5-µm-long fibers/cm^3)	Electron Microscope (EM) (EM fibers/cm^3	Mass (mg/m^3)
1 mppcf (impinger)[c]	1	6	(360)[d]	(0.2)
1 >5-µm-long fibers/cm^3 (PCLM)[e]	0.17	1	60	0.03
1 EM fiber/cm^3 (EM count)	(0.0028)	0.017	1	0.0005
1 mg/m3 (mass)	(5)	30[f]	2,000[g]	1

[a] Ratios developed by Cook and Marklund, 1982; Davis et al., 1978; Dement et al., 1982; Lynch et al., 1970; Rohl et al., 1976, and the British Occupational Hygiene Society (Walton, 1982) were used to construct the table. Some adjustment was necessary to achieve consistency.

[b] Given the base value indicated in column 1, the other columns show the equivalent value to be expected from the indicated method. Thus, 1 mppcf by impinger would be equivalent to 6 >5-µm-long fibers/cm^3 measured by PCLM or 360 fibers/cm^3 measured by the EM. Numbers have been rounded.

[c] Collected in an impinger and counted at 100X light field. mppcf = millions of particles per cubic foot.

[d] Ratios in parentheses are calculated from other ratios.

[e] Collected on membrane filters and counted by PCLM at 430X.

[f] This ratio converts to 30 LM fibers/ng versus the nominal 20 fibers/ng sometimes used.

[g] This ratio converts to 2,000 total EM fibers/ng.

The data for this table were obtained from workplace dust clouds or other environmental samples containing high concentrations of asbestos.

Fiber size/weight relationships are also presented (Table 4-3) to indicate the ratios that might be expected under various conditions. The electron microscope (EM) count/mass ratio (2,000 fibers/cm^3 per mg/m^3) in Table 4-2 is equivalent to 2,000 EM fibers per nanogram,

TABLE 4-3. The Numbers of Fibers per Nanogram for Different Size Categories (Cylindrical Fiber Shape, Density, 2.5); Diameter/Length Ratio in the Second Line[a]

	Length (μm)							
Diameter (μm)	0.625	1.25	2.5	5	10	20	40	80
0.031	819,200	409,600	204,800	102,400				
	1:20	1:40	1:80	1:160				
0.0625	204,800	102,400	51,000	25,600	12,800			
	1:10	1:20	1:40	1:80	1:160			
0.125	51,200	25,600	12,800	6,400	3,200	1,600		
	1:5	1:10	1:20	1:40	1:80	1:160		
0.25	12,800	6,400	3,200	1,600	800	400	200	
	1:2.5	1:5	1:10	1:20	1:40	1:80	1:160	
0.5		1,600	800	400	200	100	50	25
		1:2.5	1:5	1:10	1:20	1:40	1:80	1:160
1.0			200	100	50	25	12.5	6.25
			1:2.5	1:5	1:10	1:20	1:40	1:80
2.0				25	12.5	6.25	3.2	1.6
				1:2.5	1:5	1:10	1:20	1:40

[a] From Pott, 1978.

which corresponds to a distribution of fibers with a mean length of 3 μm and diameter of 0.3 μm. Such a distribution suggests the presence of substantial numbers of fibers longer than 5 μm, which would be visible under a light microscope.

The ambient air in environments far from asbestos sources have few fibers longer than 5 μm. In general, those remote ambient environments will contain many more, but smaller, fibers in a given mass than would the workplace clouds on which Table 4-2 was based (Spurny and Strober, 1981). For example, if the fibers in the remote environment had average lengths of 1 μm and diameters of 0.1 μm, there would be 70,000 EM fibers/ng (instead of the 2,000 determined for the workplace) and the ratios would be altered accordingly.

EXPOSURE TO CHRYSOTILE IN THE AMBIENT ENVIRONMENT

Chrysotile has been detected in urban air (Selikoff et al., 1972) and in lungs of urban dwellers (Langer et al., 1971; Pooley, 1972; Pooley et al., 1970). Ambient levels of chrysotile asbestos are usually expressed as mass concentrations (ng/m^3). To estimate health risks from these ambient exposures, the mass measurements need to be converted to the equivalent fiber concentrations that are used as dose measurements in workplaces, for which dose-response curves have been developed. There is no single way to do this conversion since, as explained earlier, the dust clouds are quite different, especially in regard to the sizes of fibers they contain. One approach is to convert the ambient mass data into numbers of fibers of the shortest length (5 μm) generally counted in the workplace, with an assumed diameter of 0.5 μm and aspect ratio 10:1. There are 400 fibers of this size in 1 ng.

For a mass concentration of 20 ng/m^3, which is typical of outdoor environments not near known sources, this conversion yields a concentration of 0.0080 fibers/cm^3. Even in workplaces, however, most fibers are shorter than 5 μm. Assuming that workplace fibers average 3 μm × 0.3 μm (the assumption made in Table 4-2) and applying the equivalency factors in Table 4-2, a typical equivalent concentration for 20 ng/m ^{3} would be 0.040 fibers/cm^3. However, if we were to assume an average remote ambient fiber size of 1 μm × 0.1 μm, then a concentration of 1.4 fiber/cm^3 would weigh 20 ng/m^3.

Measurements of ambient concentrations observed at single sampling locations may vary over several orders of magnitude. Seasonal changes in wind direction, especially near emission sources, account for much of this variability. For example, in studies reported by Thompson (1978), 20 specimens obtained downwind from an emission source had average asbestos fiber mass concentrations ranging from 0.03 to 8,200 ng/m3. However, for industrial cities in the continental United States from 1969 to 1970, average airborne asbestos mass concentrations ranged from 0.6 to 95.0 ng/m^3, or two orders of magnitude. During 1971 and 1972,

44 samples similarly obtained contained concentrations ranging from 0.4 to 27.7 ng/m3.

COMPLICATING FACTORS IN ENVIRONMENTAL ASSAYS

In an asbestos workplace, all the fibers may be assumed to originate from the fiber being used. However, because remote ambient environments, by definition, are distant from known asbestos sources, the identity of fibers there can neither be assumed a priori nor easily determined with any certainty, especially by light microscopy (Langer, 1979). The light microscope specified for analysis of membrane filter specimens (phase contrast microscopy) yields only size and shape information, which may allow the analyst to "identify" fibers by morphology alone. With the increased resolution of the electron microscope, the internal structure of the elementary chrysotile fibril may be visualized (Langer and Pooley, 1973). For chrysotile asbestos, morphological information and the behavior of the fiber under the electron beam are usually sufficient information for identification (see discussion in Langer et al., 1974). However, other fibers require additional diagnostic procedures. Selected area electron diffraction (SAED) yields crystal data reflecting characteristic structural elements that may enable the microscopist to distinguish among types of fibers. Chemical information may also be obtained by means of either energy dispersive x-ray analysis or crystal spectrometry probe techniques.

For fibers in remote ambient samples to be accepted as asbestiform, accurate fiber identification is needed. For example, Spurny and Strober (1981) have shown that more than 90% of "mineral fibers" in nonurban areas sampled in Europe were not asbestos, but, rather, were such materials as fibrous gypsum and even ammonium sulfate. In a study of the fibrous content of the lungs of the general population, Churg (1983) found approximately as many nonasbestos mineral fibers as asbestos fibers. Therefore, proper diagnostic tools are needed to characterize fibers in remote ambient samples as asbestiform. Furthermore, when extrapolating health risks from the workplace to such remote environments, it must be recognized not only that fiber concentrations and size distributions are different in the two environments but also that fiber types may include nonasbestiform varieties. The asbestiform properties enumerated in Chapter 2 cannot as yet be measured on microscopic samples.

FUTURE MEASUREMENT OF EXPOSURE TO ASBESTIFORM FIBERS

Walton (1982) has noted that "there is no practicable alternative to the membrane filter/phase contrast optical microscope for routine use in the occupational environment." Nonetheless, the method is too insensitive and nonspecific to yield the information needed to assess fiber exposure in the nonoccupational environment.

Several basic objectives should guide the development and eventual selection of a method for measuring fibers in nonoccupational or remote environments. First, the method should yield data that are useful in conducting epidemiological studies relating exposure and disease and in making decisions designed to reduce health risks. The ideal method should measure a characteristic, parameter, or index with biological relevance, i.e., the measurement should be related to the risk of the disease end point being studied. Possible types of measurement include fiber number, mass, length, diameter, and surface charge. Because of the great extent of environmental variability, developing accurate information about the concentrations of fibers in the air will be more dependent on the number of samples collected than on limitations of analytical techniques.

Current methods for determining ambient concentrations of fibrous particles could benefit from substantial improvement. However, sufficient standardization is needed to allow comparisons of data from various laboratories so that a data bank of ambient concentrations can be established for use by epidemiologists and other researchers.

Sensitivity and specificity improved as the light microscope was superceded by the electron microscope (EM) with its greater resolving power. One issue to be considered now concerns the relative merits of using the transmission electron microscope (TEM) and the scanning electron microscope (SEM). Other issues concern methods of preparing the fibers for the EM without disturbing them and development of improved identification techniques (Middleton and Jackson, 1982).

The SEM has been used extensively to examine environmental fibers and has produced some dramatic photographs of fibers in situ. Although the SEM direct preparation method provides little opportunity for contamination, the image resolution, contrast, and x-ray resolution of the SEM have not been sufficient for precise mineralogical identification. With an energy-dispersive x-ray attachment, the SEM can now provide analytical information for identifying minerals, but it still does not provide structural data. Because of its high resolving power, the TEM has been more generally applied to studies of environmental fibers, especially when confidence in fiber identification is required (Chatfield, 1979, 1982; Chatfield and Dillon, 1978).

Researchers do not agree on the best method of preparing representative and quantitative EM samples. The fibers in air or water must be deposited evenly and unaltered on the flat surface of an EM grid and spaced far enough apart to be readily counted and examined, yet not so far apart that there are too few to count. In most modern methods, the sample is collected either on mixed cellulose ester Millipore filters or on polycarbonate Nuclepore filters. To transfer the deposit directly onto an EM grid, the filter must be dissolved, usually by washing gently with solvent. With uncoated Millipore filters, as much as 80% of the fibers is lost.

The most satisfactory direct transfer preparation technique involves the carbon coating of particles on the surface of a Nuclepore filter. This technique is part of the current EPA interim procedure (Samudra et al., 1977). Nuclepore filters are preferred because, unlike the Millipore filters, they have a smooth, featureless surface. Because of this property, vacuum-coating with carbon produces a replicate that surrounds and traps the particles, holding them in their original position as the filter dissolves. The large amount of surface detail on Millipore filters makes them unsuitable for carbon coating.

Rigorous fiber identification is not always necessary, especially in occupational or other defined environments. Morphology alone is often adequate, especially for chrysotile. For environmental samples, which may contain many fiber-shaped particles of different minerals, selected area electron diffraction (SAED) and energy dispersive x-ray analysis (EDXA) may be used to obtain crystallographic and chemical information for more precise identifications.

RECOMMENDATIONS

Concentrations of asbestiform fibers in urban and rural locations, and at various distances from known sources, should be routinely monitored so that fiber levels and population exposures can be determined with respect to time and location. Fiber characterization is also needed. If feasible, these data should be used in conjunction with health studies to determine any effects on the exposed populations.

Characterization of fibrous dusts should include to the extent possible the length, diameter, quality, and type of all fibers present and their concentrations, both as mass and number. Direct transfer techniques and TEM examination of the preparations, or other techniques that allow examination of particles as they existed in the aerosol, should be used.

Fiber monitoring techniques for use in nonoccupational environments should be standardized so that results from various studies are comparable. Automated instrument techniques are needed to permit analysis of the large number of samples required to monitor exposure of different segments of the U.S. population over time.

REFERENCES

Addingly, C. G. 1966. Asbestos dust and its measurement. Ann. Occup. Hyg. 9:73-82.

Ayer, H. E., and J. R. Lynch. 1961. Motes and fibers in the air of asbestos processing plants and hygienic criteria for airborne asbestos. Pp. 511-522 in C. N. Davies, ed. Inhaled Particles and Vapours, Pergamon Press, Oxford.

Beattie, J., and J. F. Knox. 1961. Studies of mineral content and particle size distribution in the lungs of asbestos textile workers. Pp. 419-433 in C. N. Davies, ed. Inhaled Particles and Vapours, Pergamon Press, Oxford.

British Occupational Hygiene Society Committee on Asbestos. 1983. A study of the health experience in two U.K. asbestos factories. Ann. Occup. Hyg. 27:1-55.

Burdett, G., J. M. LeGuen, A. P. Rood, and S. J. Rooker. 1980. Comprehensive methods for rapid quantitative analysis of airborne particulates by optical microscopy, SEM and TEM with special reference to asbestos. Stud. Environ. Sci. 8:323-328.

Chatfield, E. J. 1979. Preparation and analysis of particulate samples by electron microscopy with special reference to asbestos. Scanning Electron Microsc. I:563-578.

Chatfield, E. J. 1982. Analytical procedures and standardization for asbestos fiber counting in air, water and solid samples. Pp. 91-107 in J. Small and E. Steel, eds. Asbestos Standards: Materials and Analytical Methods. NBS Spec. Pub. No. 619. National Bureau of Standards, Gaithersburg, Md.

Chatfield, E. J., and M. J. Dillon. 1978. Some aspects of specimen preparation and limitations of precision in particulate analyses by SEM and TEM. Scanning Electron Microsc. I:487-496.

Churg, A. 1983. Nonasbestos pulmonary mineral fibers in the general population. Environ. Res. 31:189-200.

Cook, P. M., and D. R. Marklund. 1982. Sample preparation for quantitative electron microscope analysis of asbestos fiber concentrations in air. Pp. 53-67 in J. Small and E. Steel, eds. Asbestos Standards: Materials and Analytical Methods. NBS Spec. Pub. No. 619. National Bureau of Standards, Gaithersburg, Md.

Davis, J. M. G., S. T. Beckett, R. E. Bolton, P. Collings, and A. P. Middleton. 1978. Mass and number of fibres in the pathogenesis of asbestos-related lung disease in rats. Br. J. Cancer 37:673-688.

Dement, J. M., R. L. Harris, Jr., M. J. Symons, and C. Shy. 1982. Estimates at dose response for respiratory cancer among chrysotile asbestos textile workers. Ann. Occup. Hyg. 26:869-882.

Dreessen, W. C., J. M. Dalla Valle, T. I. Edwards, J. W. Miller, R. R. Sayers, H. F. Eason, and M. F. Trice. 1938. A study of asbestosis in the asbestos textile industry. Public Health Bull. 241:217.

Edwards, G. H., and J. R. Lynch. 1968. The method used by the U.S. Public Health Service for enumeration of asbestos dust on membrane filters. Ann. Occup. Hyg. 11:1-6.

Holmes, S. 1965. Developments in dust sampling and counting techniques in the asbestos industry. Ann. N.Y. Acad. Sci. 132:288-297.

Holt, P. F. 1957. Pneumoconiosis: Industrial Diseases of the Lung. E. Arnold & Co., London. 268 pp.

Langer, A. M. 1979. Significance of aspect ratio in regulation of asbestos fiber exposure. Ann. N.Y. Acad. Sci. 330:601-604.

Langer, A. M., and F. D. Pooley. 1973. Identification of single asbestos fibers in human tissues. Pp. 119-225 in P. Bogovski, J. C. Gilson, V. Timbrell, and J. C. Wagner, eds. Biological Effects of Asbestos, IARC Scientific Publ. No. 8. International Agency for Research on Cancer, Lyon.

Langer, A. M., A. Sastre, and I. J. Selikoff. 1971. Chrysotile asbestos in the lungs of persons in New York City. Arch. Environ. Health 22:348-361.

Langer, A. M., A. D. Mackler, and F. D. Pooley. 1974. Electron microscopical investigation of asbestos fibers. Environ. Health Perspect. 9:63-80.

Langer, A. M., C. M. Maggiore, W. J. Nicholson, A. N. Rohl, I. B. Rubin, and I. J. Selikoff. 1979. The contamination of Lake Superior with amphibole gangue minerals. Ann. N. Y. Acad. Sci. 330:549-572.

Leidel, N. A., S. G. Bayer, K. A. Busch, and R. D. Zumwalde. 1979. USPHS/NIOSH membrane filter method for evaluating airborne asbestos fibers. NIOSH Pub. No. 79-127. National Institute for Occupational Safety and Health, Cincinnati.

Liddel, F. D. K., G. W. Gibbs, and J. C. McDonald. 1982. Radiological changes and fibre exposure in chrysotile workers aged 60-69 years at Thetford mines. Ann. Occup. Hyg. 26:889-898.

Lynch, J. R. 1965. Asbestos study proceedings and findings. Transactions of the American Conference on Governmental Industrial Hygienists, May 1965. American Conference of Governmental Industrial Hygienists, Cincinnati.

Lynch, J. R., and H. E. Ayer. 1966. Measurement of dust exposures in the asbestos textile industry. Amer. Ind. Hyg. Assoc. J. 27:431-443.

Lynch, J. R., H. E. Ayer, and D. L. Johnson. 1970. The interrelationships of selected asbestos exposure indices. Amer. Ind. Hyg. Assoc. J. 31:598-604.

Middleton, A. P., and E. A. Jackson. 1982. A procedure for the estimation of asbestos collected on membrane filters using transmission electron microscopy (TEM). Ann. Occup. Hyg. 25:381-391.

Pooley, F. D. 1972. Electron microscope characteristics of inhaled chrysotile asbestos fiber. Br. J. Ind. Med. 29:146-153.

Pooley, F. D., P. D. Oldham, H. Um-Chang, and J. C. Wagner. 1970. The detection of asbestos in tissues: Pneumoconiosis. Pp. 108-116 in H. Shapiro, ed. Proceedings of the Third International Conference. Oxford University Press, Capetown.

Pott, F. 1978. Some aspects on the dosimetry of the carcinogenic potency of asbestos and other fibrous dusts. Staub-Reinhalt Luft 38:486-490.

Rohl, A. N., A. M. Langer, M. S. Wolff, and I. Weisman. 1976. Asbestos exposure during brake lining maintenance and repair. Environ. Res. 12:110-128.

Samudra, A. U., C. F. Harwood, and J. D. Stockhalm. 1977. Electron microscope measurement of airborne asbestos concentration. EPA-600/1-77-178. Environmental Protection Agency, Research Triangle. Park, N.C.

Selikoff, I. J., W. J. Nicholson, and A. M. Langer. 1972. Asbestos air pollution. Arch. Environ. Med. 25:1-13.

Spurny, K. R., and W. Strober. 1981. Some aspects of analysis of single fibers in environmental and biological samples. Int. J. Environ. Anal. Chem. 9:265-281.

Thompson, R. J. 1978. Ambient air monitoring for chrysotile in the U.S. Pp. 355-363 in C. C. Gravatt, P. D. LaFleur, and K. F. J. Heinrich, eds. Proceedings of Workshop on Asbestos: Definitions and Measurement Methods. NBS Spec. Pub. No. 506. National Bureau of Standards, Gaithersburg, Md.

U.S. Occupational Safety and Health Administration. 1971. Occupational Safety and Health Standards, Part 1910.93 Air Contaminants (Gases, Vapors, Fumes, Dusts, and Mists). Fed. Regist. 36:10503-10506.

Walton, W. H. 1982. The nature, hazards and assessment of occupational exposure to airborne asbestos dust: A review. Ann. Occup. Hyg. 2. 5:11.5-247.

5

Effects of Asbestiform Fibers on Human Health

This chapter begins with a discussion of the types of evidence that researchers generally use in determining causes of disease. It then provides information on biodisposition of fibers and on diseases associated with exposure to asbestos. A discussion of health consequences that have Been associated with nonoccupational exposure of humans to asbestos and other asbestiform fibers is followed by a description of occupational epidemiological studies.

NATURE OF EVIDENCE

Three lines of evidence—clinical, epidemiological, and laboratory—are considered when determining whether a particular environmental agent may cause adverse effects on human health. For asbestos, as for most hazardous environmental agents, the first evidence of health effects was provided by clinical observations. Physicians observed that individual or clusters of cases of pneumoconiosis,[1] lung cancer, and finally mesothelioma were associated with exposure to asbestos.

Pneumoconiosis was the first health effect to be associated with asbestos. In 1907 Dr. Montague Murray reported his observations of such disease in a man who had worked in a carding room at an asbestos plant in England (Murray, 1907). In 1924, Cooke wrote that "medical men in areas where asbestos is manufactured have lone suspected the dust to Be the cause of chronic bronchitis and fibrosis...." (Cooke, 1924). Numerous other reports followed. Other types of pneumoconioses, such as silicosis, were also known at that time, so asbestosis, the fibrotic disease caused by asbestos, was not an entirely new type of disease. However, mesothelioma was sufficiently rare that its connection with asbestos was not accepted until 1960 (Wagner, 1960).

Clinical observations led to the hypothesis that asbestos caused the observed disease. Epidemiologists then conducted studies to ascertain whether the hypothesis was true. The association was eventually

[1] Pneumoconiosis is the pathological reaction of tissue to the inhalation and accumulation of dust in the lungs.

established primarily through cohort studies, in which the rate of disease occurrence in an exposed group is compared with the rate in a group not exposed to the material of concern (Doll, 1955; McDonald and McDonald, 1981; Selikoff and Hammond, 1979).

In laboratory studies, asbestos was administered to animals to determine whether pathological effects similar to those found in humans could be induced. These experiments followed the methodology established in the scientific study of infectious agents as causes of disease—a methodology later extended to the investigation of noninfectious agents. However, performing the experiments and interpreting the results are more complicated for diseases with long latency periods. The laboratory studies demonstrated that asbestos could cause lung cancer and mesotheliomas in animals. Fibrotic reactions, however, usually differed somewhat from the lesions observed in humans with asbestosis. This difference could be attributed to variation among species and in the nature and amount of fibers (Wagner, 1960).

Each of the three kinds of data have strengths and weaknesses. The clinician distinguishes the observed disease from similar conditions and considers the possible links to environmental and other factors. Thus the clinical contribution to understanding lies primarily in the definition of clinical entities and in suggesting possible etiological factors. Erroneous conclusions may be drawn—or new insights gained—if an atypical group of cases comes to a particular clinician's attention. Difficulties may also arise if the observed effects are confused with other syndromes with similar signs and symptoms. Misinterpretation may also occur because of the usual reliance at this stage on nonquantitative methods of assessing the relationship to environmental circumstances.

The epidemiological approach results in the quantification of risk for a defined health effect associated with exposure to particular environmental circumstances. During the application of this method, two types of errors are commonly made: (1) the findings are generalized too far beyond the population and circumstances studied and (2) there is a failure to adequately take into account the presence of other factors that may be involved in addition to, or instead of, the major factor being examined.

In laboratory experiments in animals, the investigator has the great advantage of being able to exercise control over the conditions of observation, rather than haying to rely on observations of natural phenomena as in most nonintervention clinical and epidemiological studies. Also, the laboratory investigator can make more detailed observations over time, thereby increasing the potential for ascertaining the mechanism or steps by which the agent exerts its effect. On the other hand, inference from one species to another carries some uncertainty. There is also uncertainty in extrapolating from laboratory observations to the exposures and resulting effects experienced by humans. Furthermore, laboratory animals are usually exposed to one agent, whereas humans are exposed to many.

Ultimately, the determination of a causal relationship between exposure to an environmental agent and a health effect is a judgment Based on careful evaluation of evidence. Guidelines for making such causal inferences have Been suggested and generally adopted. For example, Koch's postulates for infectious agents constituted a powerful and widely accepted framework for Judging laboratory evidence to determine whether a particular microbiological agent is responsible for a certain disuse. No such guidelines have been generally established for noninfectious agents. Perhaps the closest approximation is provided by the frequently cited criteria adopted By the Surgeon General's Advisory Committee on Smoking and Health (1964):

> The causal significance of an association is a matter of judgment which goes beyond any statement of statistical probability. To judge or evaluate the causal significance of the association between the attribute or agent and the disease, or effect upon health, a number of criteria must be utilized, no one of which is an all-sufficient Basis for Judgment. These criteria include:

(a) The consistency of the association [with diverse methods and among multiple studies]
(b) The strength of the association [ratio of rates among those exposed to rates among those not exposed]
(c) The specificity of the association [precision with which one component of the associated pair can be used to predict the other]
(d) The temporal relationship of the association [i.e., which comes first, the agent or the disease]
(e) The coherence of the association [with the natural history and biology of the disease]

The more of these criteria that are met and the stronger the evidence related to them, the more likely it is that a causal relationship exists. As another example, Hackney and Linn (1979) have updated Koch's postulates and applied them to environmental toxicology.

In evaluating relationships between exposure to hazardous environmental agents and adverse health effects, it is useful to proceed beyond identifying and confirming the hazard to quantifying the risks under various conditions. In a recent publication of the National Research Council (1983b), the authors noted that the steps of risk assessment involve (1) identification of a toxic agent and its effects, (2) determination of dose-response relationships, (3) determination of the extent of exposure, and finally (4) determination of risk.

In some situations, it is difficult to identify the effects of an agent because a given disease, such as lung cancer, may be caused by a variety of agents. Thus, exposure to cigarette smoke, asbestos, certain chromates, ionizing radiation, some chemicals, and possibly other agents may all increase the chance that a person will develop lung cancer. By contrast, for infectious diseases such as typhoid fever or tuberculosis, the microorganism is the specific and only cause, although not everyone infected by the organism gets the disease.

For most cancers, there is some chance that an individual will get the disease even with no known exposure to an identified cause. In comparing the risk of developing the disease in an exposed person to the risk for an unexposed person, it is often crucial and difficult to determine the existence and value of a "background" rate for the disease. A background rate is the rate of occurrence of a disease with no association, or no known association, with the agent(s) being considered. Exposure to an agent such as asbestos may then increase this background rate. For example, some lung cancer occurs in the absence of cigarette smoking or exposure to asbestos. In the absence of exposure to asbestos, cigarette smoking increases the chance of getting lung cancer (compared with nonsmokers) up to a factor of about 10, varying with the number of cigarettes smoked (U.S. Department of Health, Education, and Welfare, 1979). Asbestos exposure among insulation workers who do not smoke cigarettes increases the risk for lung cancer up to about 5 times (Hammond et al., 1979). Together, the cigarette smoking and asbestos exposure appear to produce a multiplicative effect, i.e., the lung cancer rate is increased up to 50-fold above background.

Expressing the relationship as an absolute risk, rather than as a relative risk, may provide information about the magnitude of the public health problem. If a relatively small risk is increased 10-fold, the resulting public health problem may still be much smaller than would result from doubling a larger risk. For example, the risk for coronary heart disease among smokers is about 1.6 times greater than the risk for nonsmokers, as contrasted with a 10-fold increase in risk for lung cancer among smokers compared with nonsmokers. However, cigarette smoking causes more deaths from coronary heart disease than it does from lung cancer, because the baseline "background" risk for heart disease is much higher than for lung cancer.

BIODISPOSITION OF FIBERS

In this section the committee briefly describes how asbestiform fibers enter the body, the properties of fibers that are important in cellular injury, and factors affecting durability of fibers after deposition and interaction with cells. Figure 5-1 shows the anatomy of the respiratory tract and the individual cell types involved in asbestos-associated diseases. The pathological effects of asbestos begin

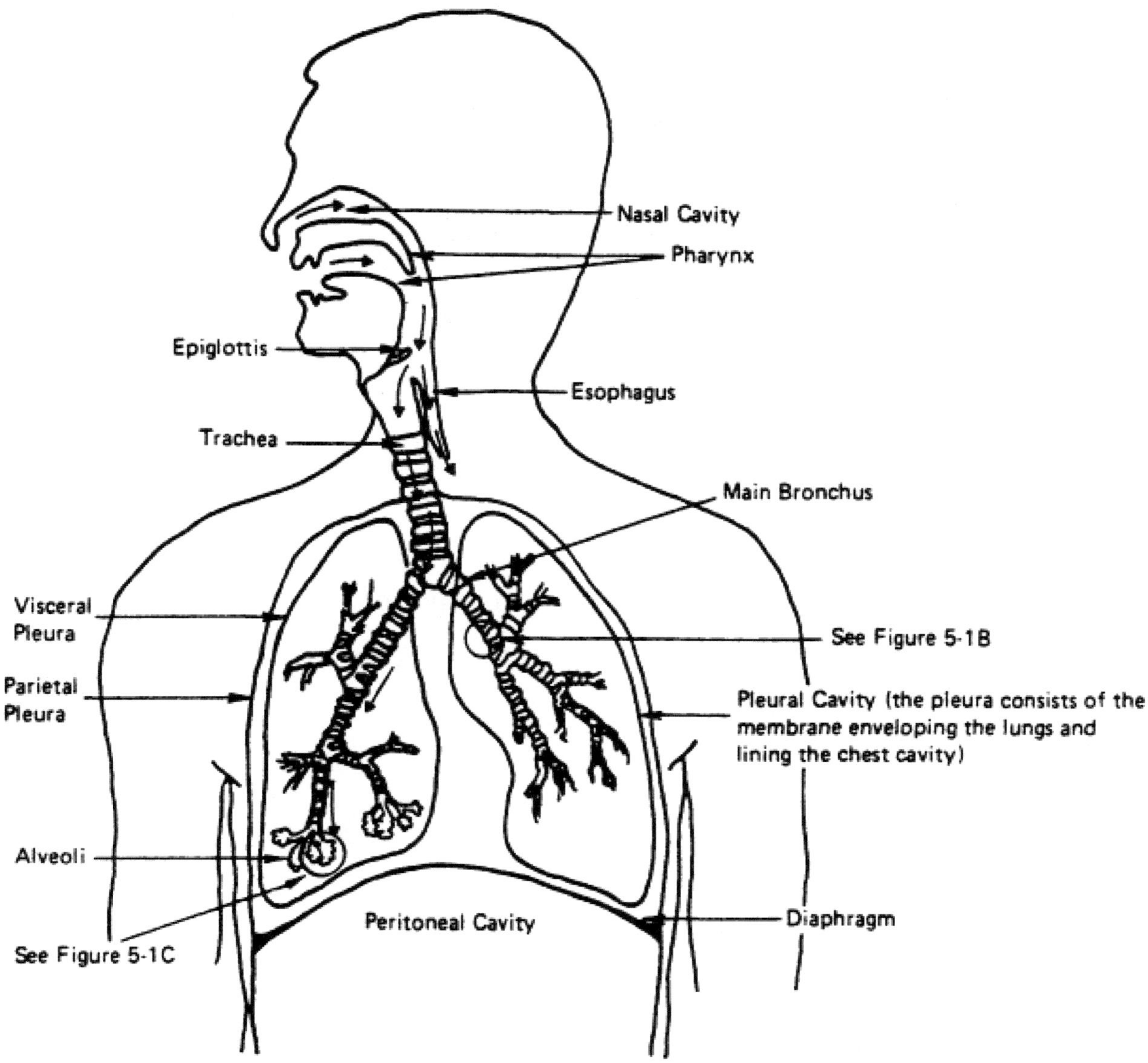

Figure 5-1A.
Routes of inhalation and ingestion of asbestiform fibers are shown by small arrows. Mesothelial cells line the outside of the lungs and the pleural and peritoneal cavities. Interaction of asbestos with these cells can result in either pleural or peritoneal mesothelioma. Adapted from Wagner, 1980.

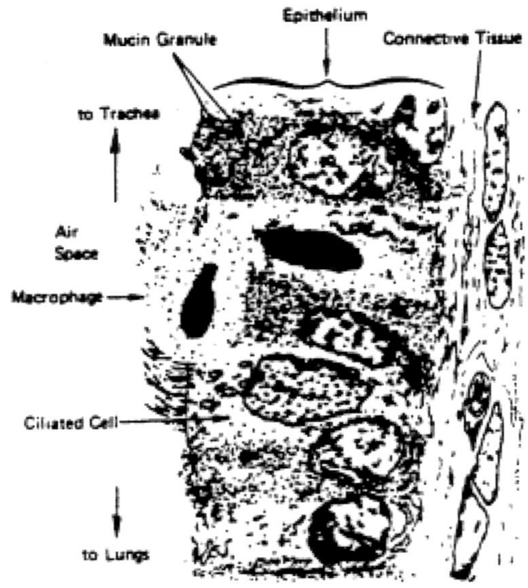

Figure 5-1B.
Cells of the bronchus, or large airways, leading from the trachea. The epithelial cell layer consists of ciliated cells, mucin-secreting goblet cells, and basal cells. The interaction of asbestos with the epithelium and with macrophages is believed to be related to the onset of asbestos-related diseases. Epithelial cells are the target for most lung cancer, whereas the macrophages serve as intermediary cells.

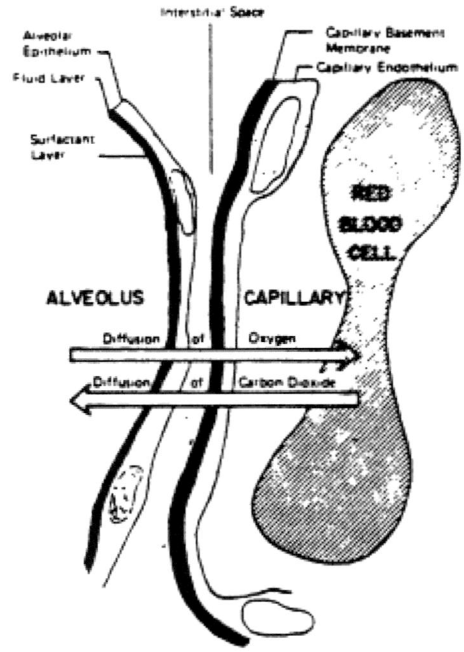

Figure 5-1C.
Cells of the alveoli, where gas exchange occurs. Interaction of asbestos with fibroblasts within the interstitial space can result in fibrosis, whereas interaction of asbestos with alveolar epithelial cells can sire rise to lung cancer. (Drawing from Guyton, 1971.)

when fibers are inhaled and ingested. Subsequently, they are deposited either in the respiratory tract or in the gastrointestinal tract. Fibers can then interact with resident cells and eventually move to the pleura and various organs. The mechanisms by which fibers reach the peritoneum are not known.

Fiber Deposition

Various factors influence the deposition of inhaled particles in the respiratory tract. When nonfibrous compact dust particles are inhaled, the ones greater than about 5 µm in diameter are generally trapped in the nasal passages before reaching the respiratory system (Walton, 1982). However, inhaled fibers align parallel to the airways and act as spheres of approximately "equivalent" diameter (Gross, 1981; Timbrell et al., 1970), where the equivalent or aerodynamic diameter of a particle is defined as the diameter of a sphere with a density of 1 g/cm^3 that has the same falling speed as the particle. There is no sharp cutoff of particle sizes determining their deposition site (Brain and Valberg, 1974).

The aerodynamic diameter of fibers depends primarily on the diameter. For fibers with aspect ratios greater than about 10:1, it is only slightly affected by length (Timbrell, 1965). From his experiments in rats, Timbrell (1965) found that the aerodynamic diameter of fibers was about 3 times the actual diameter of the fibers. Fibers with diameters greater than about 3 µm would be very unlikely to reach the alveoli.

The sizes of inhaled and deposited fibers have been compared. Morgan et al. (1979) showed the relationship between median aerodynamic diameter and alveolar deposition in rats using a variety of fibers. Hammad et al. (1982) experimented with retention of sized glass fibers in lungs of rats and found that fibers less than 1 µm in diameter accounted for most of the fibers retained (Figure 5-2). Although the count median length of fibers in the aerosol inhaled by the rats was 13 µm, the count median length found in lungs was 7 µm; for actual (as opposed to aerodynamic) diameters, the respective values were 1.2 µm and 0.5 µm. They also found that length played some role. Timbrell (1982) compared the sizes of fibers found in the air of an anthophyllite mine and mill with the sizes of fibers found in the lungs of three adult workers.

Both the configuration and dimension of asbestiform fibers determine where they impact after inhalation. Because the curlier chrysotile fiber has a relatively large cross-sectional area, its chance for interception in the airways is greater. Hence, these fibers are more likely to deposit in larger bronchioles (Morgan et al., 1973), whereas thin, rodlike fibers are carried peripherally to the terminal airways and alveoli (Timbrell, 1965; Timbrell et al., 1970; Wagner et al., 1974).

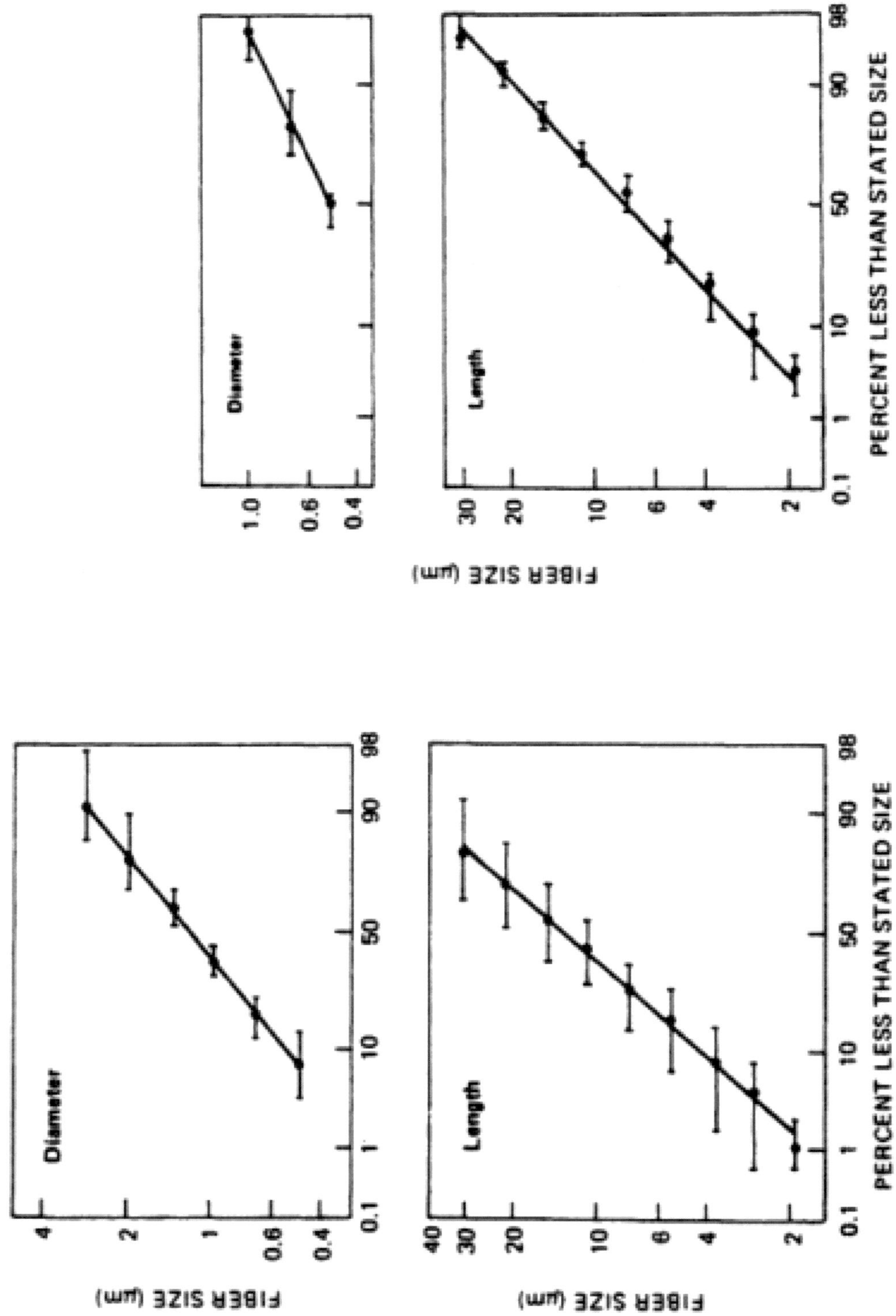

Figure 5-2.
Comparison of dimensions of man-made mineral fibers in exposure chamber and rat lung. From Hammad et al., 1982.

In addition to diameter and shape, factors such as changes in breathing rate, individual anatomic variations, smoking, and the presence of bronchitis or lung disease also influence both the extent and site of fiber deposition in humans (Brain and Valberg, 1979; Sanchis et al., 1971).

Studies in animals have demonstrated that most deposited fibers are removed from the respiratory tract within a few days. However, at least a quarter of the initial burden remains 1 month later (Evans et al., 1973; Muggenburg et al., 1981). Since much of the inhaled asbestos is not readily cleared, pulmonary tissue burden in humans may be a useful index of exposure. Attempts have been made to quantify the amount of fibers and ferruginous bodies in human and animal lungs in order to reach a better understanding of the mechanism of action of the fibers. In addition to pulmonary or other tissues, sputum and lavage samples have been studied (Di Menza, 1980).

Analyses of lung tissue samples from humans indicate that heavily exposed workers can be distinguished from those lightly exposed or from controls. Sebastien et al. (1977) reported that the number of fibers/cm^3 of lung sample, as seen by the light microscope, was approximately 106 for a heavily exposed group, 10^3 for lightly exposed workers, and 10^2 for controls.

Early researchers discovered the presence of asbestos bodies as well as asbestos fibers in pulmonary tissues of exposed workers, especially in those with asbestosis (Cooke, 1927, 1929; Cooke and Hill, 1930; Gloyne, 1929; Sebastien et al., 1979). Asbestos bodies are asbestos fibers coated with an iron-protein material that is readily visible with a light microscope. The coating, which is produced by macrophages (Suzuki and Churg, 1969), seems to prevent the fiber from interacting with cells as effectively as uncoated fibers. Because the coating may also be found on other types of fibers, the term ferruginous body is now often used instead of asbestos body. There are many reports of ferruginous bodies counted under various circumstances (Sebastien et al., 1979), but the pathological significance of these bodies is unclear. Asbestos bodies form with greater efficiency on varieties of amphibole asbestos than on chrysotile (Pooley, 1972). Because the vast majority of deposited fibers are not converted to ferruginous bodies, the presence of these bodies reflects past exposure in only a very limited way.

Electron microscope observations have provided detailed information on the deposition of fibers in animal and human tissues (Langer et al., 1973; Pooley, 1972). Chrysotile seems to degrade or be removed in vivo more readily than the amphiboles (Langer et al., 1972a, b; Wagner et al., 1974, 1982; Rowlands, 1983). Fibers found in tissue samples obtained from the general population tend to be shorter in length and diameter than those found in workers (Langer et al., 1971; Pooley et al., 1970). Fibers have also been detected in extrapulmonary tissues from both humans and animals. (For reviews, see Sebastien et al., 1979 and Cook, 1983).

Fiber burden in the lung parenchyma (the body of the lung) may be different from that in the parietal pleura (the pleura lining the chest cavity) as shown in a study of 29 persons, most of whom had pleural asbestosis (Sebastien et al., 1979). The parenchymal samples had both amphibole and chrysotile fibers. Their average length was 4.9 μm; 15% of them were longer than 8 μm. The pleural samples were predominantly chrysotile fiber, with an average length of 2.3 μm; 2% of these fibers were longer than 8 μm. Thus, short chrysotile fibers tended to predominate in the parietal pleura.

Most studies of fibers in human tissues have been conducted in workers known to have been exposed to asbestos (Churg, 1983a). However, there have been some studies of the amounts and types of fibers in the general population (Churg, 1983b; Churg and Warnock, 1980). Churg (1983b) examined mineral fibers[2] in the pulmonary tissues of 20 patients with no known occupational exposure to asbestos. He reported 13 types or groups of minerals, other than asbestos, including silica, talc, and attapulgite. More than 85% of the particles counted, and all of the attapulgite particles, were less than 5 μm long.

Clearance and Transport

Several mechanisms are involved in clearing fibrous materials from the lung. These include removal by the beating of ciliated cells and secretion of mucin (i.e., mucociliary clearance), transport by alveolar macrophages to regional lymph nodes and distal sites (Lippmann et al., 1980; Morgan et al., 1978, 1982), uptake by epithelial cells that line the airways and alveoli (Mossman et al., 1977; Suzuki, 1974), and direct translocation of fibers between epithelial cells to the interstitium and the pleura.

The physical properties (i.e., length and cross-sectional dimensions) of fibers appear to determine the mechanisms of cellular interaction and transport. For example, short fibers with fine diameters can be translocated within cells, whereas longer fibers (approximately 20 μm long) are not completely engulfed by macrophages and are cleared ineffectively (Morgan et al., 1978). Incomplete mucociliary clearance might result from discontinuities in the mucus layer or hypersecretion, a situation observed in people who smoke or have infections. Alternatively, toxic irritants such as cigarette smoke cause dysfunction and loss of ciliated and secretory cells that line the airways (Sanchis et al., 1971).

Clearance of asbestos from the gastrointestinal tract is less well understood, although it has been reported that fibers cross the mucosa of

[2] The materials detected did not necessarily have the characteristics of asbestiform fibers.

the stomach and intestines (Cook, 1983; Westlake et al., 1965). Fibers have been detected in urine and feces (Muggenburg et al., 1981). When injected into the femoral vein of pregnant rats, chrysotile crosses the placenta and has been observed in fetal liver and lung (Cunningham and Pontefract, 1974).

CLINICAL ASPECTS OF ASBESTOS-ASSOCIATED DISEASES

The four major asbestos-related diseases or changes are: (1) lung cancer; (2) mesothelioma; (3) pulmonary asbestosis; and (4) pleural plaques or diffuse thickening, calcifications, and effusion. Some other cancers may also be related to asbestos exposure (Selikoff et al., 1979). Lung cancer and mesothelioma are typically fatal cancers. Therefore, the degrees of severity are generally not relevant. Pulmonary asbestosis and the pleural changes noted above are nonmalignant pathological conditions that may range from mild to severe. They are usually related to the amount (intensity and duration) of exposure that the individual has experienced.

Although lung cancer can usually be diagnosed with reasonable certainty, mesothelioma and asbestosis are often more difficult to identify. For example, by the time a tumor is observed in a patient with mesothelioma, it may be difficult to ascertain both cell type and tissue of origin. For asbestosis, there is no complete agreement as to what constitutes a definitive diagnosis, especially for milder cases. These diagnostic uncertainties present difficulties to those analyzing results of epidemiological studies and determining incidence rates.

Inhalation is the major route by which asbestiform fibers enter the body. They may also enter the digestive tract via ingested material such as water or drugs or via asbestos-containing secretions from the lung airways that are brought up into the mouth and then swallowed (Bouhuys, 1974; Langer et al., 1979; Selikoff and Lee, 1978).

Necessary Assumptions Used in Determining Health Effects

In the absence of adequate data on the health effects of low-level and nonoccupational exposure, certain assumptions must be made in order to predict and identify possible health effects. One assumption is that clinical manifestations in nonoccupational and occupational illness will be similar in kind but not necessarily in extent or degree. In cases of lung carcinoma and mesothelioma, malignancy is usually the cause of death. Both the time from exposure to onset of symptoms and the rate of progression from time of diagnosis are assumed to be similar in nonoccupational and occupational disease.

There is little information about the rate at which pulmonary asbestosis progresses following removal from exposure (Becklake, 1976), especially brief, low-level exposure. Seidman et al. (1977) showed that even exposure of a few months and no known subsequent external exposure can increase the risk of lung cancer. It would be important to know how removal from specific exposure to asbestos modifies the risk of getting lung cancer or severe asbestosis. Day and Brown (1980) have discussed this subject with regard to cancer and asbestos.

Sensitivity and Specificity of Clinical Evidence

It is difficult to show that a disease is associated with exposure to asbestiform fibers when the exposure is nonoccupational and had not previously been suspected. One reason is that clinical symptoms and signs and underlying tissue reactions are often general and nonspecific. Although certain clinical pictures, such as bilateral pleural thickening, are typically associated with asbestiform fiber-related disease, many causes can evoke the same or a very similar response. In addition, mesothelioma is rare, and most cases investigated seem to have been associated with asbestos exposure.

The diagnostic process often begins with observations of respiratory symptoms that establish functional impairment. Then the possible morphological changes underlying the change in function are considered. Finally, the agent or factor that caused the tissue changes is sought.

The response to an inhaled agent such as asbestos is likely to include airway reactions and tissue reactions (Becklake, 1976; Craighead et al., 1982; Selikoff and Lee, 1978) that affect breathing and ventilation in a manner similar to the effect of smoking (Niewoehner, 1974). Moreover, tobacco smoking is a confounding factor in the development of asbestos-related disease, except for mesotheliomas (Hammond et al., 1979). Thus, smoking history, as well as other environmental and occupational exposures, are relevant in determining whether a disease may be related to asbestos exposure.

When diseases are observed in occupational groups exposed to asbestos, the exposure may be considered as a cause or contributing factor (Craighead et al., 1982; Goodman, 1983; Selikoff and Lee, 1978). When such diseases occur among populations not exposed in the workplace and exposure to asbestos is not suspected, the relationship may never be established. However, if mesothelioma is suspected in such nonoccupational groups, asbestos exposure will almost certainly be a diagnostic consideration. In contrast, patients believed to have lung cancer may be asked about smoking but not about asbestos exposure. For nonmalignant diseases, such as pulmonary fibrosis, nonoccupational exposure to asbestos is likely to be light and may lead to some abnormalities, mainly pleural, but to no more than mild functional impairment. Again, an association with asbestos exposure may never be established.

General Diagnostic Measures

The following general discussion of diagnosis is followed by more specific information on each disease. Depending on the disease, the patient's history often contains accounts of shortness of breath (dyspnea) upon exercise and, perhaps, at rest; a dry cough or one that produces sputum; occasional coughing up of blood; and chest pain. Other symptoms may include generalized malaise, fatigue, and weight loss. None of these complaints are pathognomonic[3] for any single illness (Becklake, 1976; Bouhuys and Gee, 1980).

Chest radiographs are an important screening and diagnostic tool. For occupational diseases with well-established exposure, the radiographic appearance may be so characteristic that it provides a diagnosis with a high degree of likelihood. For nonoccupational diseases, a characteristic chest radiograph may suggest asbestos-related changes as a possibility (Goodman, 1983; Weill et al., 1973). An international classification for the radiological assessment of asbestosis and asbestos-induced pleural disease has been recommended to help standardize diagnoses (American College of Radiology, 1982; International Labour Office, 1980).

Various abnormalities may be discovered by conducting a physical examination of a patient with an illness possibly related to exposure to asbestiform fibers. Chest auscultation[4] is noninvasive, simple, and quick to perform, and therefore lends itself to screening. However, the procedure has limitations as a clinical tool because of variability in its application among clinicians and its lack of sensitivity and specificity for asbestosis.

Lung function tests are often useful in diagnosing diseases that might be related to asbestos, although pulmonary tests alone do not lead to a definitive diagnosis. There are two basic groups of lung function tests:

Spirometric tests. These tests are performed to measure vital capacity and timed expiratory volumes, to assess restrictions on lung movement (as in fibrosis or pleural thickening) or obstructions to air flow in the airways (as in bronchitis or emphysema), and to screen for

[3] Distinctively characteristic of a specific disease, i.e., the presence of the symptom uniquely determines the diagnosis.
[4] Auscultation is the act of listening to sounds made by body organs, such as lungs.

disease. Lung volumes may also be measured, but the necessary equipment is available only in well-equipped pulmonary function laboratories.

Tests to measure diffusing capacity. In these tests, measurements are made of The lung's ability to exchange oxygen and carbon dioxide (the "blood gases") between air spaces (alveoli) and small blood vessels (capillaries). This so-called diffusing capacity measurement has been used extensively, in part because it is noninvasive. A reduced diffusing capacity results when a decreased amount of surface area is available for gas exchange, which may occur in pulmonary emphysema or in pulmonary parenchymal asbestosis. The most accurate way of assessing blood gas exchange is to measure the partial pressures of oxygen and carbon dioxide in arterial blood, but the use of this test in screening is limited because it requires sampling of arterial blood.

These pulmonary function tests give reliable information on the degree of functional impairment, and most of them are relatively simple, inexpensive, and easy to perform. Furthermore, the necessary facilities for performing these tests are generally available (Becklake, 1976; Bouhuys and Gee, 1980; Selikoff and Lee, 1978; Weill et al., 1975). More refined measurements, such as progressive exercise testing, are often helpful in assessing impairment.

Asbestos bodies have been found in sputum and in bronchoalveolar lavage samples from persons occupationally exposed to asbestos (Di Menza et al., 1980; Farley et al., 1977; McLarty et al., 1980; Smith and Naylor, 1972). Bronchoalveolar lavage has been used as a research tool to study asbestosis (Di Menza, 1980). This technique allows recovery of substantial numbers of fibers and cells and may prove in the future to be a useful clinical tool for assessing progression and developing a prognosis for disease.

As with many diseases, some individuals develop asbestos-associated diseases, whereas others, under similar or greater exposure conditions, do not. Why some individuals appear more susceptible to the effects of asbestos exposure than others is not understood. Immunological studies of persons with asbestosis were carried out to investigate possible differential susceptibility. Pernis (1965) found an increase in rheumatoid factor titer in individuals with pulmonary asbestosis. Turner-Warwick (1973, 1979) described an ongoing survey of immunological factors (including rheumatoid factor) and antinuclear antibodies (ANA). In a preliminary study, Merchant and coworkers (1975) reported asbestosis to be somewhat more frequent and severe among those with the W27 antigen (HLA system) than among those without the antigen, but subsequent studies suggest that the association is weak (Turner-Warwick, 1979) and not clinically relevant. At present there is no practical way to identify individuals immunologically or genetically susceptible to disease from asbestos exposure.

Lung Cancer. This disease accounts for approximately 100,000 deaths annually in the United States, predominantly among smokers. Lung cancer is a malignant tumor of the epithelial covering of lung airways (bronchi). Compared with lung cancers not associated with asbestos, asbestos-related cancers seem to arise more often from the lower and peripheral parts of the lung (Becklake, 1976; Craighead et al., 1982; Selikoff and Lee, 1978; Sluis-Cremer, 1980).

The tumor grows invasively through surrounding tissue and often spreads to other tissues. Local invasion is likely to obstruct airways, causing loss of ventilation, decrease in air volume, and subsequent infection behind the obstruction. Because local spread may affect blood vessels, hemorrhage is a frequent complication. Lung cancers of all the various cell types have been observed (e.g., adenocarcinoma and squamous cell carcinoma) (Kannerstein and Churg, 1972). The distribution of cell types in asbestos-exposed cases appears similar to that found in cases not associated with asbestos (Ives et al., 1983).

The earliest symptom is often the development of a persistent cough, or change in a chronic cough. Chest pain or coughing up of blood may also occur. Physical examination and pulmonary function tests often yield findings consistent with chronic bronchitis, especially in smokers, perhaps with a localized wheeze, but as tumor invasion continues, the symptoms and signs of localized airway obstruction or metastases appear. Later symptoms can include loss of appetite, weight loss, pain, general malaise, and weakness. Chest x-ray may show shadows that are consistent with tumors and enlarged lymph nodes. Where tumors arise in a background of pulmonary fibrosis, tomograms and computed tomography may be helpful in detection. The definitive diagnosis of lung cancer is based on the microscopic appearance of an appropriate tissue specimen (Adkins, 1976).

For treatment, a primary lung cancer is usually removed surgically unless metastases have occurred (Tisi, 1980). The response of lung cancer to radiotherapy or chemotherapy varies with the cell type, but, except for oat cell carcinoma, results are generally not successful. Under the most favorable circumstances, a simple squamous cell carcinoma without evidence of spread to lymph nodes offers a 40% to 50% survival after 5 years. In later stages of lung cancer of any cell type, the 5-year survival does not exceed 10% in the general population (Tisi, 1980).

Mesothelioma. Mesothelioma is also a tumor. It is of greatest concern when malignant. (There is a benign form of mesothelioma, not discussed in this report.) Malignant mesothelioma begins its development in the mesothelial cells of the pleura or peritoneum. During its early growth it causes few symptoms. By the time it is diagnosed, it is rapidly fatal, most deaths occurring in less than 2 years (Craighead et al., 1982).

Mesothelioma of the pleura often occurs first as a thickening of the pleura, first parietal (lining the chest cavity), then visceral (covering the lungs). With time, the lung becomes encapsulated and restricted in its movements. The tumor may invade the lung tissue and may spread into adjacent structures, such as the chest wall (Suzuki, 1980). Death often results from inadequate respiration or from hemorrhage (Becklake, 1976; Craighead et al., 1982; Selikoff and Lee, 1978).

Peritoneal mesothelioma may originate anywhere on the peritoneum and may initially grow without symptoms. Eventually the tumor is likely to restrict or constrict the bowel or interfere with other functions and to invade structures of the gastrointestinal tract and the retroperitoneal space. Ascites is common and recurs rapidly after tapping. The terminal event may be bowel obstruction or major hemorrhage.

Early symptoms are either lacking or vague (Becklake, 1976; Selikoff and Lee, 1978). The two common complaints of pleural mesothelioma patients are shortness of breath and dull, aching, progressive chest pain that is often unresponsive to pain relievers. A common radiological finding is a pleural effusion, which may be extensive and which recurs rapidly after tapping. This finding or a chest radiography showing asymmetrical thickening, especially in the presence of pleuritic pain, should lead one to suspect mesothelioma. Occupational history is also important. Serological tests have not been shown to be useful diagnostic tools. Histologic diagnosis, even at autopsy, may he difficult because of the polymorphic nature of the tumor.

It is more difficult to diagnose peritoneal mesothelioma than pleural mesothelioma. The diagnosis is confirmed only by microscopic examination, and even this may be difficult or impossible if the tumor is sufficiently undifferentiated. Mesothelioma may be mistaken for both carcinoma and sarcoma. Identification of the cell type in which the tumor originated is difficult. This procedure may be facilitated in the future by new techniques using cytoskeletal or other cell markers defined by antibodies.

The pathological diagnosis of mesothelioma is sufficiently difficult that special panels functioning under the auspices of the Union Internationale Contre Cancer (UICC) are often convened to assist in the diagnosis. Various studies have been conducted to assess differences in diagnosis among different pathologists or groups (Wright et al., in press).

Effective therapy for mesothelioma does not exist (Chahinian et al., 1982), although surgery, chemotherapy, and/or radiotherapy may delay death for a few months.

Fibrosis of Lung Parenchyma (Asbestosis). Asbestosis belongs to the group of illnesses called the pneumoconioses. This disease is characterized by a slowly progressing, diffuse interstitial fibrosis. The functional impairments from asbestosis fall into three groups:

(1) impaired ability to exchange gases between capillaries and alveolar air spaces, leading especially to inadequate oxygenation of blood (hypoxemia); (2) restricted breathing, leading to decreased lung volume; and (3) increased resistance in the small airways. Both (2) and (3) make the physical act of breathing more difficult.

Only the abnormalities seen in early and mild manifestations of asbestosis are considered in this section because the more severe forms would be unlikely to occur among those exposed to relatively low levels of particles (Becklake, 1976; Craighead et al., 1982; Selikoff and Lee, 1978). Animal experiments indicate that the earliest lesion is a local cellular reaction to the asbestos fiber lodged first in small airways and then in the alveoli (Brody and DeNee, 1981; Brody and Hill, 1982; Brody and Roe, in press; Brody et al., 1981, 1982, and in press). The fiber may be partially or completely surrounded or engulfed by macrophages or giant cells. A small portion of fibers may be converted to asbestos bodies. Studies of biomineralization may be able to offer additional insights into the interaction of asbestos and cells. Subsequently, fibroblasts lay down collagen, thereby initiating the fibrotic process, which is both restrictive (preventing movement) and destructive (disrupting air spaces and their blood supply). The small airways show local fibrosis with distortion and narrowing.

Classically, asbestosis has been regarded as a restrictive lung disease, but clinically one often finds evidence of obstructive lung disease, especially among smokers, or a mixed obstructive and restrictive physiological abnormality (Becklake, 1976). Results of well-designed epidemiological studies of the relative effects of smoking and asbestos exposure on small airways obstruction are not available.

The earliest patient complaint is often coughing; dyspnea (breathlessness on exertion) is usually associated with more advanced illness. Radiological changes may precede, occur simultaneously with, or follow the changes in pulmonary function. The changes observed in the chest radiograph are typically located in the lower half of the lung. The early changes include ill-defined linear opacities. Before any patient complaints, fine crepitations or rales at the lung bases may be heard by auscultation. In addition, arterial oxygenation and diffusing capacity may be decreased.

Smoking may also affect the pulmonary function tests and radiological results, especially with respect to small airways disease (Buist, 1983). The early changes seen in the chest radiograph may not be immediately associated with pulmonary asbestosis, but as the opacities become more profuse, more clearly defined linear opacities appear, septal lines become more marked, and pleural involvement is often seen. At that stage, the radiological picture alone may strongly suggest asbestosis.

The most effective prevention or treatment is early removal from exposure. Although asbestosis often continues to progress (Becklake,

1976), the progression is not inevitable and often not rapid (Gregor et al., 1979; Jones et al., 1980a).

Progressive hypoxia with cot pulmonale are common causes of death among those with advanced asbestosis, and many persons with advanced asbestosis die from lung cancer. Mild asbestosis is not necessarily associated with functional impairment.

Pleural Changes. Diffuse pleural thickening, plaques, calcification, and effusions are nonmalignant changes in the pleura that have been associated with asbestos exposure (Albelda et al., 1982; Epler et al., 1982; Weiss et al., 1981). These changes, usually detected by radiographic-examination rather than by patient symptoms, may indicate that asbestos exposure has occurred. They may develop after little apparent exposure and may result in few symptoms, or they may be associated with more extensive exposure and parenchymal asbestosis. The parietal pleura is usually more heavily involved than the visceral pleura (Becklake, 1976; Selikoff and Lee, 1978). There may be simple, benign pleural effusion, and the usually sterile fluid may contain lymphocytes, possibly erythrocytes, and albumin. Asbestos bodies and fibers are rarely found in the fluid or the plaques.

With extensive pleural involvement, the symptoms are similar to those of restrictive pulmonary disease, and may include dyspnea, a feeling of tightness, and pulmonary restriction that may occasionally result in marked impairment. Complaints of pain are rare.

Pleural changes progress slowly, and most patients experience little functional impairment. There are no well-designed studies to provide evidence on whether persons with these asbestos-induced pleural changes are at increased risk of lung cancer or mesothelioma beyond that attributable to asbestos exposure per se.

DISEASE ASSOCIATED WITH NONOCCUPATIONAL INHALATION EXPOSURES TO ASBESTIFORM FIBERS

Having described clinical manifestations of the diseases associated with asbestos exposure, the committee now discusses some observations among populations exposed to asbestiform fibers outside the workplace. In general, data on nonoccupational exposures are sparse. However, the studies that have been conducted provide information about the variety of minerals in fibrous form that may lead to asbestos-associated disease. If adequate population-based data were to become available, it might be possible in some situations to estimate exposure or to test risk-assessment models.

End points that have been used to detect health effects include overall mortality, mortality from lung cancer and mesothelioma, and nonmalignant respiratory changes such as the presence of asbestosis or pleural plaques. Exposures have occurred in the households of asbestos workers, in neighborhoods near asbestos-manufacturing facilities, and in areas with natural sources of asbestiform fibers.

Mesothelioma provides a useful end point for studying effects of exposure. This fatal tumor is rare, except in certain groups exposed to asbestiform fibers. In some worker cohorts, as many as 10% of the deaths have been caused by mesothelioma (McDonald and McDonald, 1980, 1981; Selikoff et al., 1979). Small numbers of mesotheliomas are more easily detected than small excess numbers of lung cancers, since lung cancers account for about 5% of all deaths in the United States (U.S. Department of Health and Human Services, 1983). Furthermore, unlike lung cancer, mesothelioma is not associated with smoking (Hammond et al., 1979).

The best estimates of the national incidence rate for mesothelioma have come from the National Cancer Institute's Surveillance, Epidemiology and End Results (SEER) Program, which collects data on cancer incidence in about 10% of the country. Approximately 1,600 mesothelioma cases were estimated to have occurred in 1980. For the period from 1977 to 1980, SEER reported 431 male cases and 117 female cases (Connelly and Myers, 1982). From these data, the annual incidence rate for mesothelioma was calculated as 11.8 per million per year for males and 2.6 per million for females, age-adjusted to 1970.

The incidence rate apparently varies with opportunities for past exposure to asbestos. In the United States, the lowest rate occurred in Iowa, where the incidence rate for white males during 1977-1980 was 7.4 cases/million per year. In Seattle and San Francisco-Oakland, where there was extensive shipbuilding during World War II, the annual incidence rate was about 20 cases/million, age-adjusted for 1970.

National mortality statistics for mesothelioma are not available from the National Center for Health Statistics (NCHS) because cancers are classified by site rather than by type. For 1979, malignant neoplasms of the pleura (ICD Code 163, 9th Revision) were reported to be the cause of death for 257 males and 83 females (S. Seeman, National Center for Health Statistics, personal communication, 1983).

Because of the difficulties in diagnosing mesothelioma and determining exposure to asbestiform fibers, the background rate of mesothelioma is not known. In one study of 4,539 cases from 22 countries between 1959 and 1976, there was no definite or probable history of exposure for 38% of the subjects (McDonald and McDonald, 1977). In North America, it was estimated that from 50% to 75% of male cases, but only 10% of females, are likely to have been exposed to asbestos (McDonald and McDonald, 1981). A recent review indicates that a few cases of mesothelioma have been reported in nickel workers[5] and in persons with

[5] Langer et al. (1980) reported that they found asbestos fibers contaminating some nickel ores.

some other specific exposures (Peterson et al., in press). It is thus possible that not all cases of mesothelioma are associated with exposure to asbestiform fibers. However, since the levels of general ambient exposures to asbestos were not known, the possibility that the residual cases might also be attributable to asbestos exposures cannot be discounted.

Epidemiological data have led to questions about the characteristics of fibers that are associated with mesothelioma. Some investigators have interpreted the data as indicating that exposure to chrysotile is less likely to produce mesothelioma than is exposure to the other asbestos fibers (Craighead and Mossman, 1982; McDonald and McDonald, 1981). However, because it is difficult to determine exposure and to characterize fibers adequately, it has not been possible to confirm or refute the argument.

Asbestos Exposure from Household Contacts

Anderson et al. (1979) studied household cohabitants of 1,664 asbestos workers. The workers were employed in a factory that had produced amosite asbestos products from 1941 to 1954. Controls were urban New Jersey residents living in the same community who had routine chest x-rays between January 1975 and December 1976. Asbestos-associated x-ray abnormalities were found in 35% of the 678 household contacts examined and in 51 of the controls. The abnormalities included small, irregular parenchymal opacities as well as pleural thickening, calcification, and plaques. Five of 550 deaths traced among the cohort of 3,100 household contacts were due to mesothelioma—a proportion much higher than that seen in the general population. No reliable estimates of dust levels in homes were available, but the authors assumed that asbestos was brought home on work clothes.

Other data also indicate that household exposure can lead to health effects. In New York State, 52 females with malignant mesothelioma between 1967 and 1977 were investigated to determine their occupational histories and the occupations of their fathers and husbands (Vianna and Polan, 1978). Thirty-two of the cases were pleural mesothelioma and 20 were peritoneal. Six cases and two of the 52 controls had been exposed occupationally. Eight other cases had husbands or fathers who had been occupationally exposed, but none of the controls had occupationally exposed husbands or fathers.

Neighborhood Exposure to Asbestos

A cohort of 1,779 males living within 0.8 km of a Unarco amosite factory in Paterson, New Jersey, was studied to determine if excess mortality had occurred (Hammond et al., 1979). Another neighborhood several kilometers away served as a control. None of the subjects had worked in the plant. No excess mortality or excess lung cancers were detected between 1962 and 1976 in the group living near the plant. Thus, in this study, males living in the factory neighborhood apparently were less at risk (at least for mesothelioma) than members of worker households. No estimates of neighborhood levels of asbestos fibers or other carcinogens were available for either area of study.

Natural Sources of Asbestiform Fibers

Asbestos-related diseases have been associated with exposure to naturally occurring mineral fibers in Turkey, Finland, and Bulgaria (Baris et al., 1981; Kiviluoto, 1960; Zolov et al., 1967). In most cases, quantitative exposure measurements have not been published. In the United States, no differences in mortality were found for specific cancers in counties with and without natural asbestos deposits (Fears, 1976), although the study design would not be likely to detect small effects. Coffin et al. (1983) have recently discussed the occurrence of mesothelioma and other asbestos-associated lesions in some human populations and in animals not known to be exposed to asbestos. They and others (e.g., Glickman et al., 1983) suggest that further study of these situations, such as mesothelioma in pet dogs, might help people to discover sources of exposure to harmful fibers.

Pleural plaques were found to be endemic among agricultural workers in an area of Southern Bulgaria (Zolov et al., 1967). Of 3,300 people examined, 4% of those with no mining exposure to asbestos had pleural plaques. Most of those subjects were agricultural workers. Analysis of soil samples revealed the presence of asbestiform fibers (Burilkov and Michailova, 1970) consisting of anthophyllite, tremolite, and sepiolite, the latter being a layered silicate with a triple subchain structure. No pleural plaques were found in a neighboring farming region that lacked asbestiform fibers in the soil.

In south central Turkey, several villages are located on and in tuff, a rock composed of volcanic detritus that may contain a variety of fibrous minerals (Artvinli and Baris, 1982; Baris et al., 1981; Lilis, 1981; Rohl et al., 1982). Dwellings are hollowed out of the rock. Studies of the populations of these villages have revealed mortality and disease patterns that are similar to those usually seen among asbestos workers, with respect to occurrence of fibrosis, pleural plaques, lung cancer, and mesothelioma (Artvinli and Baris, 1982). In Karain, a village with a population of about 600, 36 cases of mesothelioma were reported between 1969 and 1974 (Baris et al., 1981). The median age of death in Karain was 54, whereas it was 68 in the nearby village of Karlik. In another nearby village, Tuzkoy, malignancies accounted for 41 of 67 deaths that occurred from 1978 to 1980 among almost 2,000 residents older than 25 years (Artvinli and Baris, 1982). Of these deaths, 15 were due to pleural mesothelioma, 12 were attributed to peritoneal mesothelioma, and 8 were caused by lung cancer. The mesotheliomas were found equally among male and female residents, and the mean age of the mesothelioma cases was about 50, which is younger than that found among worker groups. These data suggest that an environmental exposure beginning at a young age might have been responsible for the diseases.

Dust and fiber levels were measured in Karain and in the "control" village Karlik (Baris et al., 1981). Dust levels in both villages were about 1 mg/m^3. Levels of fibers were higher in Karain than in Karlik, but in both villages, most air samples had less than 0.01 $fiber/cm^3$. Nonetheless, in 11 samples taken during the cleaning of the caves in which the Karain villagers lived, the concentrations ranged from less than 0.01 $fiber/cm^3$ to 1.38 $fibers/cm^3$.

Although tremolite asbestos was apparently present in the area, the most prevalent fibers appeared to be erionite. Analysis of pleural and parenchymal tissues from mesothelioma patients from Karain indicated that 90% of the fibrous particles had a composition consistent with that of erionite (a fibrous zeolite), whereas from 1% to 5% were consistent with tremolite (Rohl et al., 1982). The use of an analytical transmission electron microscope to examine lung tissue from two mesothelioma cases from Tuzkoy revealed a concentration of 108 fibers per gram of dried lung tissue (Sebastien et al., 1981). Of the uncoated fibers, 93% were erionite with a mean length of about 3.7 μm. Only 3% of the fibers were longer than 8 μm or thinner than 0.25 μm. The remaining fibers seem to have been either titanium oxide (futile) or some material resembling amphibole. The data are consistent with the hypothesis that erionite may have a role in causing the high rate of mesothelioma in these villages.

It is not clear how to account for the higher mesothelioma and lung cancer rates in these villages if the diagnoses and measured environmental exposures are correct. Possible explanations include enhanced ability of the fibers to cause cancer for reasons not yet known, the presence of other, undetected carcinogenic agents, or increased susceptibility if inhalation of the fibers starts in infancy (Baris et al., 1981), since children are known to have increased susceptibility to the effects of many environmental agents. It would be of interest to estimate the exposure necessary to account for the observed mesothelioma rates by using some of the time-dose-response models for mesothelioma that have been developed for worker populations. These models are discussed in Chapter 7 of this report. A rough calculation shows that a lifetime exposure to about 20 $fibers/cm^3$ accounts for a mesothelioma lifetime risk of 50%, based on the data presented in Table 7-3.

Rom et al. (1983) considered the possible health hazard posed by naturally occurring fibrous erionite in Arizona, Nevada, Oregon, and Utah. A review of 275 chest radiographs in one hospital near such an area in Nevada showed background levels of pleural plaques (2%) and pleural thickening (6%) and no pleural calcifications. Analysis of the fibrous materials in the various areas indicated the presence of materials of a size that would be respirable (Wright et al., 1983). Wagner (1982) has reported that erionite from Oregon is extremely potent in producing mesotheliomas in rats.

Summary

Persons residing in areas in Turkey where asbestiform fibers are present in the environment and persons living in the same household as workers exposed to asbestos develop mesothelioma at a rate in excess of that for the general population. The evidence is based primarily on clinical observations and on case-control studies that do not permit generalization. It seems likely that these mesotheliomas arise from respiratory exposure to asbestiform fibers.

EPIDEMIOLOGICAL STUDIES OF EFFECTS RESULTING FROM THE INGESTION OF ASBESTOS IN DRINKING WATER

Epidemiological studies of the effects of asbestos in drinking water in six geographical areas of the United States and Canada have been extensively reviewed and critiqued (Marsh, 1983; Workshop on Ingested Asbestos, 1983). In all these studies, a possible excess incidence of gastrointestinal (GI) cancers was evaluated as were morbidity or mortality rates for some other cancers. In addition, the National Research Council's Safe Drinking Water Committee addressed this problem and estimated the risk of excess GI cancers associated with ingesting asbestos in drinking water (National Research Council, 1983a).

Tables 5-1, 5-2, and 5-3 summarize the characteristics and results of the various studies. Duration of exposure ranged from as little as 20 years (in Duluth[6]) to more than 50 years (in Quebec); asbestos concentrations ranged from less than detectable limits to $1{,}300 \times 10^6$ fibers/liter. Except for Duluth, where taconite mine tailings were dumped into Lake Superior, the subjects were exposed to chrysotile from natural sources (in Quebec, the San Francisco Bay area, and Puget Sound) or from asbestos-cement pipes (in Utah and Connecticut).

The studies did not indicate consistent excesses of cancer. In Duluth, no consistent type of cancer occurred in excess among residents (Levy et al., 1976; Mason et al., 1974; Sigurdson et al., 1981). In Quebec, cancer mortality was evaluated in relation to asbestos in municipal water supplies. In the first study (Wigle, 1977), 22 municipalities were grouped into three categories based on level of asbestos in water supplies. In a more extensive study (Toft et al., 1981), mortality rates for two cities with high exposure ($>100 \times 10^6$ fibers/liter) were compared with 52 low exposure cities ($<5 \times 10^6$ fibers/liter). Some excess cancers in males that were noted in the two studies were attributed to probable occupational exposure. In Connecticut, tumor registry data indicated that there was no association

[6] The particles in Lake Superior were mostly acicular cleavage fragments rather than asbestiform fibers (T. Zoltai, personal communication, 1983). See also Langer et al., 1979.

between asbestos risk scores and GI tumor incidence (Harrington et al., 1978; Meigs et al., 1980). In San Francisco, there were inconsistent excesses of some cancers (Conforti et al., 1981; Kanarek et al., 1980; Tarter, 1981). In Puget Sound, a proportional incidence analysis comparing length of residence suggested an excess for some GI cancers (Polissar et al., 1982).

TABLE 5-1. Characteristics of Asbestos Exposures from Drinking Water in Different Study Populations[a]

	Exposure Characteristics			
Location of Study	Type of Asbestos	No. of Fibers per Liter (Range)	Size of Population Exposed	Maximum Duration of Exposure (Years)
Duluth	Amphibole[b]	$1\text{-}30 \times 10^6$	100,000	15-20
Connecticut	Chrysotile	BDL[c]-0.7×10^6	576,800	23-44
Quebec	Chrysotile	$1.1\text{-}1{,}300 \times 10^6$	420,000	50
Bay Area, California	Chrysotile	$0.025\text{-}36 \times 10^6$	3,000,000	40
Utah	Chrysotile	NA[d]	24,000	20-30
Puget Sound	Chrysotile	$7.3\text{-}206.5 \times 10^6$	200,000	40

[a] From Marsh, 1983.

[b] Most of these particles were probably acicular crystals rather than asbestiform fibers (T. Zoltai, University of Minnesota, personal communication, 1983). Langer et al. (1979) referred to the particles as amphibole gangue minerals and discussed the uncertainties in determining whether they are asbestiform.

[c] BDL = below detectable limit.

[d] NA = not available.

All of the epidemiological studies had limitations. Perhaps the most serious were the substantial problems in classifying exposure because population data rather than individual data were used. Errors in classification will tend to weaken any true associations that may exist between asbestos in drinking water and health effects. Given the difficulty of determining individual exposure, results of these epidemiological studies cannot be taken as strong evidence about the extent to which ingestion of drinking water containing asbestiform fibers might increase the risk of GI cancer. The NRC Safe Drinking Water.

TABLE 5-2. Hummary of Studies of Gastrointestinal Cancer in Relation to Ingested Asbestos by Cancer Site[a]

	Association of GI Cancer with Asbestos, by Site[b] (ICD 7th Revision Codes)										
Location	All Sites Combined (150-159)	Esophagus (150)	Stomach (151)	Small Intestine (152)	Colon (153)	Rectum (154)	Biliary Passages/liver (155-156A)	Gall Bladder (155.1)	Pancreas (157)	Peritoneum (158)	References
Duluth	(++)	(+-)	(++)	NS	(00)	(++)	(00)	NS	(0+)	NS	Mason et al., 1974
Duluth	(—)	(00)	(+0)	(00)	(—)	(00)	(00)	(00)	(++)	(00)	Levy et al., 1976
Duluth	(00)	(00)	(00)	(00)	(00)	(00)	(00)	(00)	(0+)	(00)	Sigurdson et al., 1976
Connecticut	NS	NS	(00)	NS	(00)	(00)	NS	NS	NS	NS	Harrington et al., 1978
Conneticut	NS	NS	(00)	NS	(00)	(00)	NS	NS	(+0)	NS	Meigs et al., 1980
Quebec	(00)	(00)	(+0)	NS	(00)	(00)	NS	NS	(0+)	NS	Wigle, 1977
Quebec	(+0)	(00)	(+0)	NS	(00)	(00)	NS	NS	(00)	NS	Toft et al., 1981
Bay Area, Calif.	(++)	(0+)	(++)	(00)	(00)	(00)	(00)	(0+)	(0+)	(++)	Kanarek et al., 1980
Bay Area, Calif.	(++)	(++)	(++)	(00)	(+0)	(00)	(00)	(00)	(++)	(0+)	Conforti et al., 1981
Bay Area, Calif.	(++)	NS	NS	NS	NS	NS	NS	NS	NS	NS	Tarter, 1981
Utah	NS	NS	(00)	(00)	(0-)	(00)	NS	(0+)	(00)	(00)	Sedler et al., in press
Puget Sound	(00)	NS	(00)	NS	(—)	NS	NS	NS	NS	NS	Severson, 1979
Puget Sound	NS	(00)	(00)	(++)	(00)	(00)	(00)	(00)	(00)	(00)	Polissar et al., 1982

[a] From Marsh, 1983.

[b] (Male, female) association with ingested asbestos.

+, positive; 0, no association;-negative; NS, not studied.

TABLE 5-3. Summary of Studies of Risk from Cancer Other Than Gastrointestinal Cancer in Relation to Ingested Asbestos, by Cancer Site[a]

	Association of Cancer Other Than GI with Asbestos, by Site[b] (ICD 7th Revision Codes)									
Location	Buccal Cavity and Pharynx (140-148)	Bronchus, Trachea and Lung (162, 163)	Pleura (162.2)	Prostate (177) (males only)	Kidney (180)	Bladder (181)	Brain/ CNS[c] (193)	Thyroid (194)	Leukemia, Aleukemia (204)	References
Duluth	NS	(+0)	NS	NS	NS	NS	(00)	NS	(00)	Mason et al., 1974
Duluth	NS	NS	NS	NS	NS	NS	NS	NS	NS	Levy et al., 1976
Duluth	NS	(00)	NS	NS	NS	NS	NS	NS	NS	Sigurdson et al., 1976
Connecticut	NS	NS	NS	NS	NS	NS	NS	NS	NS	Harrington et al., 1978
Connecticut	NS	(00)	NS	NS	(00)	(00)	NS	NS	NS	Meigs et al., 1980
Quebec	(00)	(+0)	NS	0	(00)	(00)	(00)	NS	(00)	Wigle, 1977
Quebec	(00)	(+0)	NS	0	(00)	(00)	(00)	NS	(00)	Toft et al., 1981
Bay Area, Calif.	NS	(+0)	(0+)	0	(0+)	(00)	(00)	(00)	(00)	Kanarek et al., 1980
Bay Area, Calif.	NS	(00)	(0+)	+	(00)	(00)	(00)	(00)	(00)	Conforti et al., 1981
Bay Area, Calif.	NS	NS	NS	NS	NS	NS	NS	NS	NS	Tarter, 1981
Utah	NS	NS	NS	NS	(+0)	NS	NS	NS	(+0)	Sadler et al., 1981
Puget Sound	NS	NS	NS	NS	(00)	NS	NS	NS	NS	Severson, 1979
Puget Sound	(00)	(00)	NS	+	(00)	(00)	+-)	(++)	(+-)	Polissar et al., 1982

[a] From Marsh, 1983.

[b] (Male, female) association with ingested Asbestos.

+, positive; 0, no association;-, negative; NS, not studied.

[c] CNS - central nervous system.

Committee (1983a), using a variety of assumptions, estimated the excess risk of GI cancers that might be expected from ingestion of asbestos-containing drinking water and concluded that their risk estimates are consistent with the results of the epidemiological drinking water studies considered.

OCCUPATIONAL EPIDEMIOLOGICAL STUDIES—METHODOLOGICAL CONSIDERATIONS

Evaluation of potential health effects from nonoccupational exposure to asbestiform fibers depends primarily on results of epidemiological studies of occupational groups. Most of the analyses have involved cohort[7] studies of workers exposed to asbestos of various types and in a variety of industries and occupations. Much information has been obtained from these studies. However, they also suffer from limitations common to many epidemiological studies and from some additional problems related to determining dose (exposure) and response (health end point, such as death from a specific cause). Despite the limitations of individual studies, the committee finds that, when all the studies are considered, exposure to asbestos increases the risk of developing lung cancer, mesothelioma, asbestosis, and possibly other cancers.

To quantify health risks from an exposure, it is necessary to obtain dose-response data, but exposure measurements are particularly difficult to obtain. Because of the lone latency period for asbestos-associated diseases, investigators have found it necessary to try to reconstruct past exposures. Techniques of measurement vary from place to place and over time (Acheson and Gardner, 1980; Dement et al., 1983a). For example, fiber counts obtained by light microscope in various industrial settings may need to be multiplied by a factor varying from 2 to 8 to obtain a true count of fibers longer than 5 μm.

Typically, a cumulative dose measurement is used. This does not take into account the time lapsed since last exposure nor does it distinguish between short exposures of high intensity and lone exposures to low dust concentrations. In addition, a cumulative dose measurement does not change when exposure ceases. Variability in these exposure-related

[7] The two major types of epidemiological studies are cohort studies and case-comparison studies. In a cohort study, a group with certain defined characteristics of exposure is selected and followed to determine the number of members reaching a particular end point, such as death, by a specified time. The group is called a cohort. In its purest form, the analysis of a cohort study depends entirely on within-cohort comparisons, and the results may be presented as arrays of morbidity or mortality rates or by a large variety of other expressions of association or correlation. A cohort might comprise two major groups, differentiated by their exposure experience. However, in occupational studies, especially of cancer, the rate of occurrence of death or disease in the group is often compared with the rate in some

factors affect mortality responses in occupational cohorts. In some studies, exposure surrogates, such as type of Job and duration of employment, are used to estimate exposure. These estimates may be less precise than actual measurements. (See Consumer Product Safety Commission, 1983, for a detailed assessment of exposure estimates among the various asbestos studies.)

There may also be variability in reporting causes of death, ascertainment of deaths, and diagnostic accuracy of the reported cause of death. Inaccuracies are particularly likely for mesothelioma and asbestosis (Hammond et al., 1979). In morbidity studies, asbestosis, pleural thickening and calcification, and pulmonary dysfunction may be incompletely diagnosed. For example, although the American College of Radiology has stated that certain radiographic evidence [i.e., Category 1 profusion, as defined in the International Labor Organization (ILO) 1980 Classification] together with a clear history of exposure to asbestos suffices to make a presumptive diagnosis of asbestosis, other diagnostic criteria have been suggested.

Methodological differences are a major source of variation in comparing studies (Enterline, 1976). For example, the results obtained will depend on the criteria for selecting the cohort, the choice of comparison groups, the influence of other environmental factors that may introduce competing disease risks, and the records available.

In addition, heterogeneity in the time at which onset of exposure begins can introduce additional distortion in the observed relative risks (Weiss, 1983), especially because the types of exposure experienced by some workers in the distant past may differ from exposures experienced only more recently. Weiss also discussed how the results of lung cancer studies can be affected if persons who left a job are not included in the study cohort. He found that the exclusion of these workers could affect the relative risk by a factor of 2 to 3.

An additional difficulty is encountered when comparing dose-response results from mortality and morbidity studies, particularly if the

---

other appropriate, external population, such as males of an appropriate age group, because the researchers did not have an appropriate internal comparison group. Results of mortality studies of cohorts are usually expressed as a standardized mortality ratio (SMR), which is defined as observed deaths in the cohort divided by expected deaths. An SMR of greater than 1, if statistically significant, may indicate that excess deaths have occurred in the exposed cohort. The SMR is similar to the relative risk. In a case-comparison study, the epidemiologist starts with cases of the disease of interest, such as lung cancer or meso-thelioma, and then compares exposure parameters and other risk factors between cases and appropriately selected persons without the disease to to determine whether certain exposures are seen more frequently among cases than among the noncases (sometimes called controls).

morbidity studies are confined to active workers, which is usually the case. A bias is introduced in studies of active workers, since those with severe disease have probably already left employment. However, asbestosis generally progresses after cessation of dust exposures (Becklake et al., 1979; Rubino et al., 1979b).

Numerous follow-up studies of asbestos-related mortality have been conducted on cohorts with varying intensity and duration of exposure, type of exposure, type of work, time and duration of follow-up periods, and employment status at onset of study. There have also been differences in the completeness of the cohort, completeness of mortality ascertainment, availability of smoking histories, geographic area of study, selection of comparison populations, and methods of data analysis. Because of the variations noted, it is not surprising that the standardized mortality ratios (SMRs) and dose-response results differ greatly among studies (See Appendix E, Table E-1, and Consumer Product Safety Commission, 1983.) In general, however, the same major diseases—lung cancer, mesothelioma, and asbestosis—have been observed, although not all investigators conducting these studies have reported or detected excesses of all three of those diseases.

CANCER MORTALITY IN OCCUPATIONAL COHORTS EXPOSED TO ASBESTOS

To evaluate variations in cancer mortality associated with occupational exposure to asbestos, the committee reviewed studies of 23 occupational cohorts. These are summarized in Table 5-4 and in Appendix E, Table E-1. These studies indicate the variety of occupations and industries where asbestos exposure has occurred and the types of asbestos commercially used.

The epidemiological study by Doll (1955) verified and quantified the occurrence of excess lung cancer among persons who work with asbestos. His study population consisted of 113 men who had been exposed to high levels of chrysotile in an asbestos-processing plant in England before the effective implementation of regulations in 1933. During the follow-up through 1953, there were 11 deaths from lung cancer in comparison to an expected value of 0.8 based on national death rates.

In 1980, Peto (1980a) reported on the mortality experience of 679 men who were initially employed after 1933 at the same plant studied by Doll. Among these workers, 40 deaths from lung cancer were observed compared to 23 expected. In addition, there were 10 pleural mesotheliomas. Furthermore, the risk of mesothelioma appeared to be associated with time elapsed since initial exposure.

In the United States, excess lung cancers among persons who worked with asbestos were reported by epidemiologists in 1954, 1963, and 1964 (Breslow et al., 1954; Mancuso and Coulter, 1963; Selikoff et al., 1964). Among 632 insulation workers who had been followed for at least 20 years, there were 45 deaths from lung cancer in comparison to an expected number of 6.6, based on U.S. death rates (Selikoff et al., 1964).

TABLE 5-4. Summary of Mortality Data for Mesothelioma, Lung Cancer, and Gastrointestinal Cancer in Asbestos-Exposed Occupational Cohorts[a]

			Deaths in Cohort		Total Mesothelioma/	Respiratory Cancer[b]		
Sex and Occupation of Cohort	Country[c]	Size of Cohort Traced	No.	%	Pleural-Peritoneal	Obs	Exp	O/E
MALES:								
Mining and Milling								
Chrysotile	C	9,850	3,291	33.4	10/10-0	230	184.0	1.3[f]
	C	544	178	32.7	1/1-0	28	11.0	2.5[f]
	I	933	332	35.6	0[g]/0-0	10	10.4	1.0
Anthophyllite	F	1,045[h]	384	36.7	0/0-0	44	22.0	2.0[f]
Crocidolite	Aus	1,960	526	10.6	26/26-0	60	38.2	1.6[f]
Manufacturing								
Chrysotile	US	1,261	308	23.6	1/0-1	35	11.1	3.2[f]
Amosite	US	820	528	64.4	14/7-7	83	22.8	3.6[f]
Mixed	B	2,887[k]	545	18.9	46/19-27	103	43.2	2.4[f]
	B	7,474	1,339	17.9	8/8-0	143	139.5	1.0
	B	1,071[h]	317	29.6	10/10-0	51	23.8	2.1[f]
	US	1,075	781	72.7	5/NA	63	23.3	2.7[f]
	US	5,645	601	10.6	0[g]/0-0	49	49.1	1.0
	C	241	72	22.0	11/6-5	20	3.3	6.1[f]
	D	5,686	—[l]	—	3/NA	47	27.8	1.7[f]
Insulation								
Mixed	US	632	478	75.6	38/11-27	93	13.3	7.0[f]
	US	17,800	2,271	12,8	175/63-112	429	105.6	4.0[f]
	B	162	122	75.3	13/8-5	35	5.0	7.0[f]
Shipyards								
Mixed	B	6.076	1,043	17.2	31/NA	88	100.7	0.9
	I	2,190	1,970	48.9	NA	123	54.9	2.2[f]
FEMALES:								
Manufacturing								
Crocidolite	B	578	166	28.7	17/13-4	12	6.3	1.9[f]
Mixed	B	783	200	25.5	21/13-7	27	3.2	8.4[f]
	B	3,708	299	8.1	2/2-0	6	11.3	0.5
	B	1,304	396	30.4	6/NA	22	11.0	2.0[f]

[a] Adapted from McDonald (1981) and from Consumer Product Safety Consumer Product Safety Commission (1983, p. II-57). These studies are described in more detail in Table E-1 of appendix E.

[b] Obs = observed; Exp = expected: 0/E = observed/expected; LL = lower limit; UL = upper limit.

[c] Country of study: US = United States, B = Britain, C = Canada, F = Finland, I = Italy, D = Denmark, Aus = Australia.

[d] 95% confidence intervals (two-sided) calculated assuming normal distribution for log SMR.

[e] The columns headed "power" above indicate the probability of detecting an effect, given the size of the population studied, assuming that exposure produced a minimum relstive risk of 1.5. More precisely, Statistical power is the probability that the null hypothesis of no increased relative risk (R = 1) will be rejected by a one-sided test with $\alpha = 0.05$ if the true relative risk (R) is actually 1.5 in a population of the size studied. The calculation (see Beaumont and Breslow, 1981) is based on the assumption that, under the null hypothesis, the observed number of deaths has a Poisson distribution with expected value equal to E (the expected number of deaths for persons of this age group) and that the square root transformation stabilizes the variance of the Poisson distribution. Power is calculated by computing $Z = 1.645 - 2(\sqrt{R} - 1)(\sqrt{E})$ and then determining the area to the right of Z from a table of the standard normal distribution.

Respiratory Cancer (cont.)			Gastrointestinal Cancer[b] (cont.)						
95% Confidence Limits[d]		Power to Detect O/E >1.5, α =				95% Confidence Limits[d]		Power to Detect O/E >1.5, α =	
LL	UL	0.05[e]	Obs	Exp	O/E	LL	UL	0.05[e]	References
1.1	1.4	1.00	276	272.4	1.0	0.9	1.1	1.00	McDonald et al., 1980
1.8	3.7	0.44	10	9.5	1.1	0.6	2.0	0.40	Nicholson et al., 1979
0.5	1.8	0.42	19	19.3	1.0	0.6	1.5	0.63	Rubino et al., 1979a
1.5	2.7	0.68	7	8.0	0.9[i]	0.4	1.8	0.36	Meurman et al., 1979
1.2	2.2	0.87	NA	NA	NA	—	—	—	Hobbs et al., 1980
2.3	4.4	0.44	13	9.9	1.3	0.8	2.3	0.41	Dement et al., 1983b
2.9	4.5	0.69	28	22.7	1.2	0.9	1.8	0.69	Seidman et al. 1979
2.0	2.9	0.90	40	34.0	1.2	0.9	1.6	0.84	Newhouse and Berry, 1979
0.9	1.2	1.00	103	107.2	1.0	0.8	1.2	1.00	Newhouse et al., 1982
1.6	2.8	0.71	16	15.7	1.0	0.6	1.7	0.56	Peto et al., 1977
2.1	3.5	0.70	55	39.9	1.4[f]	1.1	1.8	0.88	Henderson and Enterline, 1979
0.8	1.3	0.93	25	50.1	0.5	0.3	0.7	0.94	Hughes and Weill, 1980
3.9	9.4	0.20	4	2.5	1.6	0.6	4.3	0.18	Finkelstein, 1983
1.3	2.3	0.76	59	49.3	1.2	0.9	1.5	0.93	clemmesen and Hjalgrim-Jenson, 1981
5.7	8.6	0.50	43	15.0	2.9[f]	2.1	3.9	0.54	Selikoff et al., 1979
3.7	4.4	1.00	94	59.4	1.6[f]	1.3	1.9	0.97	Selikoff et al., 1979
5.0	9.7	0.26	13	2.2	5.9[f]	3.4	10.2	0.16	Elmes and Simpson, 1977
0.7	1.1	1.00	73	83.3	0.9	0.7	1.1	0.99	Rossiter and Coles, 1980
1.9	2.7	0.95	74	58.6	1.3	1.0	1.6	0.96	Puntoni et al., 1979
1.1	3.4	0.30	10	20.3	0.5	0.3	0.9	0.65	Jones et al., 1980
5.8	12.3	0.20	20	10.2	2.0[f]	1.3	3.0	0.42	Newhouse and Berry, 1979
0.2	1.2	0.45	29	27.4	1.1	0.7	1.5	0.76	Newhouse et al., 1982
1.3	3.0	0.44	NA	NA	NA	—	—	—	Acheson et al., 1982

[f] Statistically significant increase ($p < .05$).

[g] One possible case (Rubino et al., 1979); two cases not meeting criteria (Hughes and Weill, 1980).

[h] Males and females (Meurman et al., 1979; Peto et al., 1977).

[i] Based upon 1974 report (Meurman et al., 1974).

[j] NA = data not available.

[k] Based on males, excluding Laggers (Newhouse and Berry, 1979).

[l] Study of cancer incidence (Clemmesen and Hjalgrim-Jenson, 1981).

Since 1964, a number of investigators have documented an excess occurrence of lung cancer and/or mesothelioma among persons occupationally exposed to asbestos. Several of these studies are briefly described below, by industry and fiber type. Criteria for selecting these studies included the availability of quantitative exposure data or a qualitative exposure assessment, size of the available occupational cohort, and any unusual exposure or disease observations not reported in other studies. (See Table 5-4 and Appendix E, Table E-1 for more details on these studies.)

Mining and Milling

Chrysotile. Three cohorts occupationally exposed to chrysotile asbestos during mining and milling operations had a moderately increased risk for lung cancer (SMRs from 1.0 to 2.6). In the largest investigation, McDonald et al. (1980) studied all employees who had worked for at least 1 month in Quebec mines. From 1950 to 1975, 3,291 deaths occurred among the 9,850 male employees successfully traced and followed for 20 years or more after initial employment. An increase in lung cancer mortality was observed (SMR = 1.3, 230 observed vs. 184 expected), and the risk increased with duration of employment (SMR = 1.0 for <1 year to 1.6 for ≥ 20 years) and level of exposure (SMR = 0.9 for <30 mppcf(yr) to 2.3 for ≥ 300 mppcf(yr). Eleven cases of mesothelioma were observed.

Anthophyllite. Male and female employees of anthophyllite asbestos mines in Finland were studied by Meurman et al. (1974, 1979), who reported a twofold increase in lung cancer mortality (44 observed vs. 22.4 expected) and no mesotheliomas among the 1,045 persons successfully traced. All lung cancer deaths occurred among the male employees, and the risk was associated with estimated intensity of exposure (SMR = 1.4 vs. 3.3 for low and heavy exposures, respectively). Lung cancer risk among nonsmoking asbestos-exposed employees was 1.4 compared to a relative risk of 17.0 for the asbestos-exposed employees who smoked.

Crocidolite. For exposure associated with crocidolite mining in Western Australia, there was a similar increase in risk of lung cancer (SMR = 1.6, 60 observed vs. 38.2 expected) and a strong association with mesothelioma (Hobbs et al., 1980). Twenty-six cases of pleural mesothelioma were observed among the 526 deaths, and the mesothelioma risk increased with increased duration and intensity of exposure. Follow-up period was relatively short.

No increases in gastrointestinal cancer were observed for any of the mining and milling cohorts reviewed.

Manufacturing

Chrysotile. Most asbestos exposures associated with manufacturing processes involve mixed fiber types, but Dement et al. (1982, 1983a,b) examined the risks associated with exposure to chrysotile asbestos in textile factory workers. They observed a marked increase in lung cancer mortality (SMR = 3.2, 35 observed/11.1 expected), and the risk was strongly correlated with exposure level. There was also one peritoneal mesothelioma. Increased risks for both lung cancer and nonmalignant respiratory disease were observed at exposure levels lower than those reported in other studies.

Amosite. Mortality due to lung cancer was increased three-to four-fold (83 observed/22.8 expected) for 820 factory workers exposed to amosite asbestos (Seidman et al., 1979). The higher risks were observed for the subgroup followed 20 years or longer after initial employment (SMR = 5.1, 52 observed/10.1 expected). This cohort is a somewhat unusual population because of its limited duration of incense work exposure (1941-1945) and long period of observation. Other excess cancers, including 14 mesotheliomas, were also reported.

Mixed. Newhouse and Berry (1979) reported increased risks of lung cancer mortality for both males (SMR = 2.4, 103 observed/43.2 expected) and females (SMR = 8.4, 27 observed/3.2 expected) in a follow-up study of 4,600 male and 922 female employees of an East London asbestos factory in which crocidolite and amosite were used. Approximately 10% of all deaths resulted either from pleural or peritoneal mesothelioma.

Except for 10 cases of mesothelioma, no increased cancer mortality was observed among more than 11,000 males and females employed during 1941 or later at a British factory producing friction materials (Berry and Newhouse, 1983; Newhouse et al., 1982). In a case-control study that corrected for total asbestos exposure, 5 of 6 cases had definitely worked with crocidolite, whereas 2 of 10 controls had.

A cohort of 1,345 retired asbestos products workers employed from 1941 to 1967 had increased risks for lung cancer (SMR = 2.7, 63 observed/23.3 expected) and gastrointestinal cancer mortality (SMR = 1.4, 55 observed/39.3 expected) (Henderson and Enterline, 1979). Overall mortality among the 1,075 retirees successfully traced to 1973 was 73%. The lung cancer risk was strongly associated with amount of exposure, expressed as million particles per cubic foot multiplied by number of years of exposure (mppcf-yr), ranging from an SMR of 2.0 up to 7.8. Lung cancer risk differed by type of asbestos exposure (SMR of 2.5 for chrysotile alone vs. 5.2 for mixed chrysotile and crocidolite exposures). Five mesothelioma deaths were observed. Study results suggest that effects of asbestos exposure on lung cancer risk may continue long after the termination of exposure. Studies of a retiree cohort may result in an underestimation of actual risks, since deaths among employees under age 65 would be omitted. The Consumer Product Safety Commission (1983) suggests that the risks may be understated by as much as two-fold.

No increase in lung cancer mortality or cancer of any other site, except mesothelioma, was observed in the cohort of 5,645 employees of an asbestos-cement product manufacturing facility studied by Hughes and Weill (1980). In the high exposure subgroup, lung cancer risk was increased for employees exposed to crocidolite, and two mesothelioma deaths were reported. The low overall mortality, 10.6%, and the low tracing rate, approximately 75%, suggest that this study may have resulted in an underestimate of mortality risks.

Finkelstein (1983) studied 328 asbestos-cement workers hired before 1960 and employed for a minimum of 9 years. Mesothelioma was strongly associated with exposure level for production workers, whereas a dose-response relationship was not observed for lung cancer. Excess lung and gastrointestinal cancers were observed.

Clemmesen and Hjalgrim-Jenson (1981) studied cancer incidence among 6,372 Danish males who worked in asbestos-cement factories between 1944 and 1976. There were 55 cases of respiratory cancer compared to 33 expected, based on Danish Cancer Registry incidence rates. Three mesotheliomas were observed in addition to excess prostate, laryngeal, and stomach cancers. Cancer incidence in the unexposed employees at the same factories was not increased.

Jones et al. (1980b) studied a cohort of 578 females exposed to crocidolite from western Australia during the manufacture of gas masks. The 12 cases of lung cancer (SMR = 1.9, 12 observed/6.3 expected) and the 17 mesothelioma cases (13 pleural and 4 peritoneal) were all exposed to crocidolite, whereas no cases of mesothelioma or lung cancer occurred among the 102 females exposed only to chrysotile. Overall, 10% of deaths were due to mesothelioma. Risk of mesthelioma was strongly associated with duration of exposure, although no dose-response relationship was observed for lung cancer.

Similar results were reported among 1,304 females who manufactured gas masks at three locations followed from 1951 to June 30, 1980 (Acheson et al., 1980). Deaths from lung cancer (SMR = 2.0, 22 observed/11 expected) and ovarian cancer (SMR = 2.2, 17 observed/7.8 expected) were increased. Lung cancer excess was higher for those exposed predominantly to crocidolite compared to those exposed predominantly to chrysotile. Five of the six mesotheliomas occurred in those exposed predominantly to crocidolite.

All studies of occupational cohorts exposed to asbestos during manufacturing processes had an overall increased risk of lung cancer or a dose-response relationship in the exposure subgroups (Hughes and Weill, 1980; Peto et al., 1977). Elevated risk ratios (>1.1) for gastrointestinal cancer were observed in six of the nine cohorts reviewed (Clemmesen and Hjalgrim-Jenson, 1981; Dement et al., 1983b; Finkelstein, 1983; Henderson and Enterline, 1979; Newhouse and Berry, 1979; Seidman et al., 1979).

Insulation

Mixed. All three of the cohorts involved in end product use of asbestos as insulators were exposed to mixed types of asbestos. One of the largest studies is that of Selikoff et al. (1979), who studied 17,800 members of an insulator's union. Overall mortality in this cohort was 12.8%; 2,271 deaths were reported through 1976. Lung cancer risk was increased four-fold (429 observed/105.6 expected) and increases were observed for gastrointestinal cancer (SMR = 1.6, 94 observed/59.4 expected), cancer of the larynx, pharynx, buccal cavity (SMR = 1.7, 25 observed/14.8 expected), and kidney (SMR = 2.2, 18 observed/8.1 expected). Dose-response relationships were not examined because of the lack of exposure data. Mesotheliomas (63 pleural and 112 peritoneal) accounted for 7.7% of the deaths. Analysis of the relationship between smoking and lung cancer risk using data from the American Cancer Society indicated a consistent multiplicative effect, in that a 10-fold increase in risk of lung cancer was associated with smoking in both asbestos-exposed and unexposed groups. A five-fold increase in lung cancer risk was associated with asbestos exposure in both smokers and nonsmokers (Hammond et al., 1979).

Elmes and Simpson (1977) reported an unusually high risk of lung cancer (SMR = 7.0, 35 observed/5 expected) and gastrointestinal cancer (SMR = 5.9, 13 observed/2.2 expected) for a cohort of 162 insulators and pipe coverers employed in Northern Ireland during 1940. Overall mortality in this cohort was 75.31 by 1975; 54% of the deaths were due to cancer. Thirteen cases of mesothelioma (eight pleural and five peritoneal) were reported. No difference in cancer risk was apparent for workers first employed before or after 1933. Ascertainment bias is unlikely to explain the magnitude of the risks reported for this cohort.

Shipyards

Mixed exposures. Rossiter and Coles (1980) studied 6,076 dockyard workers employed before 1947. They reported no increase in lung cancer mortality (SMR = 0.7, 84 observed/119.7 expected) or gastrointestinal cancer (SMR = 0.8, 63 observed/83.3 expected). Mesothelioma was reported for 31 (3%) of the 1,043 deaths. However, since less than 20% of this cohort have died, excess cancers may not be fully apparent.

In a study of 2,190 Italian dockworkers, Puntoni et al. (1979) observed increased risks for lung cancer (SMR = 2.2, 123 observed/54.9 expected), gastrointestinal cancer (SMR = 1.3, 74 observed/58.6 expected), laryngeal cancer (SMR = 1.9, 15 observed/7.7 expected), and kidney cancer (SMR = 2.0, 29 observed/14.7 expected).

Relative Carcinogenicity of Different Types of Asbestos

There has been much discussion about whether certain asbestos varieties are more carcinogenic than others. The question is of practical importance, because the vast majority of asbestos used in the United States and the world is chrysotile; however, it is difficult to answer, because studies of different types of asbestos are confounded by type of industry (mining and milling vs. asbestos-cement vs. asbestos insulation vs. asbestos textiles), by fiber size characteristics within an industry, by variations in fiber and dust particle concentration and their measurement, and by variations in study methods. Therefore, direct comparisons are not easily made among epidemiological studies.

Special attention has been given to crocidolite, especially in regard to its association with mesothelioma. Some groups of workers exposed to crocidolite have had a relatively high rate of mesothelioma. Among those are black South African crocidolite miners (2% prevalence) (Tolent et al., 1980) and gas-mask workers (up to 10% of deaths) (Acheson et al., 1980; Jones et al., 1980). In a study of naval dockyard workers, Rossiter and Coles (1980) reported 31 deaths from mesothelioma and only 13 other deaths from asbestos-related disease among 1,043 deaths ascertained (Rossiter and Coles, 1980). McDonald (1980) suggested that use of crocidolite by the British navy could explain such a finding.

Data on chrysotile exposures are mixed. Canadian studies of chrysotile miners and millers have suggested that the average incidence of mesothelioma is relatively low (0.5%) (McDonald, 1980). Dement et al. (1983b) reported that only one of 308 deaths in a chrysotile asbestos textile plant was attributable to mesothelioma. Peto (1980b) reported a high risk from mesothelioma in an asbestos textile plant in which chrysotile predominated, although small amounts of crocidolite were also processed. Similarly, Robinson et al. (1979) reported that mesothelioma accounted for 4.3% of deaths among workers who processed predominantly chrysotile, and lesser amounts of crocidolite and amosite. The Consumer Product Safety Commission (1983) noted, "Epidemiological studies suggest that chrysotile has a lower potential for producing peritoneal mesotheliomas than [do] other fiber types, but there is less evidence of marked differences between fiber types in their potential to produce pleural mesothelioma and lung cancer." Acheson and Gardner (1983), in discussing mesothelioma in humans, have concluded that "exposure to chrysotile alone so far has rarely been shown to cause mesothelioma."

Many of these apparent differences may be explained by the differences in physical properties and concentrations of the fibers used by the various industries. Both of these factors would affect deposition and clearance of fibers in the lung. However, the possible role of other factors, including chemistry, has not been ruled out.

Thus, the epidemiological literature on the relative ability of different fiber types to cause disease does not present a clear picture.

Most of the studies on fiber type have been focussed on mesothelioma, which accounts for only some asbestos-related disease. Experimental and animal studies, discussed in Chapter 6, have not detected systematic differences in carcinogenicity or fibrogenicity among different types of asbestos.

Effects of Smoking

Cigarette smoking is the single most important known cause of lung cancer in humans. Because most asbestos workers have also been cigarette smokers, it has been difficult to evaluate separately the effects of asbestos and of cigarette smoke on lung cancer. The most dependable data are those of Hammond et al. (1979), described earlier, in which a large number of workers were studied. These investigators also reported that mesothelioma risk does not appear to be affected by cigarette smoking. Among male asbestos workers who never smoked cigarettes regularly, eight mesothelioma deaths were observed, the same number as expected based on the age-specific death rates for all asbestos workers.

Summary

An increased risk of lung cancer is associated with exposure to all major types of commercial asbestos (chrysotile, amosite, crocidolite, and anthophyllite), and this increase is observed for all occupational groups handling asbestos. Asbestos exposure is associated with an increase in risk (1.5- to 5-fold) for both smokers and nonsmokers.

An increased risk of mesothelioma in humans is associated with exposure to crocidolite, amosite, and chrysotile, but has not been reported for anthophyllite, possibly because anthophyllite is much less used than are the other types of asbestos. A lower risk of mesothelioma is observed for workers in chrysotile mining and milling operations as compared to chrysotile use in other industries.

Mortality due to gastrointestinal cancer was increased in 11 of the studies reviewed, but the magnitude of the increased risk and the quality of available evidence were not as strong as they were for lung cancer and mesothelioma. The excess risk for gastrointestinal cancer was statistically significant in 5 of the 11 studies with relative risks greater than 1.1; but only two of these studies had sufficient power (0.80) to detect a 50% increase in relative risk (Table 5-4; Henderson and Enterline, 1979; Selikoff et al., 1979). In addition, the increased risks for cancer of the larynx and kidney reported in some studies may, like risks for lung cancer, be partly a consequence of cigarette smoking and other environmental exposures. An increase in ovarian cancer observed in two studies was concentrated among the heavily exposed subgroups (Acheson et al., 1982; Newhouse and Berry, 1979). The association of asbestos with an increased risk of malignancies other than lung cancer and mesothelioma has not been confirmed in animal studies and has not been observed consistently in human studies.

The increased risk of lung cancer is associated with age, cumulative asbestos exposure, and smoking. In many studies, a linear dose-response has been observed for lung cancer and asbestos exposure; however, there was a delay of approximately 10 to 20 years following exposure before the increased risk became manifest. No association between mesothelioma and cigarette smoking has been observed. A delay of 20 to 40 years has been suggested as the latency period required for asbestos-induced mesothelioma.

Measurements of exposure intensity are lacking in most studies. Where such measurements have been attempted, it is still difficult to estimate earlier asbestos exposures when only dust measurements were obtained. Often one can only establish crude categories of exposure (high, moderate, and low) and cannot estimate cumulative fiber exposure levels for individuals.

There is considerable variation in the risk estimates obtained in the studies reviewed by the committee. As noted earlier, this variation may result from many factors in the studies themselves, as well as from a true asbestos effect. Particularly important is the use of different exposure-related criteria for selecting the study cohorts, such as selecting only individuals exposed for a certain minimum period, who survived for a period after initial exposure, who were employed before a specified date, or who were employed as of a specified date and had varying lengths of exposure and years since initial exposure.

Some cohorts are more heterogeneous than others with respect to exposure-related characteristics. Studies of these groups are likely to produce lower risk estimates. It is increasingly difficult to identify a consistent gradient of risk across exposure subgroups (low, medium, high) if they are extremely heterogeneous with regard to date of hire, duration of employment, and time from initial employment.

Comparisons of risk estimates from various studies are further limited by variations due to incomplete tracing of the cohort; misclassification of cause of death; use of inappropriate comparison groups; and more aggressive efforts to ascertain disease (or deaths) in the cohort than in the comparison group. Furthermore, in making comparisons among different cohorts, it is important to consider the percentage of the cohort that has died, since it is difficult to compare results from younger cohorts with 10% mortality with results from older cohorts with much higher mortality.

Some of the observed variation in risk may be due to differences in the effects of fibers of different types or dimensions and the use of these fibers in processes in which other contaminants are present. However, the magnitude of the difference in reported risks is not likely to be explained by fiber or process differences alone. Thus, on the basis of epidemiological data, it is not possible to determine the role of fiber type and fiber size in the risk of lung cancer and mesothelioma or to attribute greater or lesser risk to some types of asbestos fibers for lung cancer and mesothelioma.

ASBESTOSIS AND ASBESTOS-ASSOCIATED PLEURAL DISEASE IN OCCUPATIONAL COHORTS

This section reviews occupational mortality and morbidity studies of asbestosis and asbestos-associated pleural disease. For a more extensive review, see Dement et al. (in press).

Mortality Studies

Deaths attributable to asbestosis often are not reported as such. Instead, mortality rates are often reported for nonmalignant or chronic respiratory diseases among workers exposed to asbestos. These may include chronic bronchitis, emphysema, influenza, and pneumonia in addition to pulmonary fibrosis or asbestosis.

Mixed Fiber Exposures. Most manufacturing plants have used a variety of fiber types, usually chrysotile and one or more amphiboles. Investigators studying exposures to mixed fibers have reported mortality rates attributable to asbestosis. For example, in a study of 17, 800 insulation workers, Selikoff et al. (1979) reported that approximately 8% of 2, 271 deaths were due to asbestosis.

Mortality studies of asbestos textile workers exposed to a variety of fiber types have had mixed results. Mancuso and Coulter (1963) observed 14% of 195 deaths from asbestosis among workers producing textile and friction products. In a cohort of British asbestos textile workers, Peto et al. (1977) observed 35 deaths due to nonmalignant respiratory disease, whereas 25 were expected (SMR = 1.4), among those employed after implementation of environmental controls in 1933. Newhouse (1969, 1973) and Newhouse et al. (1972) studied 4,600 male and 922 female workers in a plant initially producing asbestos textile and later asbestos insulation products. Among those in the highest exposure group (>10 fibers/cm^3), mortality from chronic respiratory diseases was 1.8 times that expected.

Exposure to Single Types of Asbestos. Hobbs et al. (1980) studied 7,000 employees exposed to crocidolite mined at Wittenoom Gorge in Western Australia between 1938 and 1966. Of 198 pneumoconiosis cases, 59 were asbestosis, 122 silicoasbestosis, and 17 were silicosis. They reported an overall incidence rate of 3.5% for pneumoconiosis along with evidence for increased incidence among those with heavy exposure and those with a longer duration of employment. Among those heavily exposed and employed at least 5 years, the incidence rate was 65%.

Mortality among workers manufacturing amosite asbestos insulation between 1941 and 1945 was reported by Selikoff et al. (1972) and Seidman et al. (1977, 1979). Of 528 deaths observed over 35 years in a cohort of 820 men, approximately 5.6% were due to asbestosis.

In the past, anthophyllite asbestos was commercially mined and processed in areas of Finland also known to contain some chrysotile and tremolite asbestos. Meurman et al. (1974) reported that mortality from asbestosis was 5.2% in a group of 1,092 Finnish miners studied from 1936 to 1974 and that the mortality rate was similar between smokers and nonsmokers.

Several studies have been conducted on Quebec chrysotile miners and millers. The most recent report on this cohort included observations of 10, 939 men employed 9 or more months between 1926 and 1975 (McDonald et al., 1980). They found 42 deaths, or 1.3% of total deaths, to be attributable to asbestosis. Nicholson et al. (1979) studied a smaller cohort of 544 Quebec miners and millers with a least 20 years of seniority and followed them between 1962 and 1977. Thirty noninfectious, nonmalignant respiratory disease deaths were observed, whereas 6.7 had been expected.

Deaths from asbestosis have been reported to occur in cohorts exposed to chrysotile in manufacturing plants. For example, Robinson et al. (1979), who studied workers in a plant that used 99% chrysotile and 1% crocidolite and amosite, reported 76 deaths from noninfectious, nonmalignant respiratory diseases among males, whereas 16.4 had been expected.

Dement et al. (1983b) reported mortality and assessed dose-response for asbestosis in a cohort of asbestos textile workers exposed only to chrysotile. They found that 17 (5.5%) of 308 deaths were due to asbestosis or pulmonary fibrosis. A linear relationship was demonstrated between cumulative fiber dose and the risk of mortality for noninfectious respiratory disease. Although Dement and colleagues reported a much steeper slope, their findings are not inconsistent with those of McDonald et al. (1980), who reported a no threshold, linear dose-response relationship between asbestosis and doses of dust containing chrysotile.

Morbidity Studies

Morbidity studies have established that all asbestos fiber types are associated with asbestosis, asbestos-induced plaques, diffuse pleural thickening, and pleural calcification. Because of the methodological differences described above, it is difficult to compare these studies directly with each other or with mortality studies in regard to dose-response. Nonetheless, the various studies are quite consistent with regard to major health effects reported, whether ascertained by chest radiography, questionnaire on respiratory difficulties, or pulmonary function evaluation. Appendix E, Table E-2 summarizes morbidity studies of asbestos-exposed populations.

Mixed Fiber Exposure. Early cross-sectional studies of asbestos workers, which relied on chest radiography, demonstrated a prevalence of pulmonary fibrosis as high as 80% among those exposed for 20 years or longer (Donnelly, 1936; Dreessen et al., 1938; Merewether and Price, 1930; Shull, 1936). More recent studies have confirmed the general observations of these early investigators, although disease prevalence has varied from industry to industry. Selikoff and his colleagues studied insulation workers exposed to chrysotile and amosite. They reported an overall prevalence of 50% with small irregular opacities and a 90% prevalence among those with more than 30 years of exposure (Selikoff, 1965; Selikoff et al., 1965). Pleural fibrosis was observed in roughly two-thirds of those examined 40 years after first exposure. Elapsed time from first exposure was similarly found to correlate with pleural calcification, which occurred in 50% of those examined 40 years or more after their first occupational exposure. Murphy et al. (1971, 1978) studied insulation workers in shipyards and, using a more restrictive definition for asbestosis, reported an 11-fold prevalence compared to age-matched, unexposed controls.

Asbestos textile plant exposures have been studied by Lewinsohn et al. (1972), Berry et al. (1979), and Baselga-Monte and Segarra (1978). Data from this type of plant formed the basis for the British Occupational Hygiene Society (BOHS) (1968) recommendation that was used to establish occupational exposure standards. The initial BOHS analysis revealed that there was radiographic evidence of asbestosis[8] for 2.7% of the 290 workers exposed to asbestos (chrysotile with some crocidolite) after 1933, when dust control had been implemented. A risk of 1% for a worker developing basal rales was estimated to result from exposure for 50 years at an estimated average exposure of 2 fibers/cm^3 as measured by a standard membrane filter method (fibers longer than 5 μm), or a cumulative exposure of approximately 10 (fibers/cm^3)yr. The BOHS estimate of risk is the basis for occupational standards for asbestos exposure in the United Kingdom, the United States, and several other countries. Precise criteria for radiographic assessment were not given, and subsequent studies have revealed more disease in this population. In a later analysis of these data, Berry et al. (1979) estimated a prevalence of 1% for crepitations at a cumulative dose of 43 (fibers/cm^3)yr. For possible and certified asbestosis, 1% prevalences were estimated to occur at cumulative doses of 55 and 72 (fibers/cm^3)yr, respectively.

This same plant was later studied cross-sectionally by Lewinsohn (1972), who reported a much higher prevalence of "pulmonary fibrosis" and pleural thickening. Berry et al. (1979) subsequently restudied 379 men

[8] Radiological changes considered significant included increased general opacity of the lower lobes, blurring of the cardiac outline, pleural thickening, and adhesions (British Occupational Hygiene Society, 1968).

working at this same textile factory for at least 10 years. The most reliable data were judged to be those obtained for men employed after 1950; 6.6% of these were believed to have "possible asbestosis"[9] after an average follow-up of 16 years and an average exposure of 5 fiber/cm^3 as assessed by static area dust samples. As exposure increased, there was a decline in pulmonary function, as measured by spirometric techniques such as forced expiratory volume and forced vital capacity. Nonsmokers and light smokers had less crepitations, asbestosis, and small opacities than did heavier smokers with similar exposure. On the basis of these data, Berry and colleagues estimated that "possible asbestosis" would result in no more than 1% of men after 40 years of exposure to concentrations ranging from 0.3 to 1.1 fibers/cm^3. Furthermore, they noted that continued follow-up was indicated in order to refine the estimates.

Baselga-Monte and Segarra (1978) studied 1,262 Barcelona factory workers exposed to mixed-fiber asbestos and established a relationship between individual risk and cumulative dose (fibers/cm^3)yr, based on radiographic findings only. They estimated a threshold limit value (TLV) of 0.07 or 0.10 fibers/cm^3 for a 1% or 5% incidence of asbestosis for a 50-year work exposure.

Weill and colleagues (1973, 1975) correlated radiographic changes and lung function with exposure among 859 U.S. asbestos-cement workers. Cumulative dust exposures were estimated but were expressed as mppcf-yr. Both rounded and irregular opacities were observed, and there was a 4% prevalance of small opacities (reflecting a mixed dust exposure) at less than 50 mppcf-yr. Prevalence increased to 30% at exposures greater than 400 mppcf-yr. An 11% prevalence of pleural abnormalities was observed among those in the lowest exposure category. Lung volumes decreased in relation to increasing cumulative dust exposure, but pulmonary diffusing capacity was not related to dose (Weill et al., 1975).

Finkelstein (1982) recently reported asbestosis incidence rates in a cohort of 157 Canadian asbestos-cement workers exposed to both chrysotile and crocidolite. Criteria for certification of asbestosis were similar to those reported by Berry et al., (1979) and were based on the findings of a pneumoconiosis medical panel. Finkelstein found an average overall incidence rate of 0.7%, 1.6%, and 2.4% for 0-49, 50-99, and 100-149 cumulative (fibers/cm^3)yr, respectively.

Progression of radiographic abnormalities and lung function changes have been reported by Jones et al. (1980a) and Gregor et al. (1979). Jones and coworkers studied progression among 204 asbestos-cement workers

[9] The determination of "possible asbestosis" was based on basal rales, radiological changes of varying degree, a falling gas transfer factor, and restrictive lung function changes.

between 1970 and 1976. They concluded that progression (increased profusion of small opacities) depended on both average and cumulative exposure, that decline in lung function was related to both amount smoked and cumulative exposure, and that pleural changes progressed as a function of time from first exposure. Gregor et al. (1979) studied a variety of asbestos workers referred to the Brompton Hospital from the British Pneumoconiosis Panel. They documented a progression in radiographic findings without further asbestos exposure.

The relationship between lung function and radiographic findings associated with asbestos exposure was further studied by Lumley (1977), who reported highly significant decreases in lung function with pulmonary fibrosis and diffuse pleural thickening, somewhat less of a decrease when there were only plaques, and no difference if only pleural calcification was present.

Epidemiological and clinical evidence of asbestos-related disease has been found in studies of workers in some major industries not originally associated with asbestos exposure. For example, in recently reported studies of asbestos-related disease in the United States, investigators have documented that characteristic radiographic abnormalities have been found among chemical plant maintenance workers, oil refinery workers, brake workers, and railroad workers employed before 1950 during the steam locomotive era (Lilis et al., 1980; Lorimer et al., 1976; Sepulveda and Merchant, 1983).

Anthophyllite and Tremolite. In several studies of Finnish anthophyllite miners, investigators have observed increased respiratory symptoms and increased prevalence of pleural plaques (6.51-9.01 vs. 0.1% for the Finnish population) (Kilviluoto, 1960; Meurman, 1968; Meurman et al., 1974). In upper New York State, workers exposed to talc deposits containing both anthophyllite and tremolite asbestos have been studied by several investigators. Gamble et al. (1979a), reported increased respiratory symptoms, pulmonary fibrosis, and decreased lung function in exposed workers. They also noted a marked association between pleural thickening and decreased lung function, similar to that reported by Lumley (1977) among British shipyard workers. Dement and Zumwalde (1979) reported that fiber exposure in those mining and milling operations ranged from 0.8 to 16.0 fibers/cm^3, of which 121 to 19% was identified as tremolite and 30% to 45% as anthophyllite.[10]

Another tremolite exposure resulting in a relatively low prevalence of radiographic abnormalities was recently reported by Lockey et al. (1983). Among factory workers processing tremolite-contaminated vermiculite mined in Montana, 4.4% were found to have some radiographic abnormality.

[10] Not all of the fibers counted were necessarily asbestiform fibers.

Chrysotile. The most extensive morbidity studies of chrysotile exposure have been conducted in Quebec miners and millers (Becklake et al., 1972; McDonald et al., 1972, 1974). In these studies, 1,015 current employees were studied radiographically, physiologically, and by British Medical Research Council standardized questionnaire. Respiratory symptoms were associated with dust[11] exposure, and the prevalence of bronchitis reached 50% in the highest dust exposure category. Dyspnea upon exertion was also found to be associated with dust exposure, but not with smoking, and the prevalance rose to 40% among those with a cumulative dust exposure of 800 mppcf-yr. The prevalence of those with small irregular opacities (>1/0 ILO/UC 1971 Classification) differed between the two mines studied (1.8% at the Thetford mine and 6.4% at the Asbestos mine), but rose to 26.4% and 10.9%, respectively, among those exposed to more than 800 mppcf-yr. Those with significant radiographic evidence of asbestosis (ILO category 2/1 or greater) had significantly lower values for all lung function parameters studied. Lung function also deteriorated more as cumulative dose increased (McDonald et al., 1972).

Radiographic findings among chrysotile workers were also demonstrated to progress without further exposure. Rubino et al. (1979b) reported that there was progression without additional exposure among 39% of retired asbestos miners and millers with 1/0 profusion radiographs. Becklake et al. (1979) made similar observations, but they also found that those who progressed were likely to have had higher exposures to asbestos.

Summary

Morbidity studies of occupationally exposed asbestos workers have documented that asbestosis, diffuse pleural thickening, pleural plaques, dyspnea, and altered pulmonary function are associated with all types of exposure to asbestos. Generally, prevalence of these indices is lower among those who mine and mill asbestos-bearing ore than among those who subsequently produce or use asbestos products. Morbidity data support the concept of a linear cumulative dose-response relationship.

Estimates based on mixed-fiber exposures suggest that a 1% risk of developing asbestosis (differing definitions) over a 40- to 50-year work exposure occurs when exposures are somewhere between 0.07 fiber/cm^3 and 1.1 fiber/cm^3. Because of the nonspecificity in disease definition and the lack of data at very low doses, it is not clear whether there is a threshold of exposure for asbestosis. Data do suggest, however, that any incidence rate for asbestosis at the very low exposures normally found in the nonoccupational environment would be quite low.

[11] Miners and millers are exposed to dust other than just asbestos.

HEALTH EFFECTS OF OCCUPATIONAL EXPOSURE TO MAN-MADE MINERAL FIBERS[12]

Fibrous glass has some of the same physical properties as asbestos. For example, fine glass fibers are respirable and exhibit flexibility and diameter-dependent strength. However, fibrous glass may be less durable than asbestos in biological tissues and apparently behaves differently in some biological test systems (see Chapter 6). Epidemiological studies have been conducted to determine if adverse health effects occur in workers exposed to man-made mineral fibers. The major studies are reviewed below.

Morbidity

In 1976, a committee of the American College of Chest Physicians evaluated pulmonary response to fiberglass dust (Gross et al., 1976). It concluded, "There is no evidence to indicate that inhaling fiberglass is associated with either permanent respiratory impairment or carcinogenesis; however, the final verdict as far as the latter is concerned must await the findings of long-term mortality studies." In a review article on the health effects of man-made mineral fibers, Gross (1982) concluded that "exposure has not caused an increased risk of developing lung cancer or non-malignant respiratory disease."

In Table 5-5, 10 cross-sectional studies of pulmonary function and disease among workers exposed to fibrous glass or rock wool are summarized. In general, these studies were descriptive and did not permit a rigorous comparison of pulmonary status between exposed and nonexposed persons. Because only the prevalence of pulmonary disease in current workers could be assessed, it was not possible to measure the rate of occurrence (incidence) of the development of pulmonary disease. Although no evidence of pulmonary abnormalities among workers exposed to MMMF was found in the early studies, several recent studies suggest an increased prevalence of minimal small lung opacities among workers exposed for longer periods.

These studies provided only limited information on the level of exposure to man-made mineral fibers. In studies published before 1980, exposure was mainly categorized as light, medium, or heavy. The fact that no associations were found between level of exposure and prevalence of disease could reflect imprecise measurements of exposure or could indicate that there is no effect from the exposure. In the studies published since 1980, exposure has generally been given as the number of fibers/cm^3. In general, average exposure lies between 0.1 and 1.0 respirable fibers/cm^3. Another factor probably related to pathogenicity is fiber diameter, which is described as ordinary (>3 µm),

---

[12] Man-made mineral fibers (MMMF) are sometimes called man-made vitreous fibers (MMVF).

TABLE 5-5. Summary of Cross-Sectional Morbidity Studies of Populations Exposed co Man-Made Mineral fibers

Type of Fiber	Study Population	Summary of Important Findings	References
Rock and slag wool	84 workers with 7-29 years of exposure.	"No x-ray evidence of silicosis or fibrosis of the lungs."	Carpenter and Spolyar, 1945
Fibrous glass	1,389 production workers. 1,176 had 10 or u. re years in production.	"No unusual pattern of radiologic densities was observed."	Wright, 1968
Fibrous glass	232 production workers.	No "evidence that would support a hypothesis that those with dusty jobs were less healthy than those with minimal duet exposure."	Utidjian and deTrenvills, 1970
Fibrous glass	2,028 production workers who had worked an average of 14 years.	Prevalence of pulmonary abnormalities Similar in office workers and production workers.	Nasr et al., 1971
Fibrous glass	70 fibrous glass workers; 70 controls.	"No evidence of any respiratory hazard due Co glass fibre."	Hill et al., 1973
Fibrous glass	467 production workers who had worked an average of 13 years.	Based on unstable data, the prevalence of pharyngeal-laryngitis was higher in persons who had worked at least 5 years.	Maggiori et al., 1980
Fibrous glass	340 production workers of whom 81% had worked more than 10 years.	Prevalence of small opacities greater in Ben who had worked Bore than 15 years in comparison to those who had worked less (39% vs. 9%).	Hill et al., 1982
Rock wool	162 production workers with an average of 12 years of work.	Pulmonary function test values less than expected normal values.	Skuric and Stahyljak-Boritic, 1982
Rock wool	21 production workers who had worked more than 10 years and 43 controls.	"No evidence of pulmonary disease...in the group of MMMF workers studied."	Malmberg et al., 1982
Fibrous glass	1,028 production workers who had worked an average of 19 years.	Prevalence of small opacities was related to age, smoking, small diameter fiber exposure, and in smokers, various quantitative measures of exposure dose.	Weill et al., 1982

fine (1 to 3 µm), or very fine (<1 µm). Only in the study by Weill et al. (1982) is there information on fiber diameter.

Weill et al. (1982) reported that the prevalence of small opacities in exposed workers was low, increased with age and smoking, and was found predominantly in the ordinary/fine fiber (1 to 3 µm in diameter) category. In addition, risk of small opacities was correlated with several quantitative exposure estimates among current smokers. However, respiratory symptoms and pulmonary function were not associated with exposure to man-made mineral fibers.

Mortality

Table 5-6 summarizes the results of seven retrospective mortality follow-up studies among workers exposed to MMMF. In these studies, the mortality experience of persons exposed to MMMF was compared to that of a general population in the country where the study was done, usually the United States. In computing the expected numbers of deaths, the investigators took into account age, sex, ethnic group, and calendar time.

In general, no large excesses of respiratory cancer or nonmalignant respiratory disease were observed in the entire study group. However, some excesses were found upon examination of subgroups within each cohort. Because the subgroups were formed during the process of analyzing the data, the characteristics of the subgroups differ among the several studies. Also, the observed excesses were small, and the categories of causes of death were not consistent among the studies. These excesses are summarized below, by study.

Bayliss et al. (1976). When follow-up started 10 years after onset of employment and influenza and pneumonia were not included in the mortality attributed to nonmalignant respiratory disease (NMRD), there were 19 deaths observed and 9.5 expected.

Morgan et al. (1981). Among men who worked and were exposed at least 20 years and who were followed beginning at least 30 years after onset of employment, the observed/expected numbers were: lung cancer, 14/11.8; nonmalignant respiratory disease, 5/8.1.

Enterline and Marsh (1982). Among the fibrous glass workers, 129 deaths from NMRD were observed and 99.5 deaths were expected; deaths from influenza and pneumonia were not included in these figures. There was no relationship between length of exposure to fibrous glass and excess mortality or between cumulative exposure and excess mortality. However, among those followed 30 or more years after onset of employment, there were 47 lung cancers observed and 36.0 expected.

Among men exposed to mineral wool, there was no clear relationship between the excess lung cancer or NMRD and length of work or time since

TABLE 5-6. Summary of Mortality Follow-Up Studies of Populations Exposed to Man-Made Mineral Fibers

Type of Fiber	Study Population	Summary of Important Findings (O/E)[a]	References
Fibrous glass	416 U.S. men who retired between 1945 and 1972 from six plants that made fibrous glass insulation.	All causes; 111/131; all cancers: 20/24; lung cancer: 5/6; NMRD: 9/9.	Enterline and Henderson, 1975
Fibrous glass	1,448 U.S. men who worked at least 5 years in fibrous glass production between 1949 and 1972.	All causes: 376/404; all cancers: 54/64; respiratory cancer: 16/20; NARD: 25/20.	Bayliss et al., 1976
Fibrous glass	4,399 U.S. men who worked least 10 years in fibrous glass production and who were employed at some time between 1968 and 1977.	All causes: 289/340; all cancers: 76/74; respiratory cancer: 39/29; NMRD: 14/19.	Morgan et al., 1982
Fibrous glass and rock wool	2,576 Canadian men who worked at least 90 days in fibrous glass production between 1955 and 1977.	All causes: 88/113; all tancers: 20/20; lung cancer: 9/5; NMRD: 4/5.	Shannon et al., 1982
Fibrous glass, rock wool, and slag wool	16,730 U.S. men who worked at least 1 year in insulation production between 1945 and 1963.	Fibrous glass All causes: 3,262/3,391; all cancers: 612/635; respiratory cancer: 202/203; NMRD: 186/176 Mineral wool All causes: 499/468; all cancers: 109/88; respiratory cancer: 45/28; NMRD: 29/25.	Enterline and Marsh, 1982
Fibrous glass and rock wool	17,083 European men who ever worked in mineral wool production and who Mere followed at least 20 years.	All causes: 374/339; all cancers: 109/88; respiratory cancer: 33/27; NMRD: 32/31.	Saracci et al., 1982
Rock wool and slag wool	596 U.S. men who had worked at least 1 year in mineral wool production between 1940 and 1948.	All causes: 184/205; all cancers: 36/36; lung cancer: 9/10; NMRD: 10/11.	Robinson et al., 1982

[a] O/E = observed/expected deaths. Expected deaths based on age-and time-specific mortality rates for the general population, usually that of the United States, for appropriate sex and ethnic groups. NMRD = Nonmalignant respiratory disease. (NMRD data include deaths from influenza and pneumonia.)

first exposure. Furthermore, possible exposure to asbestos during the early years of the plant's operation could not be ruled out.

Saracci et al. (1982). Among men followed at least 20 years, 33 deaths from lung cancer were observed and 27.3 were expected.

Because all the mortality studies were retrospective, there was little information on exposure. Most of the workers had started work during the 1940s and 1950s, when, presumably, fiber concentrations in the air were higher than they are today. In the study by Enterline and Marsh (1982), current average exposure was approximately 0.04 fibers/cm^3 for workers in fibrous glass plants and 0.4 fibers/cm^3 for workers in mineral wool plants. This range is similar to that reported in the morbidity studies and is below the U.S. workplace standard for asbestos Of 2 fibers/cm^3, in effect since 1976.

Saracci and Simonato (1982) reviewed the papers presented at a 1982 conference on MMMF and other relevant literature. For chronic respiratory diseases, they reviewed 10 cross-sectional studies, 7 mortality studies, and 2 other studies. The cross-sectional studies were limited because "no substantial follow-up data from the longitudinal observations of cohorts of workers are as yet available." The mortality studies were limited in that no control was possible for smoking habits, previous industrial exposures, including exposure to asbestos, or concurrent industrial exposures. Of the 19 studies, 11 were interpreted as showing no association between MMMF and chronic respiratory disease. Although the remaining eight studies showed some association between MMMF and chronic respiratory disease, the associations were weak and not readily interpretable. Enterline and Marsh (1982) and McDonald (1982) concluded that, because of the low level of respirable fibers in the facilities, it was unlikely that health effects could have been detected, even if MMMF acted like asbestos.

Four of nine studies that could evaluate the association between MMMF and respiratory cancer did not show such an association. In the five studies showing some association between MMMF and respiratory cancer in population subgroups, the excesses were small and had no association with intensity or duration of exposure to MMMF. The authors concluded that "the reality of the association of the respiratory cancer with work involving man-made vitreous fibers...remains dubious."

Summary

In the studies conducted to date, man-made mineral fibers have not presented the same magnitude of health hazard to humans as has asbestos. For example, the committee is not aware of any mesotheliomas among persons occupationally exposed to MMMF but not to asbestos. There is some evidence that a small excess of respiratory cancer has occurred among persons who produce MMMF—either fibrous glass or mineral wool.

This evidence derives from mortality studies that could have detected a large excess if one were present. However, the level of exposure to MMMF has been much lower than that for asbestos. Also, exposure to MMMF was less common before approximately 1960, thereby providing only a limited period in which to assess excess risk from MMMF for effects with long latencies. With longer follow-up and greater numbers of subjects, it may be possible to detect an excess of some cancer that could reflect a causal association with MMMF.

The evidence that MMMF causes nonmalignant respiratory disease is equivocal. Although some studies have reported an excess of nonmalignant respiratory disease among fibrous glass production workers, the excess was small and was found only in a subset of the nonmalignant respiratory diseases. Very little information is available from studies of morbidity among persons exposed to MMMF.

ADDITIONAL OCCUPATIONAL EPIDEMIOLOGICAL STUDIES

Attapulgite

A study of attapulgite miners and millers in Georgia and in Florida has been performed by the National Institute for Occupational Safety and Health (R. Waxweiler, personal communication, 1983). Consistent evidence of health effects was not found, although some excess lung cancers may have occurred. The report had not been released as of January 1983.

Talc

Talc is a hydrated magnesium silicate that is often contaminated with other minerals, including those that may occur as asbestiform fibers. In addition, talc can itself be fibrous, but this form is extremely rare. Materials often found with talc include quartz, calcite, serpentine minerals, and amphiboles (both as cleavage fragments and asbestiform fibers). The fiber content of talc can vary from an undetectable level in some Montana mines to as high as 50% in some New York mines.[13] Talc is used in the ceramic, rubber, and chemical industries as well as in cosmetic powders and pharmaceuticals. It is usually placed into one of two categories: talc that contains mineral fibers and talc that does not.[14]

[13] Many of these particles may not be asbestiform as defined by this committee (T. Zoltai, University of Minnesota; R. Clifton, Bureau of Mines, personal communication, 1983).

[14] Various researchers have referred to talc that contains asbestiform fibers. Some of these fibers may be particles with 3:1 aspect ratios but without the properties of asbestiform fibers. To avoid confusion, the committee uses the more general terms "fiber" or "mineral fiber" in this section.

Workers from different geographic regions containing talc with or without fibers have been studied to determine if any adverse health effects are associated with the asbestiform fiber content of talc. Adverse effects have been found in some studies among workers exposed to talc both with and without fibers. These studies are discussed in the following paragraphs.

Epidemiological studies on workers exposed to talc containing fibers have demonstrated adverse effects on pulmonary function. In a study of 121 New York miners and millers exposed to talc containing tremolite and anthophyllite fibers, pulmonary function was found to be significantly decreased (Gamble et al., 1979b). Reductions in forced vital capacity (FVC) and 1-second forced expiratory volume (FEW_1) were associated with employment duration and the amount of fiber present. Increased pleural thickening and calcification were detected in talc workers with 15 or more years of employment (Gamble et al., 1979b).

A mortality study of 398 New York miners exposed to talc containing fibers has demonstrated excess mortality from nonmalignant respiratory disease, excluding influenza, bronchitis, or pneumonia (5 observed/ 1.3 expected) (Brown et al., 1979). An excess in lung cancer with an average latency of 20 years was also observed (9 observed/3.3 expected). Additional studies have had conflicting results. Some investigators have found no significant increases in lung cancer and nonmalignant respiratory disease (Stille et al., 1982), whereas others have reported significant increases in lung cancer (Kleinfeld et al., 1967, 1974).

Morbidity and mortality studies have also been conducted on workers exposed to talc with low or undetectable levels of fibers. A study on the respiratory function of 103 Vermont talc workers indicated that there was a reduction in pulmonary function in smokers (Wegman et al., 1982). After adjusting for smoking, the effect of the exposure to talc was not statistically significant, although there was evidence of an exposure-related effect in workers with an annual dust exposure of approximately 1.5 mg/m^3. Exposure to talc dust was also associated with small opacities seen on chest radiographs.

Gamble et al. (1982) conducted a cross-sectional study of 299 workers from Montana, Texas, and North Carolina who were exposed to talc containing low levels of silica and fiber. There was no significant difference in lung function, respiratory symptoms, or pneumoconiosis between workers and controls, although there was a significant increase in bilateral pleural thickening among the workers. Results of pulmonary pathology studies have also provided evidence of fibrosis in workers exposed to talc that does not contain fibers (Vallyathan et al., 1981).

A mortality study of 392 Vermont workers exposed to talc not containing fibers showed that there were excess deaths from nonmalignant respiratory disease, excluding influenza and pneumonia, among millers (11 observed/1.79 expected) (Selevan et al., 1979). This excess mortality was associated with small opacities seen on chest radiographs. An excess of respiratory cancer mortality among miners was also noted (5 observed/1.15 expected), but was attributed to exposures other than talc.

RECOMMENDATIONS

New detailed prospective epidemiological studies should be undertaken, and ongoing investigations continued, to examine cohorts exposed occupationally to fibrous materials. Despite the considerable number of studies reported, additional epidemiological studies of occupational groups exposed to asbestos and other fibrous materials, such as man-made mineral fibers, are needed. These studies should include reliable fiber exposure measurements and should have a high statistical power (ability to detect a true effect of a specified magnitude) at relevant lengths of latency. They should also include adequate controls for confounding factors, such as smoking and exposures to other substances in the environment. The studies should be designed to facilitate evaluation of risk over several exposure levels.

Continued follow-up of workers exposed to man-made mineral fibers is needed, especially to determine morbidity. Workers should be examined to determine current status of pulmonary function and pulmonary disease and followed for 5-20 years, with reexamination every few years to assess changes in pulmonary function. For epidemiological studies, efforts should be made to obtain detailed information about the characteristics of the respirable fibers in inhaled air. Every effort should be made to ensure that workers with long service in these industries are autopsied at death, especially for cases involving respiratory disease.

Additional case-control studies of lung cancer and mesothelioma should be conducted among nonoccupationally exposed persons. Emphasis should be placed on assessment of previous exposure to asbestiform fibers and should include use of electron microscopy and other sensitive techniques to identify and quantify exposure and body burden. The feasibility of conducting prospective studies in nonoccupationally exposed populations should be studied, and the possibility of conducting more complete surveillance for mesothelioma in the United States should be considered.

Clinical and epidemiological data indicate that a reduction in cigarette smoking should be encouraged, especially in view of its multiplicative effect in causing lung cancer in conjunction with asbestos exposure. Those in the medical profession and the general public should be informed about the possible exposures to asbestiform fibers and the health effects resulting therefrom.

REFERENCES

Acheson, E. D., and M. J. Gardner. 1980. Asbestos: Scientific basis for environmental control of fibres. Pp. 737-754 in J. C. Wagner, ed. Biological Effects of Mineral Fibres. Vol. 2. IARC Scientific Pub. No. 30. International Agency for Research on Cancer, Lyon.

Acheson, E. D., and M. J. Gardner. 1983. Asbestos: The Control Limit for Asbestos. An up-date of relevant sections of Asbestos: Vol. 2: Final Report of the Advisory Committee, Health and Safety Commission, 1979. Her Majesty's Stationery Office, London.

Acheson, E. D., M. J. Gardner, E. C. Pippard, and L. P. Grime. 1982. Mortality of two groups of women who manufactured gas masks from chrysotile and crocidolite asbestos: A 40-year follow-up. Br. J. Ind. Med. 39:344-348.

Adkins, C. 1976. Neoplasms of the lung. Chapter 18 in D. C. Sabiston and F. C. Spencer, eds. Gibbon's Surgery of the Chest. W. B. Saunders, Philadelphia.

Albelda, S. M., D. M. Epstein, W. B. Gefter, and W. T. Miller. 1982. Pleural thickening: Its significance and relationship to asbestos dust exposure. Am. Rev. Respir. Dis. 126:621-624.

American College of Radiology. 1982. Asbestos Related Diseases: Clinical, Epidemiologic, Pathologic, and Radiologic Characteristics and Manifestations. Prepared by the Asbestos Working Group, a special committee of the ACR Task Force on Pneumoconiosis. American College of Radiology, Chicago.

Anderson, H. A., R. Lilis, S. M. Daum, and I. J. Selikoff. 1979. Asbestosis among household contacts of asbestos factory workers. Ann. N.Y. Acad. Sci. 330:387-399.

Artvinli, M., and Y. I. Baris. 1982. Environmental fiber-induced pleuro-pulmonary diseases in an Anatolian village: An epidemiologic study. Arch. Environ. Health 37:177-181.

Baris, Y. I., L. Simonato, R. Saracci, J. W. Skidmore, and M. Artvinli. 1981. Malignant mesothelioma and radiological chest abnormalities in two villages in central Turkey. Lancet 1:984-987.

Baselga-Monte, M., and F. Segarra. 1978. Epidemiological Study of Asbestosis in the Barcelona Area: A Dose-Response Relationship. Presented at the XIX International Congress on Occupational Health, Dubrovnik, Yugoslavia. September 25-30.

Bayliss, D. L., J. M. Dement, J. K. Wagoner, and H. P. Blejer. 1976. Mortality patterns among fibrous glass production workers. Ann. N.Y. Acad. Sci. 271:324-335.

Beaumont, J., and N. Breslow. 1981. Power considerations in epidemiologic studies of vinyl chloride workers. Am. J. Epidemiol. 5:725-734.

Becklake, M. R. 1976. Asbestos-related diseases of the lung and other organs: Their epidemiology and implications for clinical practice. Am. Rev. Respir. Dis. 114:187-227.

Becklake, H. R., G. Fournier-Massey, C. E. Rossiter, and J. C. McDonald. 1972. Lung function in chrysotile asbestos mine and mill workers of Quebec. Arch. Environ. Health 24:401-409.

Becklake, M. R., F. D. K. Liddel, J. Manfreda, and J. C. McDonald. 1979. Radiological changes after withdrawal from asbestos exposure. Br. J. Ind. Med. 36:23-28.

Berry, G., and M. L. Newhouse. 1983. Mortality of workers manufacturing friction materials using asbestos. Br. J. Ind. Med. 40:1-7.

Berry, G., J. C. Gilson, S. Holmes, H. C. Lewinsohn, and S. A. Roach. 1979. Asbestos: A study of dose-response relationships in an asbestos textile factory. Br. J. Ind. Med. 36:98-112.

Bouhuys, A. 1974. Breathing—Physiology Environment and Lung Disease. Grune and Stratton, New York.

Bouhuys, A., and J. B. L. Gee. 1980. Environmental lung disease. Pp. 1217-1223 in K. J. Isselbacher, R. D. Adams, E. Braunwald, R. G. Petersdorf, and J. D. Wilson, eds. Harrison's Principles of Internal Medicine, Ninth Edition. McGraw-Hill, New York.

Brain, J. D. and P. A. Valberg. 1974. Models of lung retention based on ICRP task group report. Arch. Environ. Health 28:1-11.

Brain, J. D., and P. A. Valberg. 1979. Deposition of aerosol in the respiratory tract. Am. Rev. Resp. Dis. 120:1325-1373.

Breslow, L., L. Hoeglin, G. Rasmussen, and H. K. Abrams. 1954. Occupations and cigarette smoking as factors in lung cancer. Am. J. Pub. Health 44:171-181.

British Occupational Hygiene Society. 1968. Hygiene standards for chrysotile asbestos dust. Am. Occup. Hyg. 11:4769.

Brody, A. R., and P. B. DeNee. 1981. Biological activity of inorganic particles in the lung. Pp. 277-299 in C. P. Straub, ed. Critical Reviews in Environmental Control. CRC Press, Boca Raton, Fla.

Brody, A. R., and L. Hill. Hill. 1982. Interstitial accumulation of inhaled chrysotile asbestos fibers and consequent formation of microcalcifications. Am. J. Pathol. 109:107-114.

Brody, A. R., and M. Roe. Roe. In press. Deposition pattern of inorganic particles at the alveolar level in the lungs of rats and mice. Am. Rev. Resp. Dis.

Brody, A. R., L. M. Hill, B. Adkins, and R. W. O'Conner. 1981. Chrysotile asbestos inhalation in rats: Deposition pattern, and reaction of alveolar epithelium and pulmonary macrophases. Am. Rev. Resp. Dis. 123:6170-6179.

Brody, A. R., M. W. Roe, J. N. Evans, and G. S. Davis. 1982. Deposition and location of inhaled silica in rats. Lab. Invest. 47:533-542.

Brody, A. R., G. George, and L. H. Hill. In press. Interaction of chrysotile and crocidolite asbestos with red blood cell membranes: Chrysotile binds to sialic acid. Lab. Invest.

Brown, D. P., J. M. Dement, and J. K. Wagoner. 1979. Mortality patterns among miners and millers occupationally exposed to asbestiform talc. Pp. 317-324 in R. Lemen and J. M. Dement, eds. Dusts and Disease. Pathotox Publishers, Inc., Park Forest South, Ill.

Burilkov, T., and L. Michailova. 1970. Asbestos content of the soil and endemic pleural asbestosis. Environ. Res. 3:443-451.

Buist, A. S. 1983. Tests for small-airways disease. Respir. Ther. (Sept./Oct.):91-103.

Carpenter, J. L., and L. W. Spolyar. 1945. Negative chest findings in a mineral wool industry. J. Indiana State Med. Assoc. 38:389-390.

Chahinian, A. P., T. F. Pajak, J. F. Holland, L. Norton, R. M. Ambinder, and E. M. Mandel. 1982. Diffuse malignant mesothelioma. Ann. Int. Med. 96:746-755.

Churg, A. 1983a. Asbestos fiber content of the lungs of patients with and without asbestos airways disease. Am. Rev. Respir. Dis. 127: 470-473.

Churg, A. 1983b. Nonasbestos pulmonary mineral fibers in the general population. Environ. Res. 31:189-200.

Churg, A., and M. L. Warnock. 1980. Asbestos fibers in the general population. Am. Rev. Respir. Dis. 122:669-678.

Clemmesen, J., and S. Hjalgrim-Jenson. 1981. Cancer incidence among 5686 asbestos-cement workers followed from 1943 through 1976. Ecotox. Environ. Safety 5:15-23.

Coffin, D. L., L. D. Palekar, and P. M. Cook. 1983. Influence of mineral fibers from noncommercial asbestos sources on the induction of neoplasia. A talk presented at the International Conference on Environment and Lung Disease, Taormina, Italy. March 23-27, 1983.

Conforti, P. M., M. S. Kanarek, L. A. Jackson, R. C. Cooper, and J. C. Murchio. 1981. Asbestos in drinking water and cancer in the San Francisco Bay Area: 1969-1974 incidence. J. Chronic Dis. 34:211-224.

Connelly, R. R., and M. H. Myers. 1982. The incidence of mesothelioma in the United States. A talk presented at the 13th International Cancer Congress, Seattle. September 8-15, 1982.

Cook, P. M. 1983. Review of published studies on gut penetration by ingested asbestos fibers. Environ. Health Perspect. 53:121-130.

Cook, P. M., L. D. Palekar, and D. L. Coffin. 1982. Interpretation of the carcinogenicity of amosite asbestos and ferroactinolite on the basis of retained fiber dose and characteristics in vivo. Toxicol. Lett. 13:151-158.

Cooke, W. E. 1924. Fibrosis of the lungs due to the inhalation of asbestos dust. Br. Med. J. 2:147.

Cooke, W. E. 1927. Pulmonary asbestosis. Br. Med. J. 2:1024-1025.

Cooke, W. E. 1929. Asbestos dust and the curious bodies found in pulmonary asbestosis. Br. Med. J. 2:578-580.

Cooke, W. E., and C. F. Hill. 1930. Further observations on pulmonary asbestosis with special reference to asbestos dust and the curious bodies found in the lungs. J. E. Microsc. Soc. 50:15-19.

Craighead, J. E., and B. T. Mossman. 1982. The pathogenesis of asbestos-associated diseases. N. Engl. J. Med. 306:1446-1455.

Craighead, J. E., J. L. Abraham, A. Churg, F. H. Green, J. Kleinerman, P. C. Pratt, T. A. Seemayer, N. Vallyathan, and H. Weill. 1982. The pathology of asbestos associated diseases of the lungs and pleural cavities: Diagnostic criteria and proposed grading schema. Report of the Pneumoconiosis Committee of the College of American Pathologists and the National Institute for Occupational Safety and Health. Arch. Pathol. Lab. Med. 106:544-597.

Cunningham, H. M., and R. D. Pontefract. 1974. Placental transfer of asbestos. Nature 249:117-118.

Day, N. E., and C. C. Brown. 1980. Multistage models and primary prevention of cancer. J. Natl. Cancer Inst. 64:977-989.

Dement, J. M., and R. D. Zumwalde. 1979. Occupational exposures to talcs containing asbestiform minerals. Pp. 287-305 in R. Lemen and J. M. Dement, eds. Dusts and Disease. Pathotox Publishers, Inc., Park Forest South, Ill.

Dement, J. M., R. L. Harris, M. J. Symons, and C. Shy. 1982. Estimates of dose-response for respiratory cancer among chrysotile asbestos textile workers. Ann. Occup. Hyg. 26:869-887.

Dement, J. M., R. L. Harris, M. J. Symons, and C. Shy. 19833. Exposures and mortality among chrysotile asbestos workers: Part I, Exposure estimates. Am. J. Ind. Med. 4:399-420.

Dement, J. M., R. L. Harris, M. J. Symons, and C. M. Shy. 1983b. Exposures and mortality among chrysotile asbestos workers: Part II. Mortality. Am. J. Ind. Med. 4:421-434.

Dement, J. M., J. A. Merchant, and F. H. Y. Green. In press. Asbestosis. In J. A. Merchant, B. A. Boehlecke, and G. Taylor, eds. Occupational Respiratory Diseases. National Institute for Occupational Safety and Health, Washington, D.C.

Desai, R., and R. J. Richards. 1978. The adsorption of biological macromolecules by mineral dusts. Environ. Res. 16:449-464.

Di Menza, L., A. Hirsch, P. Sebastien, A. Gaudichet, and J. Bignon. 1980. Assessment of past asbestos exposure in patients: Occupational questionnaire versus monitoring in broncho-alveolar lavage. Pp. 609-614 in J. C. Wagner, ed. Biological Effects of Mineral Fibres. Vol. 2. IARC Scientific Pub. No. 30. International Agency for Research on Cancer, Lyon.

Doll, R. 1955. Mortality from lung cancer in asbestos workers. Br. J. Indust. Med. 12:81-86.

Donnelly, J. S. 1936. Pulmonary asbestosis: Incidence and prognosis. J. Ind. Hyg. 18:222-278.

Dreessen, W. C., J. M. Dalla Valle, T. J. Edwards, J. W. Miller, R. R. Soyers, H. F. Eason, and M. F. Trice. 1938. A study of asbestosis in the asbestos textile industry. Public Health Bull. 241:217.

Elmes, P. C., and M. Simpson. 1977. Insulation workers in Belfast. A further study of mortality due to asbestos exposure (1940-75). Br. J. Ind. Med. 34:174-180.

Enterline, P. E. 1976. Pitfalls in epidemiological research: An examination of the asbestos literature. J. Occup. Med. 18:150-156.

Enterline, P. E., and G. M. Marsh. 1982. The health of workers in the man-made mineral fiber industry. Presented at the Biological Effects of Man-Made Mineral Fibers, Occupational Health Conference, WHO-EURO, Copenhagen, April 20, 1982. World Health Organization.

Epler, G. R., T. C. McLoud, and E. A. Gaensler. 1982. Prevalence and incidence of benign asbestos pleural effusion in a working population. J. Am. Med. Assoc. 247: 617-622.

Evans, J. C., R. J. Evans, A. Holmes, R. F. Hounam, D. M. Jones, A. Morgan, and M. Walsh. 1973. Studies on the deposition of inhaled fibrous material in the respiratory tract of the rat and its subsequent clearance using radioactive tracer techniques. Environ. Res. 6:180-201.

Farley, M. L., S. D. Greenberg, E. H. Shuford, G. A. Hurst, C. G. Spivey, and C. S. Christianson. 1977. Ferruginous bodies in spurs of former asbestos workers. Acta Cytol. 21:693-700.

Fears, T. R. 1976. Cancer mortality and asbestos deposits. Am. J. Epidemiol. 104:523-526.

Finkelstein, M. M. 1982. Asbestosis among long-term employees of an Ontario asbestos cement factory. Ann. Rev. Respir. Dis. 125:496-501.

Finkelstein, M. M. 1983. Mortality among long-term employees of an Ontario asbestos-cement factory. Br. J. Ind. Med. 40:138-144.
Gamble, J. F., W. Fellner, and M. J. DiMeo. 1979a. An epidemiologic study of a group of talc workers. Am. Rev. Resp. Dis. 119:741-753.
Gamble, J., W. Fellner, and M. J. DiMeo. 1979b. Respiratory morbidity among miners and millers of asbestiform talc. Pp. 307-316 in R. Lemen and J. M. Dement, eds. Dusts and Disease. Pathotox Publishers, Inc., Park Forest South, Ill.
Gamble, J., A. Greife, and J. Hancock. 1982. An epidemiological-industrial hygiene study of talc workers. Ann. Occup. Hyg. 26:841-859.
Glickman, L. T., L. M. Domanski, T. G. Maguire, R. R. Dubielzig, and A. Churg. 1983. Mesothelioma in pet dogs associated with exposure of their owners to asbestos. Environ. Res. 32:305-313.
Gloyne, S. R. 1929. The presence of the asbestos fibre in the lesions of asbestos workers. Tubercle 10:404-407.
Goodman, L. R. 1983. Radiology of asbestos disease. J. Am. Med. Assoc. 249:644-646.
Gregor, A., R. W. Parker, R. du Bois, and M. Turner-Warwick. 1979. Radiographic progression of asbestos: Preliminary report. Ann. N. Y. Acad. Sci. 330:147-156.
Gross, P. 1981. Consideration of the aerodynamic equivalent diameter of respirable mineral fibers. Am. Ind. Hyg. Assoc. J. 42:449-452.
Gross, P. 1982. Man-made vitreous fibers: Present status of research on health effects. Int. Arch. Occup. Environ. Health 50:103-112.
Gross, P., P. A. Theodos, R. L. H. Murphy, W. C. Cooper, and W. K. C. Morgan. 1976. The pulmonary response to fiberglass dust. Chest 69: 216-219.
Guyton, A. C. 1971. Textbook of Medical Physiology. W. B. Saunders Co., Philadelphia.
Hackney, J. D., and W. S. Lima. 1979. Koch's postulates updated: A potentially useful application to laboratory research and policy analysis in environmental toxicology. Am. Rev. Resp. Dis. 119:849-852.
Hammad, Y., J. Diem, J. Craighead, and H. Weill. 1982. Deposition of inhaled man-made mineral fibers in the lungs of rats. Ann. Occup. Hyg. 26:179-187.
Hammond, E. C., I. J. Selikoff, and H. Seidman. 1979. Asbestos exposure, cigarette smoking and death rates. Ann. N.Y. Acad. Sci. 330:473-490.
Harington, J. S., A. C. Allison, and D. V. Badami. 1975. Mineral fibers: Chemical, physicochemical, and biologic properties. Adv. Pharmacol. Chemother. 12:291-402.
Harrington, J. M., G. F. Craun, J. W. Meigs, P. J. Landrigan, J. T. Flannery, and R. S. Woodhull. 1978. An investigation of the use of asbestos cement pipe for public water supply and the incidence of gastrointestinal cancer in Connecticut, 1935-1973. Am. J. Epidemiol. 107:96-103.
Henderson, V., and P. E. Enterline. 1979. Asbestos exposure: Factors associated with excess cancer and respiratory disease mortality. Ann. N.Y. Acad. Sci. 330:117-126.

Hill, J. W., C. E. Rossiter, and D. W. Fode. 1982. A pilot respiratory study of cancers in a MMMF plant in the United Kingdom. Presented at the Biological Effects of Man-Made Mineral Fibers, Occupational Health Conference, WHO-EURO, Copenhagen, April 20, 1982. World Health Organization.

Hobbs, M. S. T., S. D. Woodward, B. Murphy, A. W. Musk, and J. E. Elder. 1980. The incidence of pneumoconiosis, mesothelioma and other respiratory cancer in men engaged in mining and milling crocidolite in western Australia. Pp. 615-625 in J. C. Wagner, ed. Biological Effects of Mineral Fibres. Vol. 2. IARC Scientific Pub. No. 30. International Agency for Research on Cancer, Lyon.

Hughes, J., and H. Weill. 1980. Lung cancer risk associated with manufacture of asbestos-cement products. Pp. 627-635 in J. C. Wagner, ed. Biological Effects of Mineral Fibres. Vol. 2. IARC Scientific Pub. No. 30. International Agency for Research on Cancer, Lyon.

International Labour Office. 1980. International classification of radiographs of the pneumoconioses; Occupational Safety and Health Series XX. International Labour Office, Geneva, Switzerland.

Irwig, L. M., R. S. J. DuToit, G. K. Sluis-Cremer, A. Solomon, R. G. Thomas, P. P. H. Hamel, I. Webster, and T. Hastie. 1979. Risk of asbestosis in crocidolite and amosite mines in South Africa. Ann. N.Y. Acad. Sci. 330:34-52.

Ives, J. C., P. A. Buffler, and S. D. Greenberg. 1983. Environmental associations and histopathologic patterns of carcinoma of the lung: The challenge and dilemma in epidemiologic studies. Am. Rev. Resp. Dis. 128:195-209.

Jaurand, M. C., J. Bignon, P. Sebastien, and J. Goni. 1979. Leaching of chrysotile asbestos in human lungs. Correlation with in vitro studies using rabbit alveolar macrophages. Environ. Res. 14:245-254.

Jones, R. N., J. E. Diem, H. Glindmeyer, H. Weill, and J. C. Gilson. 1980a. Progression of asbestos radiographic abnormalities: Relationships to estimates of dust exposure and annual decline in lung function. Pp. 537-543 in J. T. Wagner, ed. Biological Effects of Mineral Fibres. Vol. 2. IARC Scientific Pub. No. 30. International Agency for Research on Cancer, Lyon.

Jones, J. S. P., F. D. Pooley, G. W. Sawle, R. J. Madeley, P. G. Smith, G. Berry, B. K. Wignall, and A. Aggarwal. 1980b. The consequences of exposure to asbestos dust in a wartime gas-mask factory. Pp. 637-653 in J. C. Wagner, ed. Biological Effects of Mineral Fibres, Vol. 2. ARC Scientific Pub. No. 30. International Agency for Research on Cancer, Lyon.

Kanarek, M. S., P. M. Conforti, L. A. Jackson, R. C. Cooper, and J. C. Murchio. 1980. Asbestos in drinking water and cancer incidence in the San Francisco Bay Area. Am. J. Epidemiol. 112:54-72.

Kannerstein, M., and J. Churg. 1972. Pathology of carcinoma of the lung associated with asbestos exposure. Cancer 30:14-21.

Kannerstein, M., J. Churg, and W. T. E. McCaughey. 1978. Asbestos and mesothelioma: A review. Pathol. Ann. 13:81-129.

Kilburn, K. H. 1977. Clearance mechanisms in the respiratory tract. Pp. 243-262 in D. H. K. Lee, H. Falk, and S. D. Murphy, eds. Handbook of Physiology, Section 9: Reactions to Environmental Agents. American Physiological Society, Bethesda, Md.

Kiviluoto, R. 1960. Pleural calcification as a roentgenologic sign of non-occupational endemic anthophyllite-asbestos. Acta Radiologica (Supplement) 194:1-67.

Kiviluoto, R. 1965. Pleural plaques and asbestos: Further observations on endemic and other nonoccupational asbestosis. Ann. N.Y. Acad. Sci. 132:235-239.

Kleinfeld M., J. Messire, O. Kooyman, and M. H. Zaki. 1967. Mortality among talc miners and miners in New York State. Arch. Environ. Health 14:663-667.

Kleinfeld, M., J. Messire, and A. J. Langer. 1973. A study of workers exposed to asbestiform minerals in commercial talc manufacture. Environ. Res. 6:132-143.

Kleinfeld, M., J. Messite, and M. H. Zaki. 1974. Mortality experience among talc workers: A follow-up study. J. Occup. Med. 16:345-349.

Klingholz, R. 1977. Technology and production of man-made mineral fibres. Ann. Occup. Hyg. 20:153-159.

Knox, J. F., S. Holmes, R. Doll, and I. D. Hill. 1968. Mortality from lung cancer and other causes among workers in an asbestos textile factory. Br. J. Ind. Med. 25:293-303.

Laamanen, A., L. Noro, and V. Raunio. 1965. Observations on atmospheric pollution caused by asbestos. Ann. N.Y. Acad. Sci. 132:240-254.

Langer, A. M., I. J. Selikoff, and A. Sastre. 1971. Chrysotile asbestos in the lungs of persons in New York City. Arch. Environ. Health 22:348.

Langer, A. M., I. Rubin, and I. J. Selikoff. 1972a. Chemical characterization of asbestos body uses by electron microprobe analysis. J. Histochem. Cytochem. 20:723-734.

Langer, A. M., I. B. Rubin, I. J. Selikoff, and F. D. Pooley. 1972b. Chemical characterization of uncoated asbestos fibers from the lungs of asbestos workers by electron microprobe analysis. J. Histochem. Cytochem. 20:735-740.

Langer, A. M., B. S. Ashley, V. Baden, M. S. Berkley, E. C. Hammond, A. D. Mackler, C. J. Maggiore, W. J. Nicholson, A. N. Rohl, I. B. Rubin, A. Sastre, and I. J. Selikoff. 1973. Identification of asbestos in human tissues. J. Occup. Med. 15:287-295.

Langer, A. M., C. M. Maggiore, W. J. Nicholson, A. N. Rohl, I. B. Rubin, and I. J. Selikoff. 1979. The contamination of Lake Superior with amphibole gangue minerals. Ann. N.Y. Acad. Sci. 330:549-572.

Langer, A. M., A. N. Rohl, I. J. Selikoff, G. E. Harlow, and M. Prinz. 1980. Asbestos as a cofactor in carcinogenesis among nickel-processing workers. Science 209:420-422.

Levy, B. S., E. Sigurdson, J. Mandel, E. Laudon, and J. Pearson. 1976. Investigating possible effects of asbestos in city water: Surveillance of gastrointestinal cancer incidence in Duluth, Minnesota. Am. J. Epidemiol. 103:362-368.

Lewinsohn, H. C. 1972. The medical surveillance on asbestos workers. R. Soc. Health J. 92:69-77.

Liddel, F. D. K., and J. C. McDonald. 1980. Radiological findings as predictors of mortality in Quebec asbestos workers. Br. J. Indust. Med. 37:257-267.

Lilis, R. 1981. Fibrous zeolites and endemic mesothelioma in Cappadocia, Turkey. J. Occup. Med. 23:548-550.

Lilis, R., S. Daum, H. Anderson, G. Andrews, and I. J. Selikoff. 1980. Asbestosis among maintenance workers in the chemical industry and in oil refinery workers. Pp. 795-810 in J. C. Wagner, ed. Biological Effects of Mineral Fibres. Vol. 2. IARC Scientific Pub. No. 30. International Agency for Research on Cancer, Lyon.

Lippmann, M., D. B. Yeates, and R. E. Albert. 1980. Deposition, retention, and clearance of inhaled particles. Br. J. Ind. Med. 37:337-362.

Lockey, J., S. Tasakek, S. Carson, R. McKay, T. Harber, P. Khoury, J. Morrison, J. Wiot, H. Stite, and S. Brooks. 1983. Pulmonary hazards from vermiculite exposure. Pp. 303-316 in W. L. Wagner, W. N. Rom, and J. A. Merchant, eds. Health Issues Related to Metal and Nonmetallic Miming. Proceedings of the Fourth Park City Conference on Occupational Safety and Health. Ann Arbor Press, Ann Arbor.

Lorimer, W. V., A. N. Rohl, A. Miller, W. J. Nicholson, and I. J. Selikoff. 1976. Asbestos exposure of brake workers in the United States. Mr. Sinai J. Med. 43:207-218.

Lumley, K. D. S. 1977. Physiological changes in asbestos pleural disease. Pp. 781-788 in W. H. Walton, ed. Inhaled Particles IV. Part 2. Pergamon Press, Oxford.

Maggiori, A., G. Meregalli, C. Sala, and M. Riva. 1980. Respiratory and skin diseases in glass fibre workers. Med. Lavoro 3:216-277. (In Italian, English abstract).

Malmberg P., H. Hedenstrom, B. Kolmodin-Hedman, and S. Krantz. 1982. Pulmonary function in workers in a mineral rock fiber plant. Presented at the Biological Effects of Mah-Made Mineral Fibers, Occupational Health Conference, WHO-EURO, Copenhagen, April 20, 1982. World Health Organization.

Mancuso, T. F., and E. J. Coulter. 1963. Methodology in industrial health studies. The cohort approach, with special reference to an asbestos company. Arch. Environ. Health 6:210-226.

Marsh, G. H. 1983. Review of epidemiologic studies related to ingested asbestos. Environ. Health Perspect. 53:49-56.

Mason, T. J., F. W. McKay, and R. W. Miller. 1974. Asbestos-like fibers in Duluth water supply: Relation to cancer mortality. J. Am. Med. Assoc. 228:1019-1020.

McDonald, J. C. 1980. Asbestos-related disease: An epidemiological review. Pp. 587-601 in J. C. Wagner, ed. Biological Effects of Mineral Fibres. Vol. 2. IARC Scientific Pub. No. 30. International Agency for Research on Cancer, Lyon.

McDonald, J. C. 1982. Mortality of workers exposed to man-made mineral fibers: Current evidence and future research. Presented at the Biological Effects of Kan-Made Mineral Fibers, Occupational Health Conference, WHO-EURO, Copenhagen, April 20, 1982. World Health Organization.

McDonald, J. C., and A. D. McDonald. 1977. Eptdemiology of mesotheltoma from estimated incidence. Prev. Med. 6:426-446.
McDonald, A. D., and J. C. McDonald. 1980. Malignant mesothelioma in North America. Cancer 46:1650-1656.
McDonald, J. C., and A. D. McDonald. 1981. Mesothelioma as an index of asbestos impact. Pp. 73-85 in R. Pets and M. Schneiderman, eds. Banbury Report 9. Quantification of Occupational Cancer. Cold Spring Harbor Laboratory, Cold Spring Harbor, N.Y.
McDonald, J. C., M. R. Becklake, G. Fournier-Massey, and C. E. Rossiter. 1972. Respiratory symptoms in chrysotile asbestos mine and mill workers in Quebec. Arch. Environ. Health 24:358-363.
McDonald, J. C., M. R. Becklake, G. W. Gibbs, A. D. McDonald, and C. E. Rossiter. 1974. The health of chrysotile asbestos mine and mill workers of Quebec. Arch. Environ. Health 28:61-68.
McDonald, J. C., F. D. K. Liddel, G. W. Gibbs, G. E. Eyssen, and A. D. McDonald. 1980. Dust exposure and mortality in chrysotile mining, 1910-1975. Br. J. Ind. Med. 37:11-24.
McLarty, J. W., S. D. Greenberg, and G. A. Hurst. 1980. The clinical significance of ferruginous bodies in sputa. J. Occup. Med. 22:92-96.
Meigs, J. W., S. D. Walter, J. F. Heston, J. R. Millette, and G. F. Craun. 1980. Asbestos-cement pipe and cancer in Connecticut, 1955-1974. J. Environ. Health 42:187-191.
Merewether, C. R. A., and C. W. Price. 1930. Report on the Effects of Asbestos Dust on the Lungs and Dust Suppression in the Asbestos Industry. I. Occurrence of pulmonary fibrosis and other pulmonary affections in asbestos workers. II. Processes giving rise to dust and methods for its suppression. Her Majesty's Stationary Office, London.
Merchant, J. A., P. T. Klonda, C. A. Soutar, W. R. Parkes, S. D. Lawler, and M. Turner-Warwick. 1975. The HLA system in asbestos workers. Br. Med. J. 189:191.
Meurman, L. O. 1968. Pleural fibrocalcific plaques and asbestos exposure. Environ. Res. 2:30-46.
Meurman, L. O., R. Kiviluoto, and M. Hakama. 1974. Mortality and morbidity among the working population of anthophyllite asbestos miners in Finland. Br. J. Ind. Med. 31:105-112.
Meurman, L. O., R. Kiviluoto, and M. Hakama. 1979. Combined effects of asbestos exposure and tobacco smoking on Finnish anthophyllite miners and millers. Ann. N.Y. Acad. Sci. 330:491-495.
Morgan, A. 1974. Absorption of human serum albumin by asbestiform minerals and its application to the measurement of surface areas of dispersed samples of chrysotile. Environ. Res. 7:330-341.
Morgan, A. 1979. Fiber dimensions: Their significance in the deposition and clearance of inhaled fiber dusts. Pp. 87-96 in R. Lemen and J. M. Dement, eds. Dusts and Disease. Pathotox Publishers, Inc., Park Forest South, Ill.
Morgan, A., J. C. Evans, and A. Holmes. 1973. Deposition and clearance of inhaled fibrous minerals in the rat. Studies using radioactive tracer techniques. I. UICC crocidolite asbestos. Environ. Res. 6:180-201.

Morgan, A., R. J. Talbot, and A. Holmes. 1978. Significance of asbestos fibres from lung. Br. J. Ind. Med. 35:146-153.

Morgan, E. W., S. D. Kaplan, and J. A. Bratsberg. 1981. Mortality study of fibrous glass production workers. Arch. Environ. Health 36:179-183.

Morgan, R. W., S. D. Kaplan, and J. A. Bratsberg. 1982. Mortality in fibrous glass production workers. Presented at the Biological Effects of Man-Made Mineral Fibers, Occupational Health Conference, WHO-EURO Copenhagen, April 20, 1982. World Health Organization.

Mossman, B. T., B. Ley, J. B. Kessler, and J. E. Craighead. 1977. Interaction of crocidolite asbestos with hamster respiratory mucosa in organ culture. Lab. Invest. 36:131-139.

Muggenburg, B. A., B. B. Boecker, J. H. Diel, and M. B. Smipes. 1981. Observations on the lung retention of inhaled relatively insoluble, environmentally related particles. Chest 80:19-20.

Murphy, R. L., B. G. Ferris, and W. A. Burgess. 1971. Effects of low concentrations of asbestos. Clinical, environmental, radiologic and epidemiologic observations in shipyard pipe coverers and controls. N. Engl. J. Med. 285:1271-1278.

Murphy, R. L. H., E. A. Gaensler, B. G. Ferris, M. Fitzgerald, N. Solliday, and W. Morrisey. 1978. Diagnosis of asbestosis. Observations from longitudinal survey of shipyard pipe coverers. Am. J. Med. 65:488-498.

Murray, H. M. 1907. Report of the Committee on Compensation for Industrial Diseases. Minutes of Evidence.

Nasr, A. N. M., T. Ditchek, and P. A. Scholtens. 1971. The prevalence of radiographic abnormalities in the chests of fiber glass workers. J. Occup. Med. 13:371-376.

National Research Council. 1983a. Drinking Water and Health. Vol. 5. A report of the Safe Drinking Water Committee, Commission on Life Sciences. National Academy Press, Washington, D.C. 157 pp.

National Research Council. 1983b. Risk Assessment In the Federal Government: Managing the Process. A report of the Committee on the Institutional Means for Assessment of Risks to Public Health, Commission on Life Sciences. National Academy Press, Washington, D.C. 191 pp.

Newhouse, M. L. 1969. A study of the mortality of workers in an asbestos factory. Br. J. Ind. Med. 26:294-301.

Newhouse, M. L. 1973. Cancer among workers in the asbestos textile industry. Pp. 203-208 in P. Bogovski, J. C. Gibson, V. Timbrell, and J. C. Wagner, eds. Proceedings of the Conference on Biological Effects of Asbestos. IARC Scientific Pub. No. 8. International Agency for Research on Cancer, Lyon.

Newhouse, M. L., and G. Berry. 1979. Patterns of mortality in asbestos factory workers in London. Ann. N.Y. Acad. Sci. 330:53-60.

Newhouse, M. L., G. Berry, J. C. Wagner, and M. E. Turok. 1972. A study of the mortality of female asbestos workers. Br. J. Ind. Med. 29:134-141.

Newhouse, M. L., G. Berry, and J. W. Skidmore. 1982. A mortality study of workers manufacturing friction materials with chrysotile asbestos. Ann. Occup. Hyg. 26:899-909.

Nicholson, W. J., I. J. Selikoff, H. Seidman, R. Lilis, and P. Formby. 1979. Long-tern mortality experience of chrysotile miners and millers in Thetford mines, Quebec. Ann. N.Y. Acad. Sci. 330:11-21.

Niewoehner, D. F., J. Kleinerman, and D. B. Rice. 1974. Pathologic changes in peripheral airways of young cigarette smokers. N. Engl. J. Med. 291:755-758.

Pernis, B., E. C. Vigliani, and I. J. Selikoff. 1965. Rheumatoid factor in serum of individuals exposed to asbestos. Ann. N.Y. Acad. Sci. 132:112-120.

Peterson, J. T., S. D. Greenberg, P. A. Buffler. In press. Non-asbestos-related malignant mesothelioma: A review. Cancer.

Peto, J. 1979. Dose-response relationships for asbestos related disease. Ann. N.Y. Acad. Sci. 330:195-204.

Peto, J. 1980a. The incidence of pleural mesothelioma in chrysotile asbestos textile workers. Pp. 703-711 in J. C. Wagner, ed. Biological Effects of Mineral Fibres. Vol. 2. IARC Scientific Pub. No. 30. Tnternational Agency for Research on Cancer, Lyon.

Peto, J. 1980b. Lung cancer mortality in relation to measured dust levels in an asbestos textile factory. Pp. 829-836 in J. C. Wagner, ed. Biological Effects of Mineral Fibres. Vol. 2. IARC Scientific Pub. No. 30. International Agency for Research on Cancer, Lyon.

Peto, J., R. Doll, S. V. Howard, L. J. Kinlen, and H. C. Lewinsohn. 1977. Mortality study among workers in an English asbestos factory. Br. J. Ind. Med. 34:169-173.

Peto, J., H. Seidman, and I. J. Selikoff. 1982. Mesothelioma mortality in asbestos workers: Implications for models of carcinogenesis and risk assessment. Br. J. Cancer 45:124-135.

Polissar, L., R. K. Severson, E. S. Boatman, and D. B. Thomas. 1982. Cancer incidence in relation to asbestos in drinking water in the Puget Sound region. Am. J. Epidemiol. 116:314-328.

Pooley, F. D. 1972. Asbestos bodies, their formation, composition and character. Environ. Res. 5:363-379.

Pooley, F., P. D. Oldham, Um Chang-Hyun, and J. D. Wagner. 1970. The detection of asbestos in tissues. Pp. 108-116 in H. A. Shapiro, ed. Pneumoconiosis: Proceedings of the International Conference, Johannesburg, 1969. Oxford University Press, Cape Town.

Puntoni, R., M. Vercelli, F. Merlo, F. Valerio, and L. Santi. 1979. Mortality among shipyard workers in Genoa, Italy. Ann. N.Y. Acad. Sci. 330:353-377.

Robinson, C. F., R. A. Lemen, and J. K. Wagoner. 1979. Mortality patterns, 1940-1975, among workers employed in an asbestos textile, friction, and packing products manufacturing facility. Pp. 131-143 in R. A. Lemen and J. H. Dement, ads. Dusts and Disease. Pathotox Publishers, Inc., Park Forest South, Ill.

Robinson, C. F., J. M. Dement, G. O. Ness, and R. J. Waxweiler. 1982. Mortality patterns of rock and slag mineral wool production workers: An epidemiological and environmental study. Br. J. Ind. Died. 39:45-53.

Rohl, A. N., A. M. Langer, G. Moncure, I. J. Selikoff, and A. Fischbein. 1982. Endemic pleural disease associated with exposure to mixed fibrous dust in Turkey. Science 216:518-520.

Rom, W. N., K. R. Casey, W. T. Parry, C. H. Mjaatvedt, and F. Moatamed. 1983. Health implications of natural fibrous zeolites for the intermountain west. Environ. Res. 30:1-8.

Rossiter, C. F., and R. M. Coles. 1980. H. M. Dockyard, Devonport: 1947 mortality study. Pp. 713-721 in J. C. Wagner, ed. Biological Effects of Mineral Fibres. IARC Scientific Pub. No. 30. International Agency for Research on Cancer, Lyon.

Rowlands, N., G. W. Gibbs, and S. D. McDonald. 1982. Asbestos fibres in lungs of chrysotile miners and millers—a preliminary report. Ann. Occup. Hyg. 26:411-415.

Rubino, G. F., G. Piolatto, M. L. Newhouse, G. Scansetti, G. A. Aresini, and R. Murray. 1979a. Mortality of chrysotile asbestos workers at the Balangero mine, northern Italy. Br. J. Ind. Med. 36:187-194.

Rubino, F. G., M. Newhouse, G. Murray, G. Scansetti, G. Piolatto, and G. Aresini. 1979b. Radiological changes after cessation of exposure among chrysotile asbestos miners in Italy. Ann. N. Y. Acad. Sci. 330:157-161.

Sadler, T. D., W. N. Rom, J. L. Lyon and J. O. Mason. In press. The use of asbestos-cement pipe for public water supply and the incidence of cancer in selected communities in Utah, 1967. J. Commun. Health

Sanchis, J., M. Dolovich, R. Chalmers, and M. T. Newhouse. 1971. Regional deposition and lung clearance mechanisms in smokers and nonsmokers. Pp. 183-191 in W. H. Walton, ed. Inhaled Particles III. Vol. 1. Unwin Brothers, Surrey, England.

Saracci, R., and L. Simonato. 1982. Man-made vitreous fibers and workers' health. Scand. J. Work Environ. Health 8:234-242.

Saracci, R., L. Simonato, E. D. Acheson, A. Anderson, P. A. Bertazzi, N. Charnay, J. Claude, J. Esteve, R. R. Frentzel-Beyme, M. Gardner, O. Jensen, R. Maasing, J. Olsen, L. Teppo, C. Zocchetti, and P. Westerholm. 1982. The IARC mortality and cancer incidence study of man-made mineral (vitreous) fibre (MMM(V)F) production workers in seven European countries. Presented at the Biological Effects of Man-Made Mineral Fibers, Occupational Health Conference, WHO-EURO, Copenhagen, April 20, 1982. World Health Organization.

Sebastien, P., A. Fondimare, J. Bignon, G. Monchaux, J. Desbordes, and G. Bonnaud. 1977. Topographic distribution of asbestos fibres in human lung in relation to occupational and non-occupational exposure. Pp. 435-446 in W. H. Walton and B. McGovern, eds. Inhaled Particles IV. Part 2. Pergamon Press, Oxford.

Sebastien, P., X. Janson, G. Bonnaud, G. Riba, R. Masse, and J. Bignon. 1979. Translocation of asbestos fibers through respiratory tract and gastrointestinal tract according to fiber type and size. Pp. 72-85 in R. Lemen and J. Dement, eds. Dust and Disease. Pathotox Publishers, Inc., Park Forest South, Ill.

Sebastien, P., A. Gaudichet, J. Bignon, and Y. I. Baris. 1981. Zeolite bodies in human lungs from Turkey. Lab. Invest. 44:420-425.

Seidman, H. R., R. Lilis, and I. J. Selikoff. 1977. Short-term asbestos exposure and delayed cancer risk. Pp. 943-960 in H. E. Niebergo, ed. Third International Symposium on Detection and Prevention of Cancer. Marcel Dekker, New York.

Seidman, H., I. J. Selikoff, and E. C. Hammond. 1979. Short-term asbestos exposure and long-term observation. Ann. N.Y. Acad. Sci. 330:61-89.

Selevan, S. G., J. M. Dement, J. K. Wagoner, and J. R. Froines. 1979. Mortality patterns among miners and millers of non-asbestiform talc: Preliminary report. J. Environ. Pathol. Toxicol. 2:273-284.

Selikoff, I. J. 1965. The occurrence of pleural calcification among asbestos insulation workers. Ann. N. Y. Acad. Sci. 132:351-367.

Selikoff, I. J. 1976. Lung cancer and mesothelioma during prospective surveillance of 1249 asbestos insulation workers, 1963-1974. Ann. N.Y. Acad. Sci. 271:448-456.

Selikoff, I. J., and D. H. K. Lee. 1978. Asbestos and Disease. Academic Press, New York.

Selikoff, I. J. 1977. Clinical survey of chrysotile asbestos miners and millers in Baie Verte, Newfoundland—1976, National Institute of Environmental Health Sciences, Cincinnati.

Selikoff, I. J., and E. C. Hammond, eds. 1979. Health Hazards of Asbestos Exposure. Ann. N. Y. Acad. Sci. 330:1-811.

Selikoff, I. J., J. Churg, and E. C. Hammond. 1964. Asbestos exposure and neoplasia. J. Am. Med. Assoc. 188:142-146.

Selikoff, I. J., J. Churg, and E. C. Hammond. 1965. The occurrence of asbestosis among insulation workers in the United States. Ann. N.Y. Acad. Sci. 132:139-155.

Selikoff, I. J., E. C. Hammond, and J. Churg. 1968. Asbestos exposure, smoking and neoplasia. J. Am. Med. Assoc. 204:104-110.

Selikoff, I. J., E. C. Hammond, and J. Churg. 1972. Carcinogenicity of amosite asbestos. Arch. Environ. Health 25:183-196.

Selikoff, I. J., E. C. Hammond, and H. Seidman. 1979. Mortality experience of insulation workers in the United States and Canada, 1943-1976. Ann. N.Y. Acad. Sci. 330:91-116.

Sepulveda, M. J., and J. A. Merchant. 1983. Roentgenographic evidence of asbestos exposure in a select population of railroad workers. Am. J. Ind. Med.4:631-640.

Severson, R. 1979. A study of the effects of asbestos in drinking water and cancer incidence in the Puget Sound region. M.S. thesis, University of Washington, Seattle.

Shannon H. S., M. V. Hayes, J. A. Julian, and D. C. F. Muir. 1982. Mortality studies of Canadian fibreglass workers. Presented at the Biological Effects of Man-Made Mineral Fibers, Occupational Health Conference, WHO-EURO, Copenhagen, April 20, 1982.

Shettigara, P. T., and R. W. Morgan. 1975. Asbestos, smoking and laryngeal carcinoma. Arch. Environ. Health 30:517-519.

Shull, J. R. 1936. Asbestosis. A roentgenologic review of 71 cases. Radiology 27:279-292.

Sigurdson, E. E., B. S. Levy, J. Mandel, R. McHugh, L. L. Michienzi, H. Jagger, and J. Pearson. 1981. Cancer morbidity investigations: Lessons from the Duluth study of possible effects of asbestos in drinking water. Environ. Res. 25:50-61.

Skuric Z., and D. Stahyljak-Boritic. 1982. Occupational exposure and ventilatory function changes in rock wool workers. Presented at the Biological Effects of Man-Made Mineral Fibers, Occupational Health Conference, WHO-EURO, Copenhagen, April 20, 1982. World Health Organization.

Sluis-Cremer, G. K. 1980. The relationship between asbestosis and bronchial cancer. Chest 78:380-381.

Smith, M. J., and B. Naylor. 1972. A method for extracting ferruginous bodies from sputum and pulmonary tissue. Am. J. Clin. Pathol. 58:250-255.

Startsfield, D., and J. R. Edge. 1974. Circulatory rheumatoid factor and antinuclear antibodies in shipyard asbestos workers with pleural plaques. Br. J. Dis. Chest 68:166-170.

Stell, P. M., and T. MacGill. 1973. Asbestos and laryugeal carcinoma. Lancet 2:416-417.

Stille, W. T., and I. R. Tabershaw. 1982. The mortality experience of upstate New York talc workers. J. Occup. Med. 24:480-484.

Summary Workshop on Ingested Asbestos. 1983. Proceedings of a meeting held in Cincinnati October 13 and 14, 1982, sponsored by the Environmental Protection Agency. Environ. Health Perspect. Vol. 53.

Suzuki, Y. 1974. Interaction of asbestos with alveolar cells. Environ. Health Perspect. 9:241-252.

Suzuki, Y. 1980. Pathology of human malignant mesothelioma. Seminars in Oncology 8:268-282.

Suzuki, Y., and J. Churg. 1969. Structure and development of the asbestos body. Am. J. Pathol. 55:79-107.

Tarter, M. E. 1981. Pattern recognition in the context of an asbestos cancer threshold study. Presented at the 13th Annual Symposium on the Interface: Computer Science and Statistics.

Timbrell, V. 1965. The inhalation of fibrous dusts. Ann. N.Y. Acad. Sci. 133:255-273.

Timbrell, V. 1982. Retention of fibers in human lungs. Pp. 347-369 in W. H. Walton, ed. Inhaled Particles. Vol. V. Pergamon Press, Oxford.

Timbrell, V., N. E. Beran, A. S. Davies, and D. E. Munday. 1970. Hollow cast of lungs for experimental purposes. Nature 22:97-98.

Tisi, G. M. 1980. Neoplasms of the lung. Pp. 1259-1265 in K. J. Isselbacher, R. D. Adams, E. Braunwald, R. G. Petersdorf, and J. D. Wilson, eds. Harrison's Principles of Internal Medicine. McGraw-Hill, New York.

Toft, P., D. T. Wigle, J. C. Meranger, and Y. Mao. 1981. Asbestos and drinking water in Canada. Sci. Total Environ. 18:77-89.

Tolent, J. M., W. O. Harrison, A. Soloman, and J. Webster. 1980. A survey of black mineworkers of the Cape crocidolite mines. Pp. 723-729 in T. C. Wagner, ed. Biological Effects of Mineral Fibres. Vol. 2. IARC Scientific Pub. No. 30. International Agency for Research on Cancer, Lyon.

Turner-Warwick, M. 1973. Immunology and asbestosis. Proc. R. Soc. Wed. 66:927-930.

Turner-Warwick, M. 1979. HLA phenotypes in asbestos workers. Br. J. Dis. Chest 73:243-244.
U.S. Consumer Product Safety Commission. 1983. Chronic Hazard Advisory Panel on Asbestos: Report of the U.S. Consumer Product Safety Commission. July 1983. Consumer Product Safety Commission, Washington, D.C.
U.S. Department of Health, Education, and Welfare. 1964. Smoking and Health: Report of the Advisory Committee to the Surgeon General of the Public Health Service. Department of Health, Education, and Welfare, Washington, D.C.
U.S. Department of Health, Education, and Welfare. 1979. Smoking and Health: A Report of the Advisory Committee to the Surgeon General of the Public Health Service. DHEW Pub. No. 79-50066. Department of Health, Education, and Welfare, Washington, D.C.
U.S. Department of Health and Human Services. 1983. National Center for Health Statistics. Monthly Vital Statistics Report. Vol. 32, No. 4, Supplement. August 11, 1983. U.S. Department of Health and Human Services, Washington, D.C.
Utidjian, H. M., and R. T. P. de Trenville. 1970. Fibrous glass manufacturing and health. Transactions of the 35th Annual Meeting of the Industrial Health Foundation, Inc. 44:98-111.
Vallyathan, N. V., and J. E. Craighead. 1981. Pulmonary pathology in workers exposed to nonasbestiform talc. Human Pathol. 12:28-35.
Vianna, N. J., and A. K. Polan. 1978. Non-occupational exposure to asbestos and malignant mesothelioma in females. Lancet 2:1061-1063.
Wagner, J. C. 1980. The pneumoconioses due to mineral dusts. J. Geol. Soc. London 137:537-545.
Wagner, J. C. 1982. Health hazards of substitutes. Pp. 244-266 in Proceedings of the World Symposium on Asbestos, held May 25-27, 1982 in Montreal. Canadian Asbestos Information Center, Montreal.
Wagner, J. C., C. A. Sleggs, and P. Matchand. 1960. Diffuse pleural mesothelioma and asbestos exposure in the North Western Cape Province. Br. J. Ind. Med. 17: 260-271.
Wagner, J. C., G. Berry, J. W. Skidmore, and V. Timbrell. 1974. The effects of the inhalation of asbestos in rats. Br. J. Cancer 29: 252-269.
Wagner, J. C., M. Chamberlain, R. C. Brown, G. Berry, F. D. Pooley, R. Davies, and P. M. Griffiths. 1982. Biological effects of tremolite. Br. J. Cancer 45:352-360.
Walton, W. H. 1982. The nature, hazards, and assessment of occupational exposure to airborne asbestos dust: A review. Ann. Occup. Hyg. 25:117-247.
Wegman, D. H., J. M. Peters, M. G. Boundy, and T. J. Smith. 1982. Evaluation of respiratory effects in miners and millers exposed to talc free of asbestos and silica. Brit. J. Ind. Med. 39: 233-238.
Weill, H., C. Waggenspack, W. Bailey, M. Ziskind, and C. Rossiter. 1973. Radiographic and physiologic patterns among workers engaged in the manufacture of asbestos cement products. A preliminary report. J. Occup. Med. 15:248-252.

Weill, H., M. M. Ziskind, and C. Waggenspack. 1975. Lung function consequences of dust exposure in asbestos cement manufacturing plants. Arch. Environ. Health 30:88-97.

Weill, H., J. M. Hughes, Y. Y. Hammad, H. W. Glindmeyer, G. Sharon, and R. N. Jones. 1982. Respiratory health of workers exposed to man-made vitreous fibers. Presented at the Biological Effects of Nan-Made Minerals Fibers, Occupational Health Conference, WHO-EURO, Copenhagen, April 20, 1982. World Health Organization.

Weiss, W. 1971. Cigarette smoking, asbestos and pulmonary fibrosis. Am. Rev. Reap. Dis. 104:223-227.

Weiss, W. 1983. Heterogeneity in historical cohort studies: A source of bias in assessing lung cancer risk. J. Occup. Med. 25:290-294.

Weiss, W., and P. A. Theodos. 1978. Pleuropulmonary disease among asbestos workers in relation to smoking and type of exposure. J. Occup. Med. 20:341-345.

Weiss, W., R. Levin, and L. Goodman. 1981. Pleural plaques and cigarette smoking in asbestos workers. J. Occup. Med. 23:427-430.

Westlake, G. E., H. A. Spjut, and M. N. Smith. 1965. Penetration of colonic mucosa by asbestos particles. Lab. Invest. 14:2029-2033.

Wigle, D. T. 1977. Cancer mortality in relation to asbestos in municipal water supplies. Arch. Environ. Health 32:185-190.

Workshop on Ingested Asbestos. 1983. Summary Workshop on Ingested Asbestos, October 13-14, 1982, Cincinnati. Environ. Health Perspect. 53:1-204.

Wright, G. W. 1968. Airborne fibrous glass particles. Chest roentgenograms of persons with prolonged exposure. Arch. Environ. Health 16:175-181.

Wright, W. E., W. N. Rom, and F. Moatamed. 1983. Characterization of zeolite fiber sizes using scanning electron microscopy. Arch. Environ. Health 38:99-103.

Wright, W. E., R. P. Sherwin, E. A. Dickson, L. Bernstein, J. B. Fromm, and B. E. Henderson. In press. Malignant mesothelioma: Incidence, asbestos exposure and reclassification of histopathology. Br. J. Ind. Med.

Zolov, C., T. Bourilkov, and L. Babadjov. 1967. Pleural asbestosis in agricultural workers. Environ. Res. 1:287-292.

6

Laboratory Studies of the Effects of Asbestiform Fibers

This chapter describes experimental studies that have elucidated some biological effects of asbestiform fibers and their interactions with cells.

STUDIES IN ANIMALS

In humans, inhalation of asbestos is associated with increased risks of lung tumors (bronchogenic carcinoma and peripheral adenocarcinoma), pleural and peritoneal mesothelioma, interstitial pulmonary fibrosis (asbestosis), pleural thickening, and possibly other tumors, including those of the gastrointestinal tract and kidney. Investigators have induced lung tumors, mesothelioma, and fibrosis after administration of asbestos to animals. This section summarizes the results of toxicological studies in an attempt to determine whether (1) certain physicochemical properties of asbestos are important in the induction of disease and whether (2) other asbestiform fibers exhibit pathogenic potential in animals.

Lung Cancer

In the lung, malignant tumors arise from the bronchial or alveolar epithelial cells and are classified according to their histological features (e.g., squamous cell carcinoma or adenocarcinoma; small or large cell carcinoma). Although small numbers of these types of tumors appear in rats after inhalation (Appendix F, Table F-1) or intratracheal instillation of asbestos and chemical carcinogens (Appendix F, Table F-2), benign (papilloma, adenoma) and malignant (fibrosarcoma) tumors uncommon to humans occur more frequently. In general, results are difficult to evaluate because of different experimental protocols (e.g., amounts of dusts, exposure regimens, different species or strains). For example, in inhalation studies conducted by Davis et al. (1978, 1982), Wagner et al. (1974, 1982a), and Bozelka et al. (1983) asbestos concentrations of approximately 10 mg/m^3 of air were used, whereas Reeves and colleagues (1971, 1974, 1976) used concentrations approximately fivefold higher.

Another shortcoming is the lack of dose-response information at various concentrations of asbestos. With the exception of Davis et al. (1978) and Lee et al. (1981), all investigators have used only one concentration of dust. The different size distributions of fibers in these studies also present problems to those attempting to compare the pathogenic potential of different types of asbestos. For example, inhalation studies by Davis et al. (1978) (Appendix F, Table F-1) demonstrated that clouds of chrysotile contain many more fibers longer than 20 μm than are found in aerosolized amphiboles. This phenomenon could account for the greater tumor incidence observed after exposure to chrysotile in these experiments. However, despite these general limitations in interpretation, data in Appendix F, Tables F-1 and F-2 support the following conclusions:

1. The development of lung cancers in rodents after inhalation of asbestos is species-specific. For example, rats and mice develop both benign and malignant neoplasms, whereas hamsters, guinea pigs, and rabbits develop only benign neoplasms (Botham and Holt, 1972a,b; Gardner, 19421 Gross et al., 19671 Reeves et al., 1974; Vorwald et al., 1951; Wagner, 1963). In the few studies conducted in cats (Vorwald et al., 1951) and monkeys (Wagner, 19631 Webster, 1970), fibrosis but no tumors developed. Thus, cats and monkeys seem to be inappropriate animal models for studies of asbestos-linked carcinogenesis.
2. Small numbers of benign and malignant lung tumors have been observed after inhalation of all types of asbestos (Appendix F, Table F-1). The short lifespan of rodents may not allow sufficient time for development of larger numbers of tumors.
3. A striking increase in the number of neoplasms has been observed after rodents were exposed by installation to a combination of asbestos and chemical carcinogens such as polycyclic aromatic hydrocarbons (PAHs). Thus, asbestos appears to act synergistically with PAH to induce lung tumors (Appendix F, Table F-2).
4. For unexplained reasons, a synergistic effect has not been observed in rats exposed to both asbestos and cigarette smoke by inhalation (Shabad et al., 1974; Wehner et al., 1975); however, development of fibrosis in these animals leads to reduced lifespan.
5. When asbestos is inhaled by rats simultaneously with the intratracheal instillation of sodium hydroxide, a caustic agent affecting mucociliary clearance, an increase in the number of tumors has been observed (Gross et al., 1967). The sodium hydroxide presumably leads to a greater retention of asbestos in the respiratory tract.
6. Several types of man-made mineral fibers (MMMFs) have been evaluated in inhalation studies. Among the fibers studied are fibrous glass (Gross 19741 Gross et al., 19701 Lee et al., 1981; Moorman, in press; Schepers and Delahant, 1955; Schepers et al., 1958) and insulation (Morrison et al., 1981); alumina (Piggott et al., 1981); glass wool, rock

wool, and glass microfibers (Wagner et al., 1982a); ceramic aluminum silicate glass (CASG) (Davis et al., 1982); and potassium titanate, i.e., Fybex and pigmentary potassium titanate (PKT) (Lee et al., 1981). In comparison to the various types of asbestos included as positive controls in many of these studies, these fibers are generally less carcinogenic. Tumors have been reported after exposure to CASG (Davis et al., 1982). Results with fibrous glass vary (see footnote to Table F-1 in Appendix F). Lee et al. (1981) produced two malignant lung tumors in hamsters exposed to potassium octatitanate fibers and bronchogenic tumors in rats with use of fine fiber glass. No malignant tumors were produced in hamsters, rats, or guinea pigs inhaling ball-milled fiberglass. Wagner et al. (1982a) reported small numbers of lung cancers in rats exposed to glass wool, rock wool, and glass microfibers by inhalation and no cancers in control animals, whereas in comparable studies, McConnell et al. (1982) did not detect such an increase.

7. In comparison to amosite asbestos, more bronchogenic tumors developed in rats after intratracheal instillation of ferroactinolite—an unusual and impure asbestiform fiber (Coffin et al., 1982; Cook et al., 1982). Ferroactinolite appears to undergo longitudinal splitting as a result of dissolution in the respiratory tract, thereby producing an increased dose of extremely thin fibers. When the animals were exposed to nonfibrous grunerite, no carcinomas were observed.

Mesothelioma

Pleural and peritoneal mesotheliomas originate in the serosal cells lining the body cavities occupied by the lungs and digestive organs, respectively. They occur in small numbers after inhalation of asbestiform fibers by animals, but in larger numbers after intrapleural and intraperitoneal injection of the fibers. The injection technique has been used most frequently in reported studies because of its reproducibility. However, injection of fibers bypasses normal lung clearance mechanisms and is criticized as a nonphysiological method of exposure. Table F-3 in Appendix F summarizes the results of experiments in animals injected with asbestiform fibers. From these data and the results of inhalation studies (Table F-1 in Appendix F), the following observations can be made:

1. Mesotheliomas have been observed in rats after injection of all types of asbestos and a number of nonasbestos fibers, including fibrous glass, ceramic fibers, attapulgite (palygorskite) from the USSR, brucite, and erionite. Fever mesotheliomas occurred in rats after inhalation of UICC chrysotile, amosite, and crocidolite, but none appeared after inhalation of respirable fibrous glass, alumina, and ceramic aluminum silicate glass fibers.
2. The incidence of fiber-induced mesothelioma in hamsters is lower than in rats and in mice, but tumors appear earlier, perhaps because of the shorter lifespan of the hamster.

3. Tumor response was related directly to the dosage of fiber administered in experiments by Smith and Hubert (1974) and by Wagner et al. (1973). Other investigators (e.g., Port and Friedrichs, 1972; Stanton and Wrench, 1972) have not observed such dose-response relationships.
4. Exposure to either long (>10 μm) or short (milled) fibers results in the appearance of mesotheliomas. Nonfibrous particles, including cleavage fragments, do not generally cause tumors (see Appendix F).
5. Alteration of crocidolite by leaching (a process that can cause fragmentation of fibers) reduces its ability to cause mesothelioma (Monchaux et al., 1981; Morgan et al., 1977), but removal of PAH or trace metals does not affect the development of tumors (Wagner et al., 1973).
6. In studies to evaluate various injected samples, no one type of asbestos has appeared to be more pathogenic than others (see Appendix F). Wagner (1982) has reported erionite from Oregon readily induces mesotheliomas in rats by inhalation or injection.
7. Inhalation of potassium octatitanate fibers (average size 6.7 × 0.2 μm) produced three mesotheliomas in 59 hamsters surviving 21 months or more. No such tumors were produced in guinea pigs and rats exposed to these fibers, or in smaller numbers of rats, guinea pigs, and hamsters inhaling amosite asbestos or ball-milled fiberglass (Lee et al., 1981).

Fibrosis

Asbestos-associated fibrosis is an irreversible disease characterized as an excessive deposition of fibrous tissue. This cellular response is thought to occur as a reparative or reactive process. All types of asbestos cause pulmonary fibrosis of the lung (also called pulmonary interstitial fibrosis, or PIF) after relatively long periods of administration (Appendix F, Table F-4). A range of morphological alterations are observed after exposure to other fibers. The important features of these experiments can be summarized as follows:

1. There are species and strain differences in fibrogenic response. After inhalation of chrysotile by rats, guinea pigs, and mice, granulomas (distinctive focal lesions formed as the result of an inflammatory reaction) and focal fibrosis have been observed in the rat and guinea pig but not in the mouse (Reeves et al., 1974). Moreover, studies by Lee et al. (1981) show a direct relationship between dosage of fibers and development of fibrosis in the rat, whereas less prominent changes occur in the hamster and guinea pig.
2. Studies with fibrous glass in a diversity of size ranges suggest that responses are minimal in comparison to those induced by asbestos of comparable dimensions. Morphological changes in exposed animals include

mild macrophage infiltration without fibrosis (Gross et al., 1970; Moorman, in press), minimal peribronchiolar fibrosis (Kuschner and Wright, 1976), alveolitis (inflammation of the alveoli) (Begin et al., 1982), and alveolar proteinosis (alveolar accumulation of granular proteinaceous material) (Lee et al., 1979). No abnormal pathology has been observed with use of fibrous glass in inhalation experiments by Lee et al. (1981), Schepers (1959), and Schepers et al. (1958).

3. Inhalation and pleural injection studies implicate the increased fibrogenic potential of longer (>10 μm) fibers of both asbestos and fibrous glass. Minimal or no change has been observed after exposure of animals to smaller fibers or particles of chrysotile (Gardner, 1942), other types of UICC asbestos (Vorwald et al., 1951), fibrous glass, and a synthetic fluoro-amphibole (Kuschner and Wright, 1976).
4. Other fibers evaluated in rodents by inhalation include alumina, which produced no fibrosis (Piggott et al., 1981); PKT and Fybex, which caused fibrosis, but to a lesser extent than amosite (Lee et al., 1981); and ceramic aluminum silicate glass, which induced alveolar proteinosis (Davis et al., 1982). These fibers tended to fall within the same size dimensions as asbestos.
5. Davis and Coniami (1973) evaluated pleural fibrosis in mice after injection of the material resulting from heating chrysotile to temperatures exceeding 600°C. Compared with control material, fiber length was reduced and the fibrotic changes in animals diminished.
6. Pleural plaques have not been observed in laboratory animals after exposure to asbestos (Craighead and Mossman, 1982).

Events in the Gastrointestinal Tract After Exposure to Asbestos

A number of investigators have attempted to induce gastrointestinal tumors in animals by administering oral doses of asbestos (Gross et al., 1974; Smith et al., 1965, 1980a; Workshop on Ingested Asbestos, 1983). Thus far, these studies have yielded negative results, as have three National Toxicology Program bioassays (McConnell et al., 1983 a,b). Moreover, asbestos was not found to be cocarcinogenic when administered to rats with azoxymethane—a documented intestinal carcinogen (Ward et al., 1980). After being ingested by rodents, asbestos has been observed in mucosal cells of the gut (Westlake et al., 1965). In guinea pigs, epithelial injury has been observed (Jacobs et al., 1978) but erosion and degenerative changes regressed by 24 hours after administration of an oral 500-mg dose (Saxena et al., 1982). The acid environment of the stomach and the secretion of mucin by gastrointestinal cells could contribute to the modification of fibers as a result of the leaching or adsorbance of mucin. Moreover, the rat gut may be resistent to asbestos. Studies by Reiss et al. (1980b) show that asbestos is toxic to intestinal and colonic cells in culture. Leaching of chrysotile in 1 N hydrochloric acid ameliorates cytotoxicity.

IN VITRO STUDIES

Investigators using suspensions of red blood cells (RBCs), monolayers of cells, and organ cultures have contributed to the understanding of the mechanisms by which cytotoxicity and carcinogenicity are induced by asbestiform fibers. Results of these studies have been discussed in various proceedings and reviews (e.g., Brown et al., 1980; Harington et al., 1975; Mossman and Craighead, 1981; Mossman et al., 1983a). The types of studies and experimental information of most importance in elucidating the interactions of fibers with cells are summarized below.

Hemolytic Assays

The mechanisms of particle-induced cytotoxicity are complex. A critical part of this process appears to be the ability of particles and fibers to bind to and damage cellular membranes (Chamberlain et al., 1982; Craighead et al., 1980; Harington et al., 1971, 1975; Jaurand et al., 1979a, 1980; Woodworth et al., 1982). The disruption of the membranes can result in hemolysis, which is the leakage of hemoglobin from the RBCs. Hemolysis can be quantified spectrophotometrically and often is used to define:

- mechanisms of membrane damage by particles (Chamberlain et al., 1982; Craighead et al., 1980; Desai et al., 1975; Jaurand et al., 1979a, 1980; Harington et al., 1971, 1975; Light and Wei, 1977a,b; Manyai et al., 1969; Zitting and Skytta, 1979) and
- the fibrogenic potential of particles (Hefner and Gehring, 1975). The degree of hemolysis by particles, however, does not correlate directly with their fibrogenic or carcinogenic effects.

The hemolytic activity of fibers relates to physicochemical properties such as size (Schnitzer and Pundsack, 1970), magnesium content (Harington et al., 1971), crystallinity (Palekar et al., 1979; Zitting and Skytta, 1979), and surface charge (Harington et al., 1971, 1975; Light and Wei, 1977a,b). A large surface area also facilitates interactions with the RBC membrane. For example, hemolysis is enhanced as the number of fibers (Desai and Richards, 1978; Schnitzer and Pundsack, 1970) and the degree of their dispersion (Schnitzer and Pundsack, 1970) increase. Particle shape is not critical since certain fibers, such as crocidolite asbestos and fibrous glass, or particles with sharp edges, such as carborundum, are only marginally hemolytic (Harington et al., 1975). Moreover, some nonfibrous particles, such as montmorillonite, are as hemolytic as chrysotile asbestos (Woodworth et al., 1982).

The importance of surface charge in hemolysis by chrysotile and crocidolite has been suggested by Light and Wei (1977a,b). Other investigators have reported that chrysotile is both hemolytic and cytotoxic in a variety of cell systems, whereas crocidolite is relatively inactive (Chamberlain and Brown, 1978; Miller and Harington, 1972; Mossman et al., 1980b; Woodworth et al., 1982). The magnitude of the surface charge on the fibers (e.g., chrysotile, +44.5 mV, and crocidolite, -43.5 mV, in distilled water, as measured by their zeta potential)[1] is directly related to their hemolytic potential. For example, when chrysotile fibers are leached in acid, their zeta potential decreases as does their hemolytic activity. In contrast, the hemolytic ability of crocidolite increases after leaching as the fibers become more negatively charged. Adsorption of components of surfactant or serum to fibers also renders them less hemolytic (Craighead et al., 1980; Desai and Richards, 1978; Jaurand et al., 1979a; Light and Wei, 1977a).

Harington et al. (1971, 1975) hypothesized that negatively charged residues of sialic acid from membrane glycoproteins bind to positively charged sites on minerals. This ionic interaction might result in the aggregation of integral membrane proteins and leakage of hemoglobin. To test this hypothesis, sialic acid was removed enzymatically from RBCs before hemolysis by chrysotile was measured. The treated RBCs were resistant to hemolysis, suggesting the importance of sialic acid in this process. Experiments with tracheobronchial epithelial cells have suggested that chrysotile also interacts with other carbohydrates on the cell surface (Mossman et al., 1983c).

Cytotoxicity Studies

Cytotoxicity is the ability of an agent to interfere with cellular function to the extent that the cell is either damaged or killed. Because asbestos and other particles are believed to play a role in the pathogenesis of respiratory tract diseases, the mechanisms whereby these substances induce cytotoxicity have been investigated in cell culture (Chamberlain et al., 1982; Harington et al., 1975; Mossman et al., 1983a). Although some researchers have attempted to correlate the cytotoxicity of fibers with their ability to cause pulmonary fibrosis and mesothelioma (Hefner and Gehring, 1975; Kaw et al., 1982; Wade et al., 1980), the validity of this correlation is not accepted in general, and one must conclude that cytotoxicity is not related directly to pathogenicity. For example, crocidolite is less damaging to red blood cells and less cytotoxic than chrysotile in macrophages and in cultures of tracheobronchial epithelia (Doll et al., 1982a,b; Haugen et al., 1982; Landesman and Mossman, 1982; Miller and Hatington, 1972; Mossman et al., 1980b; Woodworth et al., 1982). Reiss and colleagues (1980a,b) and Wade et al. (1979) have suggested that sensitivity to asbestos differs among

[1] Zeta potential is a measure of surface charge. A zeta potential of zero indicates no measurable surface charge.

the various cell types (e.g., epithelial cells, fibroblasts, and macrophages).

Cytotoxicity is dependent on both the geometry and the length of asbestos fibers. In macrophagelike cells, chrysotile is toxic, whereas its nonfibrous analog, platy serpentine, is not (Frank et al., 1979). Lone fibers of various minerals are more cytotoxic than comparable amounts of short fibers (Beck et al., 1972; Brown et al., 1978; Chamberlain and Brown, 1978; Kaw et al., 1982). There is overwhelming evidence that short fibers are phagocytized completely, whereas long fibers are only partially enveloped by cells. Uptake of fibers by cells results in the release of lysosomal enzymes (Beck et al., 1972; Davies et al., 1974) and oxygen free radicals (Mossman and Landesman, 1983), reactive species that cause peroxidation of membranes and damage to macromolecules (Freeman and Crapo, 1982). Cell injury in tracheal epithelial cell cultures can be prevented by the addition of superoxide dismutase—a scavenger of superoxide (Mossman and Landesman, 1983).

Cell death occurs rapidly when fibers are added to culture media without serum, but is inhibited or delayed when serum is present (Hatington et al., 1975; Mossman et al., 1980b). Serum proteins adsorb to fibers (Desai and Richards, 1978), and this protective coating is believed to be removed by lysosomal hydrolases after phagocytosis of the particles (Allison, 1971; Heppleston, 1979).

Alterations in Cells of the Immune System After Exposure to Asbestiform Fibers

Aberrations of humoral and cellular immunity have been reported in individuals exposed to asbestos (Kagan et al., 1977; Lange, 1980; Stansfield and Edge, 1974; Turner-Warwick and Parkes, 1973). These studies suggest activation and/or loss of normal immunoregulatory mechanisms in asbestos-associated diseases. Because macrophages may play a role as an intermediate in pulmonary defense, in vitro studies have been conducted to examine the responses of these cells to asbestos. After exposure to asbestos, macrophages release potent inflammatory factors (Hamilton et al., 1976) and synthesize prostaglandins (Sirois et al., 1980), chemotactic factors for neutrophils (Schoenberger et al., 1982), and substances that increase replication of fibroblasts (Bitterman et al., 1981).

Results of other in vitro experiments indicate that asbestos affects both cell-mediated (Barbers et al., 1982; Bozelka et al., in press) and antibody-mediated (Lawrence et al., 1982) immunity. In addition, both amphibole and serpentine types of asbestos depress viral induction of interferon—a glycoprotein that confers antiviral defense—thereby resulting in increased multiplication of the virus (Hahon and Eckert, 1976). Conversely, the mineral wollastonite enhances the induction of interferon by influenza virus in cultured cells, but the mineral per se does not induce interferon (Hahon et al., 1980). Finally, in addition to obvious modulatory effects on cells of the immune system, asbestos can activate complement, a complex in serum that is destructive to certain bacteria and cells that have been sensitized with antibody (Hasselbacher, 1979; Saint-Remy and Cole, 1950; Wilson et al., 1977).

Effects on Fibroblasts In Vitro

Although the macrophage appears to be a key cell in the induction of tissue injury by asbestos, the affected cell in the fibrotic process is the fibroblast—a cell associated with the production of collagen. It is not clear whether fibrosis results from increased production of collagen by individual cells, or from an increase in the proliferation of fibroblasts, or from both. Some investigators have suggested that these synthetic responses are elicited by fibrogenic factors released by macrophages (reviewed in Vigilani, 1968).

When noncytolytic amounts of asbestos are added to cultures of fibroblasts, abnormal and accelerated production of collagen and reticulin are observed (Hext and Richards, 1976; Richards and Jacoby, 1976). Fibroblasts undergo a maturation process leading to rapid cellular aging. Surviving cells phagocytize fibers avidly and undergo morphological and biochemical changes such as alterations in secretion of proteoglycans (Richard and Morris, 1973), metabolism of RNA, and enhancement in cell mat collagen deposition (Hext and Richards, 1976). Fibrous glass is less cytotoxic, producing minimal but similar alterations. Long fibrous glass provides a substrate for the attachment of cultured fibroblasts and acts as a stimulus to promote cell division (Maroudas et al., 1973).

INITIATION-PROMOTION MODEL OF CARCINOGENESIS

This brief discussion of the initiation-promotion model of carcinogenesis is provided as a basis for subsequent sections describing possible carcinogenic properties of asbestiform fibers. It is possible that cancers induced by asbestiform fibers result from the same fundamental mechanisms as cancers induced by other physical and chemical agents. Carcinogenesis is a complex, multistep process that has been extensively reviewed by Becker (1981), Foulds (1969, 1975), Farher (1982), and Farber and Cameron (1980).

Multiple focal proliferations of cells (hyperplasia) in target organs are common early features of carcinogenesis and serve as sites for subsequent premalignant changes (Farber, 1982). Such focal alterations give cell populations selective growth and invasive properties (Cairns, 1975; Fialkow, 1976; Foulds, 1954; Nowell, 1976). The concepts of initiation and promotion have been developed to explain this process in many experimental models and organ systems, including skin, liver, mammary gland, colon, urinary bladder, and brain (Berenblum, 1941; Boutwell, 1974; Pitot and Sirica, 1980).

Initiation is a change in the DNA of a cell induced by exposure to a carcinogen. This heritable alteration can be promoted ultimately to malignancy.

Promotion is the process whereby an initiated cell develops focal proliferations, one or more of which may act as precursors for subsequent steps in the process of carcinogenesis. Promotion creates a mitogenic environment that differentially affects initiated cells. Some investigators suspect that many tissues or organs create a physiological promoting or selecting environment. In the early stages, promotion can be reversible, but it eventually brings about the phenotypic changes needed to stabilize the characteristics exhibited by cancer cells (Trosko and Chang, 1980). By stimulating a premalignant or initiated cell to proliferate, the process of promotion also enhances the probability that additional genetic errors will occur (Potter, 1981; Trosko and Chang, 1980).

Promotion appears to occur after removal of cells, e.g., as the result of a surgical procedure or the infliction of a wound (Pound and McGuire, 1978); after physical irradiation (Argyris and Slaga, 1981); after cell death (Frei, 1976); or upon exposure to exogenous noncytotoxic chemicals (Trosko and Chang, 1980), endogenous chemicals, e.g., hormones (Yager and Yager, 1980), or solid objects, e.g., small plastic squares (Brand, 1982). Some current views on promotion and promoters have been shaped by studies in which croton oil and its active agent, 12-0-tetradecanoylphorbol-13-acetate (TPA) were used in a mouse skin test system.

Both chemical and physical tumor promoters have been shown to induce a constellation of biochemical and cellular responses (Diamond et al., 1978). Depending on the cell type, chemical tumor promoters can induce or inhibit normal differentiation (Diamond et al., 1978) or alter the proliferation of cells in a given tissue (Yuspa et al., 1982).

One of the important biochemical markers of cell division is increased synthesis of polyamines, which is often detected as an increase in the activity of ornithine decarboxylase (ODC)—a rate-limiting enzyme in the biosynthesis of polyamines. The induction of ODC is related directly to tumor-promoting activity of a number of compounds in mouse skin (O'Brien, 1976).

When applied to the skin of rodents, classical tumor promoters (e.g., phorbol esters) also cause inflammatory changes and infiltration of polymorphonuclear leukocytes (PMNs) and macrophages. These cells release oxygen free radicals—reactive by-products of oxygen that cause peroxidation of membranes and other macromolecules (McCord and Wong, 1979).

Detailed reviews of tumor promotion have been prepared by Hecker et al. (1982) and by Slaga et al. (1978).

Interaction of Asbestiform Fibers with DNA

Mutagenicity is the ability of a chemical or physical agent to induce permanent, transmissible changes in the character of a gene by modifying the DNA. This event is believed by many to be an initiating step in the process of carcinogenesis.

Daniel (in press) has prepared a review of in vitro tests that have been conducted with asbestiform fibers to determine their potential for mutagenicity and other types of interaction with DNA. In bacterial assays, such as the Ames Salmonella microsome assay, UICC reference samples of asbestos, superfine Canadian fibers, and fibrous glass have not shown mutagenic activity (Chamberlain and Tarmy, 1977; Light and Wei, 1980). The investigators believe that these negative results may be attributable to the lack of fiber uptake by bacterial cells.

Chromosome aberrations and chromatid breaks have been observed after chrysotile and crocidolite asbestos have been added to rodent cell lines (Lavappa et al., 1975), but not after the addition of fibrous or powdered glass (Sincock and Seabright, 1975). Huang (1979) demonstrated that chrysotile, crocidolite, and amosite are mutagenic to the hypoxanchine-guanine phosphoribosyltransferase (HGPRT) locus of Chinese hamster lung fibroblasts. However, the rates of induced mutation were low, and the conclusions drawn by Huang are strongly dependent on the method of statistical analysis used in this study. Moreover, neither chrysotile, crocidolite, nor amosite was mutagenic in rodent liver epithelial cells (Reiss et al., 1982). Although amosite and crocidolite produced small increases in sister chromatid exchange (SCE) in Chinese hamster ovary cells (Livingston et al., 1980), the V79-4 Chinese hamster lung cell line and cultured mesothelial cells did not exhibit altered SCE levels after exposure to crocidolite and chrysotile, respectively (Kaplan et al., 1980; Price-Jones et al., 1980). Furthermore, in tracheal epithelial cells, chrysotile and crocidolite did not cause breakage of DNA, as measured by alkaline elution (Mossman et al., 1983b).

Results of studies by Sincock (1977) and Lechner and colleagues (1983) suggest that human cells are relatively resistent to DNA damage by asbestos. Neither crocidolite, SFA chrysotile, nor glass fibers induces chromosome aberrations in human lymphocytes or fibroblasts (Sincock, 1977), although the number of chromatid and chromosome breaks increases in freshly isolated human lymphocytes exposed to Rhodesian chrysotile (Valerio et al., 1980). In another study, UICC chrysotile, amosite, and crocidolite did not appear to cause DNA strand breakage in human bronchial organ cultures (Lechner et al., 1983).

Tumor Promotion

Properties of tumor promoters have been extensively reviewed and discussed (Farber, 1982; Hecker et al., 1982; Slaga et al., 1978). In studies of cultured tracheal epithelial cells from hamsters, Mossman et al. (1977, 1980a,b, 1983a,b), Mossman and Craighead (1981), and Woodworth et al. (1983a,b) have demonstrated that several different types of asbestiform fibers exhibit the properties of tumor promoters. Both long (>10 μm) and short (<2 μm) chrysotile and crocidolite fibers interact with the membranes of differentiated superficial epithelial cells in organ culture. Short fibers are phagocytized successfully and are observed thereafter in basal epithelial cells (presumably the progenitors of carcinoma); longer asbestos fibers are enveloped by membranes, but appear incapable of being phagocytized (Mossman et al., 1977; Woodworth et al., 1983). This latter phenomenon occurs concomitantly with release of the oxygen free radical, superoxide, into culture medium (Mossman and Lands smart, 1983).

After exposure to amosite or crocidolite asbestos, there are increases in the incorporation of ^{3}H-thymidine (an indication of DNA synthesis) and basal cell hyperplasia in tracheal epithelial cells in vitro. The morphological changes were prevented by the addition of vitamin A, which has been associated with the reduction of cancer incidence in a number of studies in rodents (Mossman et al., 1980a). Enhanced uptake of ^{3}H-thymidine and morphologic changes have also been observed in monolayers of tracheal epithelial cells exposed to either crocidolite or chrysotile (Landesman and Mossman, 1982).

Some asbestiform fibers have been observed to alter normal epithelial cell function. For example, crocidolite, amosite, and fibrous glass facilitate the progression of basal cell hyperplasia to squamous metaplasia, i.e., the conversion of a differentiated epithelium to a squamous cornified layer resembling skin (Mossman et al., 1978, 1980b; Woodworth et al., 1983a,b). Chrysotile fibers induce significant increases in squamous metaplasia, but high concentrations of long fibers cause permanent destruction of the mucosa. Ground glass, attapulgite, and nonfibrous analogs of asbestos (e.g., riebeckite and antigorite) neither cause squamous metaplasia nor stimulate DNA synthesis (Woodworth et al., 1983a).

Chrysotile, crocidolite, and fibrous glass induce ODC and stimulate cell division in tracheal epithelial cells in a dosage-dependent fashion (Landesman and Mossman, 1982), whereas these changes do not occur after exposure to nonfibrous crocidolite (e.g., riebeckite), chrysotile (e.g., antigorite), glass particles, or hematite (Mossman, personal communication, 1983). These experiments suggest that fibrous glass exhibits some promoterlike features in vitro, but experiments exploring this phenomenon in whole animals are lacking.

In Vitro Studies with Mesothelial Cells

The interaction of mesothelial cells and asbestos fibers has been studied in vitro to investigate the genesis of mesothelioma (Allison, 1973; Domagala and Koss, 1977; Jaurand et al., 1979c; Rajan and Evans, 1973; Rajah et al., 1972; reviewed in Whitaker et al., 1982). Chrysotile asbestos (1-2 µm length) is ingested by cultured mesothelial cells in both organ and monolayer cultures, whereas it is unclear whether larger fibers are phagocytized (Allison, 1973; Jaurand et al., 1979c). After introduction into cultures of pleura, crocidolite causes proliferation of cells in a manner similar to that observed in tracheal organ cultures (Rajan et al., 1972).

Interactions Between Fibers and Polycyclic Aromatic Hydrocarbons (PAHs)

Because PAHs are incomplete products of combustion, they are ubiquitous in the urban environment and are found in association with various types of atmospheric aerosols (Pierce and Katz, 1975). A number of investigators have explored the possibility that fibers and particles may act as "carriers" of these PAHs into the cells of the respiratory tract.

Equal milligram amounts of crocidolite asbestos, carbon, hematite, and kaolin have been compared for their ability to bind and release the radiolabeled PAH, 3-methylcholanthrene (3MC), into culture medium (Mossman and Craighead, 1982). Asbestos neither adsorbed more 3MC nor eluted greater amounts of the hydrocarbon than did the other materials. However, when tested for release of PAH to artificial membranes or microsomas, asbestos fibers appear to be more effective than the nonfibrous materials tested (Lakowicz and Bevan, 1980; Lakowicz et al., 1978a,b).

The association of PAH with the fiber surface before the fibers are added to tracheal epithelial cell culture appears to be critical to fiber-induced cellular uptake of the hydrocarbon. For example, increased uptake and retention of radiolabeled benzo(a)pyrene (BP) have not been observed with fibrous glass, a poorly adsorptive fiber, or when BP is added 1 hour after the addition of asbestos (Eastman et al., 1983; Mossman et al., 1983b).

CONCLUSIONS

Asbestiform Fibers: Initiators and/or Promoters of Lung Tumors?

Asbestiform fibers do not seem to damage DNA directly (Fornace, 1982; Hart et al., 1979; Haugen et al., 1982; Mossman et al., 1983b) or to act as mutagens (Chamberlain and Tarmy, 1977; Reiss et al., 1982). Thus, the role of asbestos in the initiation of lung tumors is questionable. Some investigators have observed a weak mutagenic reaction (Huang, 1979; Huang et al., 1978) that could also be interpreted as indicating an epigenetic reaction (Isobe et al., 1982). The term epigenetic is used here to define the alteration of the expression, not the information, of genes. In other words, it is the repression or derepression of genetic in format ion ·

One possible explanation of asbestos-facilitated carcinogenesis is that PAHs (known initiators of carcinogenesis) are more efficiently transferred to the target cells because they adhere to the asbestos fibers (Eastman et al., 1983; Mossman et al., 1983b). Lung tumors generally do not appear after asbestos is intratracheally instilled into rodents, but they do appear when PAHs are adsorbed to fibers before instillation (Miller et al., 1965; Shabad et al., 1974; Smith et al., 1968). However, small numbers of tumors of the respiratory tract have been observed after inhalation of UICC samples of asbestos by rats (Wagner et al., 1974). The interpretation of these studies is complicated by the finding that these reference standards of asbestos may be contaminated with PAH (Harington, 1962).

The stimulation of cell proliferation by asbestiform fibers may result in the promotion of initiated epithelial cells lining the airways. In support of the hypothesis that asbestos is a tumor promoter, Topping and Nettesheim (1980) have shown that asbestos has a promoting effect in rodent tracheal grafts exposed sequentially to an initiating PAH and then to chrysotile. In these studies, asbestos increased the incidence of tumors obtained with small amounts of the PAH, although the asbestos was not carcinogenic when administered by itself. However, when asbestos was applied to tracheal grafts in 10-fold higher amounts, a low incidence (5%) of squamous cell carcinoma was observed (Topping et al., 1980). Although this latter observation might be interpreted as indicating a weak initiating or carcinogenic potential of asbestos, it seems to be a common feature of many promoters (Iversen and Iversen, 1979).

Additional evidence that asbestos acts as a promoter is provided by histological observations of hyperplasia and metaplasia in organ cultures of the respiratory tract after exposure to asbestiform fibers (Landesman and Mossman, 1982; Mossman and Craighead, 1974; Mossman et al., 1980b; Woodworth et al., 1983a,b,c). In addition, the dosage-dependent induction of ODC in tracheal epithelial cells has been seen after addition of chrysotile and crocidolite, but not after exposure to the nonasbestiform particle hematite (Landesman and Mossman, 1982). The increase in enzyme induction occurs concomitantly with a mitogenic response as measured by uptake of ^{3}H-thymidine.

The accumulation of macrophages and inflammatory cells in the air spaces of rodents after inhalation of asbestos appears to be similar to effects observed in the skin after application of phorbol esters (Gee, 1980; Hamilton, 1980). Isolated macrophages and polymorphonuclear leukocytes emit oxygen free radicals into medium and are chemiluminescent after exposure to asbestos in vitro (Gaumer et al., 1979). One might assume that these reactive species are injurious to mucosal airways. Again, the length of the fiber appears to be critical to the cellular response in that addition of superoxide dismutase (an enzyme converting the superoxide radical to H_2O_2 and O_2) to tracheal epithelial cells prevents the membrane damage caused by long (>10 μm), but not short (<2 μm), chrysotile fibers (Mossman and Landesman, 1983). Retinyl methyl ether, a synthetic vitamin A that blocks the action of at least some promoters (Verma et al., 1982), inhibits asbestos-induced epithelial changes in organ culture of hamster trachea (Mossman et al., 1980a).

Taken together, these results are consistent with the hypothesis that certain asbestiform fibers may act in lung cancer in a manner similar to other known chemical and physical agents that have the properties of tumor promoters. Some experiments have suggested that promoters may exhibit a threshold concentration below which they do not exert their tumor-promoting effects (Peraino et al., 1980; Verma and Boutwell, 1980). However, there is no experimental evidence of a threshold for carcinogenic effects of asbestos. In Chapter 7, a linear nonthreshold model is used for risk assessment.

Initiated cells in the lung could be stimulated to proliferate after exposure to asbestiform fibers either by a membrane-triggered response or by a cytotoxic response. Fibers lodged in cells might act as continuous promoting stimuli.

Asbestiform Fibers: Initiators and/or Promoters of Malignant Mesothelioma?

The pathogenesis and etiology of mesothelioma, a tumor arising from the membranes enclosing the body cavities, differ from those of lung cancer. There is no positive association between smoking and the development of mesothelioma in asbestos workers (Craighead and Mossman, 1982; Hammond et al., 1979), and prior extraction of PAH from asbestos does not appear to diminish tumor incidence after injection of fibers into the body cavities of rodents (Wagner et al., 1973). Studies by Brand and colleagues (Brand, 1982; Brand et al., 1975a,b) and by Davis (1971, 1974a,b) provide some insight into the development of this lesion.

After injection into the pleural or peritoneal cavity of rodents, longer fibers cause an immediate but chronic foreign body response, presumably because of their inability to be phagocytized by resident macrophages. Abnormal mesothelial cells with an increased mitotic index have been observed within a thickened fibrotic pleura (Jagatic et al., 1967). Studies by Davis (1974b) suggest that tumors arise from undifferentiated mesenchymal cells just below the mesothelium. These cells retain their normal pleiomorphic appearance or differentiate into either epithelial-like (mesothelial) cells or spindle-shaped cells. This hypothesized origin could explain the histological variability of tumors in humans and animals, since mesotheliomas commonly contain cells of both epithelial and mesenchymal tissue origin. Other investigators have suggested that tumors arise from multipotential mesothelial cells that can express all the variable structural patterns observed in these neoplasms (Maximov, 1927; Stout and Hurray, 1942, Whitaker et al., 1982).

Asbestiform Fibers: Possible Mechanisms of Fibrosis

During development of fibrosis (i.e., asbestosis), the normal architecture of the terminal airways and air spaces is altered by excessive deposition of fibrous tissue. Fibrosis can also occur in the pleura.

The sequence of cellular events that appear to trigger the onset of fibrosis has been hypothesized on the basis of observations in animals after inhalation or intratracheal instillation of asbestos. Deposition of fibers in the terminal bronchioles and alveolar ducts—the sites where fibrosis first appears in humans (Craighead and Mossman, 1982)—occurs with a rapid infiltration of macrophages and an acute inflammatory response (Gee, 1980). These observations suggest that asbestos and possibly other asbestiform fibers disrupt the normal proliferation and differentiation of lung fibroblasts either by direct interaction of the fibers with fibroblasts or via effects on an intermediary cell type, the macrophage (or by both mechanisms). Again, the observations summarized above are similar to those reported for the mouse skin after exposure to chemical tumor promoters: infiltration of macrophages is observed, and hyperplasia and/or abnormal differentiation occurs in some cell types (Yuspa et al., 1982).

SUMMARY

Elucidation of the pathogenicity and mechanisms of asbestiform fiber-induced disease is complicated by the complexity, diversity of sizes, and variety of these materials. The experimental results described above served as a basis for Table 6-1, which summarizes the relationships between properties of fibers, their effects on cells, and diseases associated with asbestos.

Fibers greater than approximately 3 μm in diameter are not respirable; they do not gain access to the respiratory tract but may be ingested.

TABLE 6-1. Possible Mechanisms of Disease Induction by Fibrous Materials at the Cellular Level

Disease[a]	Relevant Fiber Property[b]	Effect on Target Cells and/or Macrophages
A	1, 2, 6	Adsorbance and transfer of polycyclic aromatic hydrocarbons (PAHs) to cell membranes
A, C, D	1-7	Disruption of cell membranes (i.e., lysis and hemolysis) and release of cell enzymes
A, C	1, 2, 5	Release of oxygen free radicals
A, B, C, D	1, 2, 3	Induction of proliferative alterations (e.g., in DNA, RNA, or protein synthesis)
A, B, C, D	1, 2, 3	Alterations in cell differentiation
A, B, C, D	1, 3, 7	Interaction with DNA (e.g., chromosomal changes or alteration in normal DNA repair)
B, C	1, 2, 5, 7	Effects on immune system (e.g., activation of complement or chemotactic factors)

[a] The letters in this column represent diseases associated with exposure to fibrous materials:
A = Lung cancer
B = Mesothelioma
C = Fibrotic lung disease
D = Gastrointestonal tumors
[b] The numbers in this column represent the biologically relevant fiber properties:
1 = Respirability (<3 μm diameter)
2 = Size and aspect ratio
3 = Durability
4 = Flexibility and tensile strength
5 = Chemical composition
6 = Surface area
7 = Surface charge

Although data from the majority of investigators show an increased risk of mesothelioma with long, thin fibers in comparison to short, thick fibers, there does not appear to be a critical length below which fibers have no carcinogenic potential. For example, studies by Kolev (1982) and by Pott and colleagues (1972, 1976) suggest that amorphous asbestos and fibers shorter than 5 µm are capable of inducing mesothelioma in rodents.

The results of inhalation experiments to determine the importance of aspect ratio in inducing lung cancer are difficult to interpret because the fibers in the aerosols are heterogeneous with regard to size. The specific effects of long versus short asbestos fibers of one type have not been evaluated in comparative experiments.

Although studies by Gardner (1942), Vorwald et al. (1951), and Kuschner and Wright (1976) suggest that asbestiform fibers longer than approximately 10 µm are more active than shorter ones in inducing pulmonary fibrosis, not all long fibers (e.g., Saffil, fibrous glass) are fibrogenic. Moreover, some nonfibrous minerals (kaolin, silica) are fibrogenic in humans (Heppleston, 1979).

Asbestos fibers may fragment longitudinally during processing or within the lung and thus increase in both number and surface area. This property may enable more interaction of fibers with cells. Since direct cell contact appears essential to asbestiform fiber-induced diseases, the greater the surface area, the greater the likely pathogenic potential of a fiber. Furthermore, if polycyclic aromatic hydrocarbons (PAHs) adsorb to fibers as a function of surface area, fibers comprised of many fibrils (assuming all were accessible to the PAH) would present a greater surface for adsorption than would a single fiber. Under these circumstances, their (co) carcinogenic ability might be increased.

Longer fibers (>ca 10 µm), which tend to be more pathogenic, cannot be removed effectively by phagocytic macrophages. Thus, their time of residence in the respiratory tract might be greater than that of shorter fibers. Moreover, longer fibers appear to be more cytolytic than the shorter fibers, which can be phagocytized completely.

Durability is another factor that could account for prolonged retention of asbestos within the lung and other tissues in comparison with a variety of other asbestiform materials. Although leaching may alter the composition of the fiber, asbestos does not tend to dissolve as does glass. It is unclear whether the chemistry of asbestos plays a direct role in pathogenicity. However, since chemistry determines both durability and surface charge, the latter a feature directly related to cytotoxicity, chemistry may play at least an indirect role.

Both inhalation and in vitro studies indicate that asbestos is more pathogenic than a number of man-made mineral fibers (fibrous glass, glass wool, rock wool). However, they fail to identify one type of asbestos as more potent than others. Moreover, there have been few experiments to identify precise dose-response relationships. One obvious conclusion is that there is interspecies variability in response to asbestos. Thus, certain rodents, such as rats and mice, appear to be appropriate models for the study of carcinogenesis and fibrosis, whereas others (e.g., guinea pigs) have developed no obvious pathological effect from exposures to asbestos. Different cultured cell types (e.g., epithelial. mesothelial, fibroblastic cells) also differ in their susceptibility to the toxic effects of asbestos. Unfortunately, no in vitro model studied to date has been predictive of the fibrogenic or carcinogenic potential of fibers. However, in vitro systems have been helpful in elucidating possible mechanisms of action of asbestos. The evidence that asbestos may act as a gene or chromosomal mutagen is weak and inconclusive, but its ability to function as a tumor promoter at noncytolytic amounts and as a cytotoxic agent at higher levels is well documented.

RECOMMENDATIONS

To increase our understanding of the health hazards of asbestiform fibers, a necessary first step is to study the common physical properties of these fibers in relation to their pathogenicity in animals and ability to injure cells. A number of experiments are needed to relate the physicochemical features to biological effects.

- In vitro and inhalation studies should be conducted to test whether the biological effects of asbestiform fibers are related to their size and shape. These studies should include as controls appropriate nonfibrous analogs of similar or identical chemical composition. "Positive" responses with nonfibrous analogs would be evidence to support the view that the chemical composition of asbestos is important in the development of disease. All preparations should contain fibers of comparable and respirable size.
- Investigators comparing the pathogenic potential of various fibers and particles should define completely the characteristics (i.e., chemical constitution, surface charge, crystallization habit, crystallography, and geometry) of their source materials. Different preparations of fibers should be sized to obtain comparable size distributions, thus controlling for this important variable.
- Where possible, concentrations of particles should be documented in all experimental systems.

There are also gaps in knowledge about such important subjects as the basic molecular mechanisms by which asbestiform fibers induce cell killing, alter differentiation, or cause gene and chromosomal mutations in various cells. The following experiments would be advantageous:

- Dose-response curves for asbestiform fiber-induced cytotoxicity, altered function, and possible mutagenicity in various human cell types in vitro.
- Experiments both in vivo and in vitro to determine how various asbestiform fibers act synergistically with other environmental and host factors.
- Testing of various asbestiform fibers as initiators or promoters in lung tissue. Protocols might include:

1. Single inhalation exposure to asbestos at various doses, followed by administration of substances known to be physical or chemical promoters in lung tissue. These experiments could define fibers as "initiators" or as complete carcinogens (those not requiring exogenous promoters).
2. Investigations in animals to examine the effects of single and multiple inhalation exposures to fibers in air, water, and foods after treatment with initiators (e.g., documented chemical and physical carcinogens). These experiments would test the ability of asbestiform fibers Co act as promoters, after single or multiple exposures.
3. Studies to examine single and multiple inhalation exposures in a range of dust concentrations with adequately large numbers of animals in each experimental group. These animals should be followed through their lifespan, and a complete pathological examination should be performed at time of death. One would hope to establish whether there are dose-response relationships for fibrosis, mesothelioma, and lung tumors.

Results from these three types of studies should improve our understanding of the relationship between health effects and physicochemical properties of asbestiform fibers. This could lead to physicochemical modification of asbestos and related fibers to minimize their undesirable biological effects or, alternatively, to the synthesis of substitutes that possess the useful physicochemical properties of asbestos but that lack its known adverse health effects.

REFERENCES

Allison, A. C. 1971. Lysosomes and the toxicity of particulate pollutants. Arch. Intern. Mad. 128:131-139.

Allison, A. C. 1973. Experimental methods-cell and tissue culture: Effects of asbestos particles on macrophages, mesothelial cells and fibroblasts. Pp. 89-93 in P. Bogovski, J. C. Gilson, V. Timbrell, and J. C. Wagner, ads. Biological Effects of Asbestos. IARC Scientific Pub. No. 8. International Agency for Research on Cancer, Lyon.

Ames, B. N., W. E. Durston, E. Yamaski, and F. D. Lee. 1973. Carcinogens are mutagens: A simple test system combining liver homogenates for activation and bacteria for detection. Proc. Natl. Acad. Sci. USA 70: 2281-2285.

Argyris, T. S., and T. J. Slaga. 1981. Promotion of carcinogenesis by repeated abrasion in initiated skin of mice. Cancer Res. 41:5193-5195.

Barbers, R. G., W. W. H. Shiff, and A. Saxon. 1982. In vitro depression of human lymphocyte mitogen response (phytohaemoagglutinin) by asbestos fibers. Clin. Exp. Immunol. 48:602-610.

Beck, E. G., P. F. Holt, and C. Manojlovic. 1972. Comparison of effects on macrophage cultures of glass fiber, glass powder, and chrysotile asbestos. Br. J. Ind. Med. 29:280-286.

Becker, F. F. 1981. Recent concepts of initiation and promotion in carcinogenesis. Am. J. Pathol. 105:3-9.

Begin, R., S. Masse, and M. A. Bureau. 1982. Morphologic features and function of the airways in early asbestosis in the sheep model. Am. Rev. Respir. Dis. 126:870-876.

Berenblum, I. 1941. The cocarcinogenic actions of croton resin. Cancer Res. 1:44-48.

Bitterman, P., S. Rennard, C. Schoenberger, and R. Crystal. 1981. Asbestos stimulates alveolar macrophages to release a factor causing human lung fibroblasts to replicate. Chest 80:38.

Botham, S. K., and P. F. Holt. 1972a. The effects of inhaled crocidolites from Transvaal and North-west Cape mines on the lungs of rats and guinea pigs. Br. J. Exp. Pathol. 53:612-620.

Botham, S. K., and P. F. Holt. 1972b. Asbestos-body formation in the lungs of rats and guinea pigs after inhalation of anthophyllite. J. Pathol. 107:245-252.

Boutwell, R. K. 1974. The function and mechanism of promoters of carcinogenesis. Crit. Rev. Toxicol. 2:419-443.

Bozelka, B. E., P. Sestini, H. R. Gaumer, Y. Hammad, C. J. Heather, and J. E. Salvaggio. 1983. A murine model of asbestosis. Am. J. Pathol. 112:326-337.

Bozelka, B. E., H. R. Gaumer, J. Nordberg, and J. E. Salvaggio. In press. Asbestos-induced alterations of human lymphoid cell mitogenic responses. Environ. Res. Vol. 30.

Brand, K. G. 1982. Cancer associated with asbestosis, schistosomiasis, foreign bodies and scars. Pp. 661-692 in F.F. Becker, ed. Cancer: A Comprehensive Treatise. Vol. I. Second Edition. Plenum Press, New York.

Brand, K. G., L. C. Busen, and I. Brand. 1975a. Foreign-body tumorigenesis induced by glass and smooth and rough plastic—Comparative study of preneoplastic events. J. Natl. Cancer Inst. 55:319-322.

Brand, K. G., L. C. Buoen, K. H. Johnson, and I. Brand. 1975b. Etiological factors, stages, and the role of the foreign body in foreign body tumorigenesis: A review. Cancer Res. 35:279-286.

Brown, R. C., M. Chamberlain, D. M. Griffiths, and V. Timbrell. 1978. The effect of fibre size on the in vitro biological activity of three types of amphibole asbestos. Int. J. Cancer 22:721-727.

Brown, R. C., I. P. Gormley, M. Chamberlain, and R. Davies, eds. 1980. The In Vitro Effects of Mineral Dusts. Academic Press, London and New York.

Cairns, J. 1975. Mutation, selection and natural history of cancer. Nature 225:197-200.

Chamberlain, M., and R. C. Brown. 1978. The cytotoxic effects of asbestos and other mineral dust in tissue culture cell lines. Br. J. Exp. Pathol. 59:183-189.

Chamberlain, M., and E. M. Tarmy. 1977. Asbestos and glass fibers in bacterial mutation tests. Mutat. Res. 43:159-164.

Chamberlain, M., R. Davies, R. C. Brown, and D. M. Griffiths. 1982. In vitro tests for the pathogenicity of mineral dusts. Ann. Occup. Hyg. 26:583-592.

Coffin, D. L., L. D. Palekar, and P. M. Cook. 1982. Tumorigenesis by a ferroactinolite mineral. Toxicol. Lett. 13:159-165.

Cook, P. M., L. D. Palekar, and D. L. Coffin. 1982. Interpretation of the carcinogenicity of amosite asbestos and ferroactinolite on the basis of retained fiber dose and characteristics in vivo. Toxicol. Lett. 13:151-158.

Craighead, J. E., and B. T. Mossman. 1982. The pathogenesis of asbestos-associated diseases. N. Engl. J. Med. 306:1446-1455.

Craighead, J. E., B. T. Mossman, and B. J. Bradley. 1980. Comparative studies on the cytotoxicity of amphibole and serpentine asbestos. Environ. Health Perspect. 34:37-46.

Daniel, F. B. In press. In vitro assessment of asbestos gene toxicity. Environ. Health Perspect.

Davies, P., A. C. Allison, J. Ackerman, A. Butterfield, and S. Williams. 1974. Asbestos induces selective release of lysosomal enzymes from mononuclear phagocytes. Nature 251:423-425.

Davis, J. M. C. 1971. Epithelial outgrowths from lung tissue following intrapleural injection of asbestos dust in experimental animals. Int. J. Cancer 7:238-248.

Davis, J. M. G. 1974a. An electron microscope study of the response of mesothelial cells to the intrapleural injection of asbestos dust. Br. J. Exp. Pathol. 55:64-70.

Davis, J. M. G. 1974b. Histogenesis and fine structure of peritoneal tumors produced in animals by injections of asbestos. J. Natl. Cancer Inst. 52:1823-1837.

Davis, J. M. G. 1976. Pathological aspects of the injection of glass fiber into the pleural and peritoneal cavities of rats and mice. Pp. 141-149 in Occupational Exposure to Fibrous Glass—Proceedings of a Symposium. Pub. No. 76-151. National Institute for Occupational Safety and Health, Washington, D. C.

Davis, J. M. G., and S. W. Coniami. 1973. Experimental studies on the effects of heated chrysotile asbestos and automobile brake lining dust injected into the body cavities of mice. Exp. Mol. Pathol. 19:339-353.

Davis, J. M. G., S. T. Beckett, R. E. Bolton, P. Collings, and A. P. Middleton. 1978. The importance of fibre mass and fibre number in the pathogenesis of asbestos-related disease in rats. Br. J. Cancer 37:678-688.
Davis, J. M. G., J. Addison, R. E. Bolton, K. Donaldson, A. Jones, and A. Wright. 1982. The pathogenic effects of fibrous ceramic aluminum silicate glass administered to rats by inhalation or peritoneal injection. Presented at the Biological Effects of Man-Made Mineral Fibers, Occupational Health Conference, Copenhagen, April 20, 1982. World Health Organization.
Desai, R., and R. J. Richards. 1978. The adsorption of biological macromolecules by mineral dusts. Environ. Res. 16:449-464.
Desai, R., P. Hext, and R. Richards. 1975. The prevention of asbestos-induced hemolysis. Life Sci. 16:1931-1938.
Diamond, L., T. G. O'Brien, and G. Rovera. 1978. Tumor promoters: Effects of proliferation and differentiation of cells in culture. Life Sci. 23:1979-1988.
Doll, N. J., B. E. Bozelka, S. Goldbach, E. Anorve-Lopez, and J. E. Salvaggio. 1982a. Asbestos-induced alteration of human peripheral blood monocyte activity. Int. Arch. Allergy Appl. Immunol. 69:302-305.
Doll, N. J., R. P. Stankus, S. Goldbach, and J. E. Salvaggio. 1982b. In vitro effect of asbestos fibers on polymorphonuclear leukocyte function. Int. Arch. Allergy Appl. Immunol. 68:17-21.
Domagala, W., and L. G. Koss. 1977. Scanning electron microscopic study of human carcinoma and mesothelioma cells treated with cytochalasin B. Acta Med. Pol. 18:301-310.
Donna, A. 1970. Experimental asbestos tumors induced by chrysotile, crocidolite and amosite in Sprague-Dawley rats. Med. Lay. 61:1-32.
Eastman, A., B. T. Mossman, and E. Bresnick. 1983. The influence of asbestos on the uptake of benzo(a)pyrene and DNA alkylation in hamster tracheal epithelial cells. Cancer Res. 43:1251-1258.
Father, E. 1982. Sequential events in chemical carcinogenesis. Pp. 485-506 in F. F. Becker, ed. Cancer: A Comprehensive Treatise. Vol. 1. Second Edition. Plenum Press, New York.
Farber, E., and R. Cameron. 1980. Sequential analysis of cancer development. Adv. Cancer Res. 31:125.
Fialkow, P. J. 1976. Clonal origin of human tumors. Biochem. Biophys. Acta 458:384-421.
Fornace, A. J. 1982. Detection of DNA single-strand breaks produced during the repair of damage by DNA protein cross-linking agents. Cancer Res. 42:145-149.
Foulds, L. 1954. The experimental study of tumor progression: A review. Cancer Res. 14:317-339.
Foulds, L. 1969. Neoplastic Development. Vol. 1. Academic Press, New York.
Foulds, L. 1975. Neoplastic Development. Vol. 2. Academic Press, New York.

Frank, A. L., A. N. Robl, M. J. Wade, and L. E. Lipkin. 1979. Biological activity in vitro of chrysotile compared to its quarried parent rock (platy serpentine). J. Exp. Pathol. Toxicol. 2:1041-1046.
Freeman, B. A., and J. D. Crapo. 1982. Biology of disease: Free radicals and tissue injury. Lab. Invest. 47:412-426.
Frei, J. V. 1976. Some mechanisms operative in carcinogenesis: A review. Chem. Biol. Interact. 12:1-25.
Gardner, L. V. 1942. Chrysotile asbestos as an indicator of subtle differences in animal tissues. Am. Rev. Tuberc. 45:762.
Gaumer, H. R., J. Hro, and J. E. Salvaggio. 1979. Chemiluminescent response to asbestos fibers. Clin. Res. 27:37A.
Gee, J. B. L. 1980. Cellular mechanisms in occupational lung disease. Chest 78:384-387.
Gross, P., and R. T. P. de Treville. 1967. Experimental asbestosis studies on the progressiveness of the pulmonary fibrosis caused by chrysotile dust. Arch. Environ. Health 15:638-649.
Gross, P., and R. A. Harley. 1973. Asbestos-induced intrathoracic tissue reactions. Arch. Pathol. 96:245-250.
Gross, P., R. T. P. de Treville, E. B. Tolker, M. Kaschak, and M. A. Babyak. 1967. Experimental asbestosis: The development of lung cancer in rats with pulmonary deposits of chrysotile asbestos dust. Arch. Environ. Health 15:343-355.
Gross, P., R. T. P. de Treville, L. J. Cralley, W. T. Granquist, and F. L. Pundsack. 1970. The pulmonary response to fibrous dusts of diverse compositions. Am. Ind. Hyg. Assoc. J. 125:125-132.
Gross, P., R. A. Harley, L. M. Swinburne, J. M. G. Davis, and W. B. Greene. 1974. Ingested mineral fibres. Do they penetrate tissue or cause cancer? Arch. Environ. Health 29:341-347.
Gross, P. G., R. J. Koeiba, G. L. Sparschu, and J. M. Norris. 1977. The biologic response to titanium phosphate. Arch. Pathol. Lab. Med. 101:550-554.
Hahon, N., and H. L. Eckert. 1976. Depression of viral interferon in cell monolayers by asbestos fibers. Environ. Res. 11:52-65.
Hahon, N., J. A. Booth, B. A. Boehlecke, and J. A. Merchant. 1980. Enhanced vital interferon induction by the mineral wollastonite. J. Interferon Res. 1:49-60.
Hamilton, J. A. 1980. Macrophase stimulation and the inflammatory response to asbestos. Environ. Health Perspect. 34:63-74.
Hamilton, J., J. D. Vassalli, and E. Reich. 1976. Macrophage plasminogen activator: Induction by asbestos is blocked by anti-inflammatory steroids. J. Exp. Med. 144:1689-1694.
Hammond, E. C., I. J. Selikoff, and H. Seidman. 1979. Asbestos exposure, cigarette smoking and death rates. Ann. N.Y. Acad. Sci. 330:473-490.
Harington, J. S. 1962. Occurrence of oils containing 3,4-benzpyrene and related substances in asbestos. Nature 193:43-45.
Hatington, J. S., A. C. Allison, and D. V. Badami. 1975. Mineral fibers: Chemical, physicochemical, and biologic properties. Adv. Pharm. Chemother. 12:291-402.
Harington, J. S., K. Miller, and G. Macnab. 1971. Hemolysis by asbestos. Environ. Res. 4:95-117.

Hart, R. W., R. Fertel, H. A. I. Newman, F. B. Daniel, and J. R. Blakeslee. 1979. Effects of selected asbestos fibers on cellular and molecular parameters. EPA-600/1-79-021. Environmental Protection Agency, Washington, D.C.

Hart, R. W., F. B. Daniel, O. R. Kindig, C. A. Beach, L. B. Joseph, and R. C. Wells. 1980. Elemental modifications and polycyclic aromatic hydrocarbon metabolism in human fibroblasts. Environ. Health Perspect. 34:59-68.

Hasselbacher, P. 1979. Binding of immunoglobulin and activation of complement by asbestos fibers. J. Allergy Clin. Immunol. 61:294-297.

Haugen, A., P. N. Schafer, J. F. Lechner, G. D. Simer, B. F. Trump, and C. C. Harris. 1982. Cellular ingestion, toxic effects and lesions observed in human bronchial epithelial tissue and cells cultured with asbestos and glass fibers. Int. J. Cancer 30:265-272.

Hecker, E., N. E. Fusenig, W. Kurtz, F. Marks, and H. W. Thielmann. 1982. Cocarcinogenesis and Biological Effects of Tumor Promoters. Raven Press, New York.

Hefner, R. E., and P. J. Gehring. 1975. A comparison of the relative rates of hemolysis induced by various fibrogenic and non-fibrogenic particles with washed rat erythrocytes in vitro. Am. Ind. Hyg. Assoc. J. 36:734-740.

Heppleston, A. G. 1979. Silica and asbestos: Contrasts in tissue response. Ann. N. Y. Acad. Sci. 330:725-744.

Hext, P. M., and R. J. Richards. 1976. Biochemical effects of asbestiform minerals on lung fibroblast cultures. Br. J. Exp. Pathol. 57:281.

Huang, S. L. 1979. Amosite, chrysotile, and crocidolite asbestos are mutagenic in Chinese hamster lung cells. Mutat. Res. 68:265-274.

Huang, S. L., D. Saggioro, H. Michelmann, and H. V. Mailing. 1978. Genetic effects of crocidolite asbestos in Chinese hamster lung cells. Mutat. Res. 57:225-232.

Isobe, M., L. Ogita, M. Yoshida, M. Tosu, and T. Sekiguchi. 1982. Epigenetic modulation of the mouse HGPRT gene in interspecific reconstituted cells and cybrids. FEBS Lett. 144:293-298.

Iversen, U. M., and O. H. Iversen. 1979. The carcinogenic effect of TPA (12-0-tetradecanoyl phorbol-13-acetate) when applied to the skin of hairless mice. Virchows Arch. B. Cell Pathol. 30:33-42.

Jacobs, R., J. Humphrys, K. S. Dodgson, and R.J. Richards. 1978. Light and electron microscope studies of the rat digestive tract following prolonged and short-term ingestion of chrysotile asbestos. Br. J. Exp. Pathol. 59:443-453.

Jagatic, J., M. E. Rubnitz, M. C. Godwin, and W. Weiskopf. 1967. Tissue response to intraperitoneal asbestos with preliminary report of acetate toxicity of heat-treated asbestos in mice. Environ. Res. 1:271-230.

Jaurand, M. C., L. Magne, and J. Bignon. 1979a. Inhibition of phospholipids of hemolytic action of asbestos. Br. J. Indust. Med. 36:113-116.

Jaurand, M. C., J. Bignon, P. Sebastien, and J. Goni. 1979b. Leaching of chrysotile asbestos in human lungs. Correlation with in vitro studies using rabbit alveolar macrophages. Environ. Res. 14:245-254.

Jaurand, M. C., H. Kaplan, J. Thiollet, M. C. Pinchon, J. F. Bernaudin, and J. Bignon. 1979c. Phagocytosis of chrysotile fibers by pleural mesothelial cells in culture. Am. J. Pathol. 94:529-538.

Janrand, M. C., J. H. Thomassin, P. Baillif, L. Hagne, J. C. Touray, and J. Bignon. 1980. Chemical and photoelectron spectrometry analysis of the adsorption of phospholipid model membranes and red blood cell membranes on to chrysotile fibres. Br. J. Indust. Med. 37:169-174.

Kagan, E., A. Solomon, J. C. Cochrane, K. Petra, P. H. Rocks, and I. Webster. 1977. Immunological studies of patients with asbestoses. II. Studies of circulating lymphoid cell numbers and humoral immunity. Clin. Exp. Immunol. 28:268-275.

Kaplan, H., A. Renier, M. C. Jaurand, and J. Bignon. 1980. Sister chromatid exchanges in mesothelial cells cultured with chrysotile fibres. Pp. 251-254 in R.C. Brown, M. Chamberlain, R. Davies, and I.P. Gormley, eds. The In Vitro Effects of Mineral Dusts. Academic Press, London and New York.

Kaw, J. L., F. Tilkes, and E. G. Beck. 1982. Reaction of cells cultured in vitro to different asbestos dusts of equal surface area but different fibre length. Br. J. Exp. Pathol. 63:109-115.

Klosterkotter, W., and K. Robock. 1970. Experimentelle Untersuchungen zum Wirkungsmechanismus yon Asbest unter besonderer Berücksichtigung der Faserlànge. Schriftenr. Arbeitsmed. Sozialmed. Arbeitshyg. 36:111-130.

Kolev, K. 1982. Experimentally induced mesothelioma in white rats in response to intraperitoneal administration of amorphous crocidolite asbestos: Preliminary report. Environ. Res. 29:123-133.

Kuschner, M., and G. W. Wright. 1976. The effects of intratracheal instillation of glass fiber of varying size in guinea pigs. Pp. 151-168 in Occupational Exposure to Fibrous Glass—Proceedings of a Symposium, No. 76-151, National Institute for Occupational Safety and Health, Washington, D.C.

Lakowicz, J. R., and D. R. Bevan. 1980. Benzo(a)pyrene uptake into rat liver microsomes: Effects of adsorption of benzo(a)pyrene to asbestos and non-fibrous mineral particulates. Chem. Biol. Interact. 29:129-138.

Lakowicz, J. R., F. England, and A. Hidmark. 1978a. Particle-enhanced membrane uptake of a polynuclear aromatic hydrocarbon: A possible role in cocarcinogenesis. J. Natl. Cancer Inst. 61:1155-1159.

Lakowicz, J. R., M. McNamara, and L. Steenson. 1978b. Particle-mediated membrane uptake of chemical carcinogens studied by fluorescence spectroscopy. Science 199:305-306.

Landesman, J. M., and B. T. Mossman. 1982. Induction of ornithine decarboxylase in hamster tracheal epithelial cells exposed to asbestos and 12-0-tetradecanoyl phorbol-13-acetate. Cancer Res. 42:3669-3675.

Lange, A. 1980. An epidemiological survey of immunological abnormalities in asbestos workers. 1. Non-organ and organ-specific autoantibodies. Environ. Res. 22:162-175.

Lavappa, K. S., M. M. Fu, and S. S. Epstein. 1975. Cytogenetic studies on chrysotile asbestos. Environ. Res. 10:165-173.

Lawrence, E. C., H. W. McClung, R. K. Wilson, M. M. Kex, R. M. Dodgson, and G. A. Hurst. 1982. Alteration of in vitro immunoglobulin secretion by amosite asbestos. J. Immunol. 129:1931-1935.
Lechner, J. F., A. Haugen, T. Tokiwa, B. F. Trump, and C. C. Harris. 1983. Effects of asbestos and carcinogenic metals on cultured human bronchial epithelium. In C. C. Harris and H. Autrup, eds. Human Carcinogenesis. Academic Press, New York.
Lee, K. P., C. E. Barras, F. D. Griffith, and R.S. Waritz. 1979. Pulmonary response to glass fiber by inhalation exposure. Lab. Invest. 40:123-133.
Lee, K. P., C. E. Barras, F. D, Griffith, R. S. Waritz, and C. A. Lapin. 1981. Comparative pulmonary responses to inhaled inorganic fibers with asbestos and fiberglass. Environ. Res. 24:167-191.
Leong, B. K. J. 1978. Induction of pulmonary carcinoma in rats by chronic inhalation of dust from pulverized asbestos pipe covering. J. Toxicol. Environ. Health 4:644-659.
Light, W. G., and E. T. Wei. 1977a. Surface charge and hemolytic activity of asbestos. Environ. Res. 13:135-145.
Light, W. G., and E. T. Wei. 1977b. Surface charge and asbestos toxicity. Nature 265:537-539.
Light, W. G., and E. T. Wei. 1980. Surface charge and a molecular basis for asbestos toxicity. Pp. 139-145 in R. C. Brown, I. P. Gormley, M. Chamberlain, and R. Davies, eds. The In Vitro Effects of Mineral Dusts. Academic Press, New York.
Livingston, G. K., W. N. Rom, and M. V. Morris. 1980. Asbestos-induced sister-chromatid exchanges in cultured hamster ovary fibroblast cells. J. Environ. Pathol. Toxicol. 4:373-382.
Maher, V. M., and J. J. McCormick. 1977. Effect of DNA repair on the cytotoxicity and mutagenicity of UV irradiation of chemical carcinogens in normal and xeroderma pigmentosum cells. Pp. 129-145 in J. M. Yukus, R. M. Tennent, and J. D. Regan, eds. Biology of Radiation Carcinogenesis. Raven Press, New York.
Manyai, S., J. Kebai, J. Kis, E. Suoeges, and M. Timor. 1969. The in vitro hemolytic effect of various clay minerals. Med. Lav. 60:331-343.
Maroudas, N. G., C. H. O'Neil, and M. F. Stanton. 1973. Fibroblast anchorage in carcinogenesis by fibres. Lancet 1:807-809.
Marx, J. L. 1978. Tumor promoters: Carcinogenesis gets more complicated. Science 201:515-516.
Marx, J. L. 1983. Do tumor promoters affect DNA after all? Science 219:158-159.
Maximov, A. 1927. Über das Mesothel (Deckzellen der serosen Hàute) und die Zellen der serosen Exsudate. Untersuchungen an entzündetem Gewebe und an Gewebskulturen. Arch. Exp. Zellforsch. 4:1-36.
McConnell, E. E., H. Rutter, B. Ulland, and J. A. Moore. 1983a. Chronic effects of dietary exposure to amosite asbestos and tremolite in Fischer 344 rats. Environ. Health Perspect. 53:27-44.
McConnell, E. E., A. M. Shefner, J. Rust, and J. A. Moore. 1983b. Chronic effects of dietary exposure to amosite and chrysotile asbestos in Syrian golden hamsters. Environ. Health Perspect. 53:11-26.

McConnell, E. E., J. C. Wagner, J. W. Skidmore, and J. A. Moore. 1982. Two Inhalation studies: A comparison. Presented at the Biological Effects of Man-Made Mineral Fibers, Occupational Health Conference, Copenhagen, April 20, 1982. World Health Organization.

McCord, J. M., and K. Wong. 1979. Phagocyte-produced free radicals: Roles in cytotoxicity and inflammation. Pp. 343-367 in I. Fridovich, ed. Oxygen Free Radicals and Tissue Damage. Excerpta Medics, New York.

McLemore, T., M. Corson, M. Mace, M. Arnett, T. Jenkins, D. Shodgrass, R. Martin, N. Wray, and B. R. Brinkley. 1979. Phagocytosis of asbestos fibers by human pulmonary alveolar macrophages. Cancer Lett. 6:183-192.

Miller, K., and J. S. Harington. 1972. Some biochemical effects of asbestos on macrophages. Br. J. Exp. Pathol. 53:397-405.

Miller, L., W. E. Smith, and S. W. Berliner. 1965. Tests for effect of asbestos on benzo(a)pyrene carcinogenesis in the respiratory tract. Ann. N. Y. Acad. Sci. 132:489-500.

Monchaux, G., J. Bignon, M. C. Jaurand, J. Lafuma, P. Sebasten, R. Masse, A. Hirsch, and J. Goni. 1981. Mesotheliomas in rats following inoculation with acid-leached chrysotile asbestos and other mineral fibers. Carcinogenesis 2:229-236.

Moorman, W. J. In press. A chronic inhalation toxicology study in monkeys and rats exposed to fibrous glass. Battelle Columbus Laboratories Contract No. 210-78-0037. National Institute for Occupational Safety and Health, Washington, D.C..

Morgan, A., P. Davies, J. C. Wagner, G. Berry, and A. Holmes. 1977. The biological effects of magnesium-leached chrysotile asbestos. Br. J. Exp. Pathol. 58:465-473.

Morrison, D. G., J. Daniel, F. T. Lynd, M. P. Moyer, R. J. Esparza, R. C. Moyer, and W. Rogers. 1981. Retinyl palmitate and ascorbic acid inhibit pulmonary neoplasms in mice exposed to fiberglass dust. Nutr. Cancer 3:81-85.

Mossman, B. T., and J. E. Craighead. 1974. Topical application of polycyclic hydrocarbons to differentiated respiratory epithelium in long-term organ cultures. Pp. 514-520 in E. Karbe and J. F. Park, eds. Experimental Lung Cancer, Carcinogenesis and Bioassays. Springer-Verlag, New York.

Mossman, B. T., and J. E. Craighead. 1979. Use of hamster tracheal organ cultures for assessing the cocarcinogenic effects of inorganic particulates on the respiratory epithelium. Prog. Exp. Tumor Res. 24:37-47.

Mossman, B. T., and J. E. Craighead. 1981. Mechanisms of asbestos carcinogenesis. Environ. Res. 25:269-280.

Mossman, B. T., and J. E. Craighead. 1982. Comparative cocarcinogenic effects of crocidolite asbestos, hematite, kaolin, and carbon in implanted hamster tracheal organ cultures. Pp. 572-585 in A. Critchlow, ed. Inhaled Particles. Vol. 5. Pergamon Press, London.

Mossman, B. T., and J. M. Landesman. 1983. Importance of oxygen-free radicals in asbestos-induced injury to airway epithelial cells. Chest. 83 (Supp.):50-51.

Mossman, B. T., B. Ley, J. B. Kessler, and J E. Craighead. 1977. Interaction of crocidolite asbestos with hamster respiratory mucosa in organ culture. Lab. Invest. 36:131-139.

Mossman, B. T., K. B. Adler, and J. E. Craighead. 1978. The interaction of carbon particles with tracheal epithelium in organ culture. Environ. Res. 16:110-118.

Mossman, B. T., J. E. Craighead, and B. V. MacPherson. 1980a. Asbestos-induced epithelial changes in organ cultures of hamster trachea: Inhibition by retinyl methyl ether. Science 207:311-313.

Mossman, B. T., K. B. Adler, and J. E. Craighead. 1980b. Cytotoxic and proliferative changes in tracheal organ and cell cultures after exposure to mineral dusts. Pp. 241-250 in R. C. Brown, I. P. Gormley, M. Chamberlain, and R. Davies, eds. The In Vitro Effects of Mineral Dusts. Academic Press, London and New York.

Mossman, B. T., K. B. Adler, L. J. Jean, and J. E. Craighead. 1982. Mechanisms of hypersecretion in rodent tracheal explants after exposure to chrysotile asbestos. Chest 81S:23S-25S.

Mossman, B., W. Light, and E. Wei. 1983a. Asbestos: Mechanisms of toxicity and carcinogenicity in the respiratory tract. Ann. Rev. Pharm. Toxicol. 23:595-615.

Mossman, B. T., A. Eastman, J. M. Landesman, and E. Bresnick. 1983b. Effects of crocidolite and chrysotile asbestos on cellular uptake, metabolism and DNA after exposure of hamster tracheal epithelial cells to benzo(a)pyrene. Environ. Health Perspect. 51:331-336.

Mossman, B. T., L. J. Senn, and J. M. Landesman. 1983c. Studies using lectins to determine mineral interactions with cellular membranes. Proceedings of the Second International Conference on In Vitro Effects of Mineral Dusts. Environ. Health Perspect. 51:23-26.

Nowell, P. C. 1976. The clonal evolution of tumor cell populations. Science 194:23-28.

O'Brien, T. G. 1976. The induction of ornithine decarboxylase as an early, possibly obligatory event in mouse skin carcinogenesis. Cancer Res. 36:2644-2646.

Palekar, L. D., C. M. Spooner, and D. L. Coffin. 1979. Influence of crystalline habit of minerals on in vitro cytotoxicity. Ann. N.Y. Acad. Sci. 330:673-686.

Peraino, C., E. F. Staffeldt, D. A. Haugen, L. S. Lombard, F. J. Stevens, and R. J. M. Fry. 1980. Effects of varying the dietary concentration of phenobarbital on its enhancement of 2-acecylamino fluorene-induced hepatic tumorigenesis. Cancer Res. 40:3268-3273.

Pierce, R. C., and M. Katz. 1975. Dependency of polynuclear aromatic hydrocarbon content on size distribution of atmospheric aerosols. Environ. Sci. Technol. 9:347-353.

Piggott, G. H., B. A. Gaskell, and J. Ishmael. 1981. Effects of long term inhalation of alumina fibres in rats. Br. J. Exp. Pathol. 62:323-331.

Pitot, H. C., and A. E. Sirica. 1980. The stages of initiation and promotion in hepatocarcinogenesis. Biochem. Biophys. Acta 191-215.

Pott, F., and K. H. Friedrichs. 1972. Tumoren der Ratte nach i.p.: Injektion faserformiger Staube. Naturwissenschaften 59:318.

Pott, E. F., F. Huth, and K. H. Friedrichs. 1972. Tumoren der Ratte nach i.p.-Injektion von gemahlenem Chrysotil und Benzo(a)pyrene. Zentralbl. Bakteriol. Parasitenk. Infektionskr. Hyg. Abt. 1 Orig. Reihe B 155:463-469.

Pott, F., F. Huth, and K. H. Friedrichs. 1974. Tumorigenic effect of fibrous dusts in experimental animals. Environ. Health Perspect. 9:313-315.

Pott, F., F. Huth, and K. H. Friedrichs. 1976. Results of animal carcinogenesis studies after application of fibrous glass and their implications regarding human exposure. Pp. 183-191 in Occupational Exposure to Fibrous Glass—Proceedings of a Symposium. HEW Publ. No. 76-151, National Institute for Occupational Safety and Health, Washington, D.C.

Pott, F., H. W. Schlipkoter, U. Ziem, K. Spurny, and F. Huth. 1982. New results from implantation experiments with mineral fibres. Presented at the Biological Effects of Man-Made Mineral Fibers, Occupational Health Conference, Copenhagen, April 20, 1982. World Health Organization.

Potter, V. R. 1981. A new protocol and rationale for the study of initiation and promotion of carcinogenesis in rat liver. Carcinogenesis 2:1375-1379.

Pound, A. W., and L. J. McGuire. 1978. Repeated partial hepatectomy as a promoting stimulus for carcinogenesis response of liver to nitrosamines in rats. Br. J. Cancer 37:585-594.

Price-Jones, M. J., G. Gubbings, and H. Chamberlain. 1980. The genetic effects of crocidolite asbestos: Comparison of chromosome abnormalities and sister-chromatid exchanges. Mutat. Res. 79:331-336.

Pylev, L. N., and L. M. Shabad. 1973. Some results of experimental studies in asbestos carcinogenesis. Pp. 99-105 in P. Bogovski, J.C. Gilson, and V. Timbrell, eds. Biological Effects of Asbestos. IARC Scientific Pub. No. 8. International Agency for Research on Cancer, Lyon

Rajan, K. T., and P. H. Evans. 1973. Pp. 94-98 in P. Bogovski, J.C. Gilson, V. Timbrell, and J.C. Wagner, eds. Biological Effects of Asbestos. IARC Scientific Pub. No. 8. International Agency for Research on Cancer, Lyon, France.

Rajan, K. T., J. C. Wagner, and P. H. Evans. 1972. The response of human pleura in organ culture to asbestos. Nature 238:346-347.

Reeves, A. L. 1976. The carcinogenic effect of inhaled asbestos fibers. Ann. Clin. Lab. Sci. 6:459-466.

Reeves, A. L., H. E. Puro, R. G. Smith, and A. J. Vorwald. 1971. Experimental asbestos carcinogenesis. Environ. Res. 4:496-511.

Reeves, A. L., H. E. Puro, and R. G. Smith. 1974. Inhalation carcinogenesis from various forms of asbestos. Environ. Res. 8:178-202.

Reiss, B., S. Solomon, J. Weisburger, and G. M. Williams. 1980a. Comparative toxicities of different forms of asbestos in a cell culture assay. Environ. Res. 22:109-129.

Reiss, B., J. R. Millette, and G. N. Williams. 1980b. The activity of environmental samples in a cell culture test for asbestos toxicity. Environ. Res. 22:315-321.

Reiss, B., S. Solomon, C. Tong, M. Levenstein, S. H. Rosenberg, and G. M. Williams. 1982. Absence of mutagenic activity of three forms of asbestos in liver epithelial cells. Environ. Res. 27:389-397.

Richards, R. J., and F. Jacoby. 1976. Light microscope studies on the effects of chrysotile asbestos and fiberglass on the morphology and reticulin formation of cultured lung fibroblasts. Environ. Res. 11:112-121.

Richards, R. J., and T. G. Morris. 1973. Collagen and mucopolysaccharlde production in growing lung fibroblasts exposed to chrysotile asbestos. Life Sci. 12:441-451.

Roe, F. J. C., R. L. Carter, M. A. Walters, and J. S. Harington. 1967. The pathological effects of subcutaneous injections of asbestos fibres in mice: Migration of fibers to submesothelial tissues and induction of mesotheliomata. Int. J. Cancer 2:628-638.

Saint-Remy, J. M. R., and P. Cole. 1980. Interactions of chrysotile asbestos fibers with the complement system. Immunol. 41:431-437.

Saxena, K. C., L. Srivastava, and R. K. S. Dogra. 1982. Biochemical and histopathological response to chrysotile ingestion in guinea pigs. Ind. Health 20:19-25.

Schepers, G. W. H. 1959. Pulmonary histologic reactions to inhaled fiberglass-plastic dust. Am. J. Pathol. 35:1169-1187.

Schepers, G. W. H., and A. B. Delahant. 1955. An experimental study of the effects of glass wool on animals' lungs. Arch. Ind. Health 12: 276-286

Schepers, G. W. H., T. M. Durkan, and A. B. Delahant. 1958. The biological action of fiberglass-plastic dust. Arch. Ind. Health 18:34-56.

Schnitzer, R. J., and F. L. Pundsack. 1970. Asbestos hemolysis. Environ. Res. 3:1-13.

Schoenberger, C., G. Hunninghake, O. Kawanaki, V. J. Farrams, and R. G. Crystal. 1982. Role of alveolar macrophages in asbestoses: Modulation of neutrophil migration to the lung following asbestos exposure. Thorax 37:803-809.

Shabad, L. M., L. N. Pylev, L. V. Krivosheeva, T. F. Kulagina, and B. A. Nemenko. 1974. Experimental studies on asbestos carcinogenicity. J. Natl. Cancer Inst. 52:1175-1187.

Sincock, A. M. 1977. Preliminary studies on the in vitro cellular effects of asbestos and fine glass dusts. Pp. 941-954 in H.H. Hiat, J. D. Watson, and J. A. Winsten, ads. Origins of Human Cancer, Cold Spring Harbor Conferences on Cell Proliferation. Cold Spring Harbor Laboratory, Cold Spring Harbor, N.Y..

Sincock, A., and M. Seabright. 1975. Induction of chromosome changes in Chinese hamster cells by exposure to asbestos fibers. Nature 257:56-58.

Sirois, P., M. Rola-Pleszczynski, and R. Begin. 1980. Phospholipase activity and prostaglandin release from alveolar macrophages exposed to asbestos. Prostaglandins Med. 5:31-37.

Slaga, T. J., A. Sivak, and R. K. Boutwell. 1978. Carcinogenesis, A Comprehensive Survey. Mechanisms of Tumor Promotion and Cocarcinogenesis. Raven Press, New York.

Slags, T. J., S. M. Fischer, C. E. Weeks, K. Nelson, M. Mamrack, and A. J. P Klein-Szanto. 1982. Specificity and mechanism(s) of promoter inhibitors in multistage promotion. Pp. 19-34 in E. Hecker, N. E. Fusenig, W. Kunz, F. Marks, and H. W. Thielman, eds. Carcinogenesis: Co-Carcinogenesis and Biological Effects of Tumor Promoters, Volume 7. Raven Press, New York.

Smith, D. M., L. W. Ortiz, and R. F. Archuleta. 1982. Long-term exposure of Syrian hamsters and Osborne-Mendel rats to aerosolized 0.45 μm Mean diameter fibrous glass. Presented at the Biological Effects of Man-Made Mineral Fibers, Occupational Health Conference, Copenhagen, April 20, 1982. World Health Organization.

Smith, W. E., and D. D. Hubert. 1974. The intrapleural root as a means for estimating carcinogenicity. Pp. 93-100 in E. Karbe and J. F. Park, eds. Experimental Lung Cancer, Carcinogenesis and Bioassays. Springer, New York.

Smith, W. E., L. Miller, R. E. Elsasser, and D. D. Hubert. 1965. Tests for carcinogenicity of asbestos. Ann. N.Y. Acad. Sci. 132:456-488.

Smith, W. E., L. Miller, and J. Churg. 1968. Respiratory tract tumors in hamsters after intratracheal benzo(a)pyrene with and without asbestos. Proc. Am. Assoc. Cancer Res. 9:65.

Smith, W. E., D. D. Hubert, and H. J. Sobel. 1980a. Health of experimental animals drinking water with and without amosite asbestos and other mineral particles. J. Environ. Pathol. Toxicol. 3:277-300.

Smith, W. E., D. D. Hubert, and H. J. Sobel. 1980b. Dimensions of fibres in relation to biological activity. Pp. 357-360 in J.C. Wagner, ed. Biological Effects of Mineral Fibres. IARC Scientific Pub. No. 30. International Agency for Research on Cancer, Lyon.

Stansfield, D., and J. R. Edge. 1974. Circulating rheumatoid factor and antinuclear antibodies in shipyard asbestos workers with pleural plaques. Br. J. Dis. Chest 68:166-170.

Stanton, M. F., and M. Layard. 1978. The carcinogenicity of fibrous materials. Pp. 142-151 in Proceedings of the Workshop on Asbestos: Definitions and Measurement Methods. NBS Spec. Pub. No. 506. National Bureau of Standards, Gaithersburg, Md.

Stanton, M. F., and C. Wrench. 1972. Mechanisms of mesothelioma induction with asbestos and fibrous glass. J. Natl. Cancer Inst. 48:797-816.

Stanton, M. F., M. Layard, A. Tegaris, E. Miller, M. May, and E. Kent. 1977. Carcinogenicity of fibrous glass: Pleural response in the rat in relation to fiber dimension. J. Natl. Cancer Inst. 58:587-603.

Stanton, M. F., M. Layard, A. Tegaris, E. Miller, M. May, E. Morgan, and A. Smith. 1981. Relation of particle dimension to carcinogenicity in amphibole asbestos and other fibrous minerals. J. Natl. Cancer Inst. 67:165-175.

Stout, A. P., and M. R. Murray. 1942. Localized pleural mesothelioma. Investigation of its characteristics and histogenesis by the method of tissue culture. Arch. Pathol. 34:951-964.

Suzuki, Y. 1982. Carcinogenic and fibrogenic effects of zeolites: Preliminary observations. Environ. Res. 27:433-445.

Suzuki, Y., A. N. Rohl, A. M. Langer, and I. D. Selikoff. 1980. Mesothelioma following intraperitoneal administration of zeolite. Fed. Proc. 39:640.

Topping, D.C., and P. Nettesheim. 1980. Two-stage carcinogenesis studies with asbestos in Fischer 344 rats. J. Natl. Cancer Inst. 65:627-630.

Topping, D., P. Nettesheim, and D. Martin. 1980. Toxic and tumorigenic effects of asbestos on tracheal mucosa. J. Environ. Pathol. Toxtcol. 3:261-275.

Trosko, J. F.., and C. C. Chang. 1980. An integrative hypothesis linking cancer, diabetes and atherosclerosis. The role of mutations and epigenetic changes. Med. Hypoth. 6:455-468.

Turner-Warwick, M., and W. R. Parkes. 1973. Immunological mechanisms in occupational disorders. Proc. R. Soc. Med. 66:13-16.

Valerio, F., M. De Ferrari, L. Ottaggio, F. Repetto, and L. Santi. 1980. Cytogenetic effects of Rhodesian chrysotile on human lymphocytes in vitro. Pp. 485-489 in J.C. Wagner, ed. Biological Effects of Mineral Fibres. Vol. 1. IARC Scientific Pub. No. 30. International Agency for Research on Cancer, Lyon.

Verma, A. K., E. A. Conrad, and R. K. Boutwell. 1982. Differential effects of retinoic acid and 7,8-benzoflavone on the induction of mouse skin tumors by the complete carcinogenesis process and by the initiation-promotion regimen. Cancer Res. 42:3519-3525.

Vigliani, E. 1968. The fibrogenic response to asbestos. Med. Lav. 59:402-410.

Vorwald, A. J., T. M. Dunkan, and P. C. Pratt. 1951. Experimental studies of asbestosis. Arch. Ind. Hyg. Occup. Meal. 3:1-83.

Wade, M. J., L. E. Lipkin, and A. L. Frank. 1979. Studies of in vitro asbestos cell interaction. J. Environ. Patbol. Toxicol. 2:1029-1039.

Wade, M. J., L. E. Lipkin, M. F. Stanton, and A. L. Frank. 1980. 'In vitro' cytotoxicity assay as applied to asbestos and other minerals: Its possible relevance to carcinogenicity. Pp. 351-357 in R. C. Brown, I. P. Gormley, M. Chamberlain, and R. Davies, eds. The In Vitro Effects of Mineral Dusts. Academic Press, New York.

Wagner, J. C. 1963. Asbestosis in experimental animals. Br. J. Ind. Med. 20:1-12.

Wagner, J. C. 1982. Health hazards of substitutes. Pp. 244-266 in Proceedings of the World Symposium on Asbestos, held May 25-27, 1982 in Montreal. Canadian Asbestos Information Center, Montreal.

Wagner, J. C., and G. Berry. 1969. Mesotheliomas in rats following inoculation with asbestos. Br. J. Cancer 23:567-581.

Wagner, J. C., G. Berry, and V. Timbrell. 1973. Mesotheliomata in rats after inoculation with asbestos and other materials. Br. J. Cancer 28:173-185.

Wagner, J. C., G. Berry, J. W. Skidmore, and V. Timbrell. 1974. The effects of the inhalation of asbestos in rats. Br. J. Cancer 29:2.52-269.

Wagner, J. C., G. B. Berry, R. J. Hill, D. E. Munday, and J. W. Skidmore. 1982a. Animal experiments with man-made mineral (V) fibres. Effects of inhalation and intrapleural inoculation in rats. Presented at the Biological Effects of Man-Made Mineral Fibers, Occupational Health Conference, Copenhagen, April 20, 1982. World Health Organization.

Wagner, J. C., M. Chamberlain, R. C. Brown, G. Berry, F. D. Pooley, R. Davies, and P. M. Griffiths. 1982b. Biological effects of tremolite. Br. J. Cancer 45:352-360.

Wagner, J. C., G. Berry, and F. D. Pooley. 1982c. Mesotheliomas and asbestos type in asbestos textile workers: A study of lung contents. Br. Med. J. 285:603-606.

Ward, J. H., A. L. Frank, M. Wenk, D. Devor, and R. E. Tarone. 1980. Ingested asbestos and intestinal carcinogenesis in F344 rats. J. Environ. Pathol. Toxicol. 3:301-312.

Webster, I. 1970. The pathogenesis of asbestosis. Pp. 117-119 in H.A. Shapiro, ed. Proceedings of the International Conference on Pneumoconiosis, Johannesburg, 1969. Oxford University Press, New York.

Webner, A. P., R. H. Busch, R. J. Olson, and D. K. Craig. 1975. Chronic inhalation of asbestos and cigarette smoke by hamsters. Environ. Res. 10:368-383.

Westlake, G. E., H. A. Spjut, and M. N. Smith. 1965. Penetration of colonic mucosa by asbestos particles. Lab. Invest. 14:2029-2033.

Weymouth, L. A., and L. A. Loeb. 1978. Mutagenesis during in vitro DNA synthesis. Proc. Natl. Acad. Sci. USA 75:1924-1928.

Whitaker, D., J. M. Papdimittiou, and M. N. J. Walters. 1982. The mesothelium and its reactions: A review. Pp. 81-144 in CRC Critical Review of Toxicology. CRC Press, Cleveland.

Whitfield, J. F., A. L. Boynton, J. P. MacManus, M. Sikorska, and B. K. Tsang. 1979. The regulation of cell proliferation by calcium and cyclic AMP. Nol. Cell. Biochem. 27:155-179.

Wilson, M. R., H. R. Gaumer, and J. E. Salvaggio. 1977. Activation of the alternate complement pathway and generation of chemotactic factors by asbestos. J. Allergy Clin. Immunol. 60:218-222.

Woodworth, C. D., B. T. Mossman, and J. E. Craighead. 1982. Comparative effects of fibrous and nonfibrous minerals on cells and liposomes. Environ. Res. 27:190-205.

Woodworth, C. D., B. T. Mossman, and J. E. Craighead. 1983a. Induction of squamous metaplasia in organ cultures of hamster trachea by naturally occurring and synthetic fibers. Cancer Res. 43:4906-4912.

Woodworth, C. D., B. T. Mossman, and J. E. Craighead. 1983b. Squamous metaplasta of the respiratory tract—Possible pathogenic role in asbestos-associated bronchogenic carcinoma. Lab. Invest. 48:578-584.

Woodworth, C. D., B. T. Mossman, and J. E. Craighead. 1983c. Comparative interaction of asbestos with normal mucociliary and squamous tracheobronchial epithelium. Environ. Health Perspect. 51:27-34.

Workshop on Ingested Asbestos. 1983. Summary Workshop on Ingested Asbestos, October 13-14, 1982, Cincinnati. Environ. Health Perspect. 53:1-204.

Yager, J. D., and R. Yager. 1980. Oral contraceptive steroids as promoters of hepatocarcinogenesis in female Sprague-Dawley rats. Cancer Res. 40:3680-3685.

Yuspa, S. H., T. Ben, H. Henings, and U. Lichti. 1982. Divergent responses in epidermal basal cells exposed to the tumor promoter, 12-0-tetradecanoyl-phorbol-13-acetate. Cancer Res. 42:2344-2349.

Zitting, A., and E. Skytta. 1979. Biological activity of titanium dioxides. Int. Arch. Occup. Environ. Health 43:93-97.

7

Risk Assessment

Exposure, laboratory, and epidemiological data provided earlier in this report are used in this chapter to make quantitative and qualitative (or comparative) assessments of risks from exposure to asbestiform fibers. To place the discussion in context, the chapter begins with a brief general discussion of risk assessment and a few special considerations concerning asbestos and related fibrous materials.

Various difficulties often limit the accuracy and precision with which risk to human health can be estimated. Nevertheless, when the data base is good, the risk estimates can be sufficiently informative to aid policy judgments. Some of the factors that enhance the usefulness of the data include dose-response information based on several accurately known exposure levels; knowledge of physiologic and metabolic factors that affect exposure of body tissues; an understanding of the mechanism by which the substance results in toxicity; knowledge of the extent to which experimental systems mimic the human response; and an understanding of the properties of a complex and variable substance that account for its toxicity.

Many of these issues apply in the assessment of risk from asbestiform fibers, which have varying physical and chemical properties. Some members of the class, the commonly used naturally occurring forms of asbestos, have been clearly shown to cause fibrosis of the lung and pleura as well as cancer of the lung, mesothelium, and possibly the gastrointestinal tract in humans. Some occupational data on other fibers are also available, and considerable numbers of experimental studies have been conducted. It is reasonable from a biological viewpoint to use data from occupational studies to derive estimates of risk from nonoccupational exposure. However, differences in route of exposure, type and characteristics of fiber, exposure levels, and time patterns must be considered. Moreover, because working populations are generally healthier than the public at large, the latter may contain a higher proportion of more susceptible individuals.

THE PROCESS OF RISK ASSESSMENT

The principles guiding the assessment of health risks from environmental substances were recently reviewed by a committee of the

National Research Council (1983). These principles are summarized here to provide a framework for assessing the health risks from exposure to asbestiform fibers.

The numerous terms used to describe different aspects of risk assessment include "hazard assessment," "hazard identification," "risk assessment," "qualitative risk assessment," "dose-response assessment" "comparative risk assessment," "quantitative risk assessment," and "risk characterization." The use of these terms has not been standardized.

Three concepts are generally incorporated into the risk assessment process. First is the identification of the kinds of harmful health effects, e.g., anemia, birth defects, or cancer, that can result from sufficient exposure to a substance. Second is the dose-response curve for a particular effect, i.e., the severity of damage and/or the percentage of people or animals likely to be at various exposure levels. Third is the number of people in a particular population, e.g., residents of the United States or yorkers in a particular industry, likely to be harmed under past, present, or projected levels and conditions of exposure.

In this report, the committee has used "risk assessment" as a broad term encompassing all three of these concepts. "Hazard identification" refers to the first concept, "dose-response" curves or relationships are used in discussions of particular sets of data, and "quantitative risk assessment" refers to the estimates of risk to humans derived by mathematical extrapolations from these data. "Population risk estimates" describe the expected frequency or incidence of a harmful effect in a specific group of humans under defined conditions of exposure.

The amount and complexity of information needed increase as we progress from hazard identification to dose-response assessment to population risk estimation, although each step builds on the preceding one. Hazard identification characterizes the nature of toxic effects that a substance is capable of causing in laboratory animals or humans. Dose-response curves based on experimental or epidemiological observations define the frequency and sometimes the severity of these toxic effects at several levels of exposure.

The dose-response information is used in quantitative risk estimation. Through mathematical modeling and application of known biological principles, attempts are often made to estimate risk for dose levels, exposure conditions, or species other than those for which dose-response data have been obtained. For example, quantitative risk assessments often rely on dose-response data from studies of laboratory animals exposed to relatively high exposure levels in order to estimate the risk to humans exposed to lower levels. Assumptions and uncertainties involved in the application of quantitative risk assessment to cancer induction have been discussed extensively (Food

Safety Council, 1980; International Regulatory Liaison Group, 1979; Office of Technology Assessment, 1981). Population risk estimates bring together quantitative risk estimates and data on exposure of a specific group of humans to identify their risk under actual or anticipated exposure conditions.

The most relevant information for categorizing the hazard or the dose-response for humans is derived from studies of exposed humans. Unfortunately, evidence from this source is often unavailable or inconclusive at times when decisions about acceptable exposure must be made. Humans are exposed to so many different substances through food, medicines, air, water, household materials, and occupational environments that sorting out the causes of harmful effects on health is often difficult. Perhaps of most importance is the fact that evidence of human health hazards from substances introduced into our environment cannot be obtained directly from observations in humans until people have been harmed.

For these reasons, evidence from laboratory animals or from other biological test systems is often used as an alternative or as a supplement to data on humans. A substantial body of evidence has demonstrated the utility of these experimental systems (Doull et al., 1980; National Research Council, 1977; Richmond et al., 1981). A variety of mathematical models have been developed for using data at high doses, usually only available from studies in animals, to estimate risks for humans at low doses (Armitage, 1982; Cornfield et al., 1978; Crumpet et al., 1976; Fishbein, 1980; Food Safety Council, 1980; Krewski and Van Ryzin, 1981; Van Ryzin, 1980). Because there are extensive data on the effects of asbestos and some other fibers in humans, the quantitative risk assessments in this chapter are based exclusively on data from epidemiological studies in humans, whereas the comparative risk assessments also take into consideration data from laboratory studies.

Every scientific study or technique has some lower limit to its sensitivity. A sensitive method in analytical chemistry may be capable of detecting a few molecules of a particular chemical among a billion other kinds of molecules but incapable of detecting a few among a trillion. The sensitivity of an animal test for toxicity is limited by many factors, such as the number of animals that it is practical to study, the subtlety of the effect of interest, the occurrence of similar effects in animals not exposed to the material under test, and limitations on the amounts of material that can be administered and on the methods used to administer them.

Other difficulties limit the power of epidemiological studies. For example, it is often difficult to select appropriate control groups, estimate exposure, or detect health effects from the exposures of concern, especially if the exposures are much lower than those that occur among occupational groups.

Several kinds of information are useful for estimating risks at low exposure levels on the basis of observations at higher exposures. These include the shape of the dose-response curve in the range of exposures studied, knowledge of the mechanism by which the type of toxic effect occurs, and information on dose-related changes in the uptake, distribution, chemical or physical modification, and excretion of the substance, i.e., pharmacokinetics.

Substances vary markedly both in the quantity required to produce a toxic effect and in the rapidity with which the incidence of toxic effects decreases with decreasing dose, i.e., the shape of the dose-response curve. In an experiment covering a sufficiently wide range of exposure levels, it is possible to find some levels that are toxic and some lower levels at which no toxicity is observed. The highest dose at which no toxicity is seen is often called the "no-observed-effect level," or NOEL (Klaassen and Doull, 1980). However, any experiment will have some limit in its sensitivity to small effects, and the true no-effect-level, if any, may be below the NOEL in a particular experiment.

The fundamental assumption underlying the NOEL safety factor approach is that some minimal level of a toxic substance is required to cause damage and that the substance is not toxic below that level. The NOEL type of experiment is used to find that level.

The maximum dose at which no toxicity would occur is called the "threshold" for that substance. However, several mathematical models for quantitative estimation of cancer risk assume that there is no threshold; risk diminishes with decreasing dose, but some risk is assumed to remain as long as there is any exposure.

The determination of which of these two assumptions is correct will probably depend on the nature of the toxic effect. Thus, understanding the mechanism of toxicity can provide guidance in setting acceptable exposure levels. For a substance that exerts its toxic effect by inactivating an enzyme present in abundance in each cell, it is reasonable to assume that a threshold would exist. Inactivation of a few molecules of the enzyme is unlikely to damage the cell. On the other hand, a chemical that is mutagenic or carcinogenic because it damages some critical site on a DNA molecule that starts the carcinogenic process can reasonably be assumed not to have a threshold. The likelihood that a critical site would be damaged would decrease with decreasing dose, but the possibility that this damage could occur remains at any exposure above zero.

For many effects, the severity of the toxic effect, as well as the probability that it will occur, also decreases with dose. For example, a dose that damages a high proportion of cells in the liver may be lethal; one that damages a moderate number may cause severe illness but not death; a small dose that causes damage to a few cells may not lead to any clinical symptoms. The error in assuming a threshold if none truly existed would generally not be expected to lead to serious cases of disease in this situation.

By contrast, the severity of cancer and of mutations is not related to the dose of the substance causing them. Low dose exposure to x-rays or cigarette smoke causes fewer cancers than does high dose exposure, but the resulting cancers are just as lethal. Thus, although there may be some substances that show a threshold for cancer induction (Hoel et al., 1983), an error in assuming a threshold when none really exists would severely harm those persons who got the disease despite a low exposure.

Accurate documentation of exposure is important for determining the dose-response curves for toxicity in animals or humans and also for estimating population risks. Errors in the estimation of exposure will lead to errors in defining the dose-response curve and in making quantitative risk estimates for individuals or specific populations. The amount of a toxic substance or its active metabolite that reaches the body site that is susceptible to its effect is the exposure that accounts for toxicity, but such measures are almost never available (Hoel et al., 1983). Other measurements, such as amounts in the blood, amounts entering the body, or concentrations in the air or water of a community, are often useful surrogates, but as noted earlier in this report, they are also often unavailable.

The sensitivity of the exposed population is another consideration in the risk estimation process. Some individuals may be more sensitive than others to specific environmental insults because of nutritional deficiencies, genetic predisposition, and for children, small body size, developmental immaturity, and increased metabolic and respiratory rates (Calabrese, 1978, 1980).

With their rapid metabolic rate, children consume proportionately more food and inhale greater volumes of air than an adult for a given body weight. Thus, they would also consume or inhale proportionately more of any contaminants that are present (Babich and Davis, 1981). Human infants do not have mature hepatic detoxification systems until they reach 2 to 3 months of age (Pelkonen et al., 1973; Rane and Ackerman, 1972). Serum immunoglobulin does not attain adult levels until children are 10 to 12 years old (Calabrese, 1978). Studies in animals have also demonstrated a greater sensitivity among the young after exposure to chemicals by a variety of routes (Goldenthal, 1971). Children's lungs may also be especially sensitive to environmental pollutants. Tager et al. (1983) have observed measurable differences in lung function between children of smoking mothers and children whose mothers did not smoke.

Population risk estimation is based on all the preceding steps. First, the exposure of the study population must be known. Heterogeneity of the population with respect to level of exposure or sensitivity to the toxic material should also be considered in the calculations. Exposure, dose-response curves, distribution of sensitivity factors, and the size of the population are then used to estimate the number of people likely to suffer toxic effects from the substance of interest. If the material causes more than one type of toxic effect, each effect requires separate calculations.

Ideally, calculation of risk is an objective, scientific activity devoid of policy judgments. The latter are made separately when deciding the acceptable level of exposure. However, policy decisions can seldom be divorced completely from the process of risk assessment. The reason for this lies in the uncertainty of many of the scientific judgments required. For example, if one experimental species is more susceptible to the toxicity of a material than another and data on humans are unavailable, which species should be used for estimating human risk? Which mathematical model should be applied to the data? These and many other questions of judgment were discussed in the recent National Research Council (1983) report.

In the following sections, the committee has used epidemiological data, mostly from occupational settings, to develop a quantitative model of the relationship between fiber dose and carcinogenic response for a generalized "asbestos" exposure resulting in either lung cancer or mesothelioma. That dose-response relationship is then applied to a hypothetical, but reasonable, exposure level to show potential population risk levels in populations of arbitrary size. In the final section, the committee assesses risks for other types of fibers and, in some cases, for other diseases by qualitative comparisons with the base case of a generalized asbestos exposure.

QUANTITATIVE RISK ASSESSMENT

In the previous chapters, the committee extensively reviewed information on the health effects of asbestos and other asbestiform fibers. In preparing this section, it also reviewed several risk assessments for asbestos in the open literature and in government documents. On the basis of its evaluation of the quality and coverage of the information and the assessment techniques, the committee decided that a quantitative assessment of the risks for mesothelioma and lung cancer from nonoccupational exposures to asbestos would be meaningful. It also concluded that the information base was insufficient for useful quantitative assessments for other fiber types and diseases, but that in some cases a qualitative, comparative assessment was feasible and useful. These decisions do not mean that the asbestos assessment is without major uncertainties nor does it mean that the comparative assessments are of poor quality. In both cases, the objective is to present information useful for evaluating the health risks of asbestiform fibers in nonoccupational settings.

First, an overview of mathematical models for carcinogenic risk assessment is presented to provide a context for the assessments for lung cancer and mesothelioma, which are of principal interest. Next, there is a review of several assessments for asbestos that were based on such models. Finally, these assessments and the committee's own analyses are applied to the information presented in earlier chapters to produce quantitative risk estimates for nonoccupational exposures to asbestos in ambient air.

Mathematical Model For Carcinogenic Risk Estimate

As explained earlier, it is not necessary to use data on asbestos exposure from animal experiments to estimate risks for humans, but it is necessary to extrapolate from the health effects observed at high occupational levels of exposure to much lower nonoccupational exposures. Occupational epidemiology makes it possible to describe the probability of dying from a particular type of cancer as a function of age at first exposure, level and duration of exposure, and current age. Mathematical extrapolation models based on the multistage theory of carcinogenesis make it possible to estimate the probability of dying from that type of cancer for different ages at first exposure, different (lower) exposure levels, and different (often longer) duration of exposure, also as a function of current age. By considering the cumulative probability throughout a lifetime, the "lifetime risk" of cancer mortality can be computed.

At any age, an individual faces some probability of reaching an end point that is related to cancer in the next year, for example, dying of lung cancer. Suppose that at a given age, a, the probability is given by p(a,d), where d is the dose of the carcinogen—in this case, asbestos. When d = 0, p(a,0) is the probability of the end point for unexposed people. If t is some age of interest, then the cumulative probability P(t,d) of reaching the end point before that age is given by the sum of the annual probabilities up to that age:

$$P(t,d) = \text{the sum of } p(a,d) \text{ over all ages, } a, \leq t. \qquad (1)$$

Reaching the end point by time t is analogous to the "failure time" for a generalized system that is no longer effective after time t. General mathematical analysis can be used to show that the probability of failure as a function of time can be written as follows:

$$P(t,d) = 1 - e^{-I(t,d)}, \qquad (2)$$

where I(t,d) represents the cumulative incidence function (or cumulative hazard function) of occurrence of the observable failure prior to time t.

Armitage and Doll (1961), Peto et al. (1982), Kalbfleisch and Prentice (1980), Hartley and Sielken (1977), Hartley et al. (1981), and Kalbfleisch et al. (1983) have applied this model to carcinogenesis. If the cumulative incidence I(t,d) is small, then equation (2) may be simplified to

$$P(t,d) \doteq I(t,d), \quad (3)$$

where $\doteq$ means approximately.

In carcinogenic risk assessment, attention is usually focussed on the cumulative incidence function I(t,d) rather than on the probability function P(t,d). The Armitage-Doll (1961) multistage theory of carcinogenesis suggests that I(t,d) can be written as a product of two terms—g(d), depending only on dose, and h(t), depending only on time. That is,

$$I(t,d) = g(d)\ h(t). \quad (4)$$

If there are k dose-dependent stages in the process of carcinogenesis and the rate of transformation from one stage to the next is assumed to be a linear function of dose, the function g(d) would be a polynomial of degree k in the dose. The function h(t) depends only on time. This model and its generalization and justification have been discussed by Crump et al. (1976), Hartley et al. (1981), and Kalbfleisch et al. (1983).

To determine the values of the constants in the polynomial g(d) and the functional form for h(t), the cumulative incidence function must be fitted to data—preferably to data based on observations in human populations. The multistage model described above has been fitted successfully to many sets of cancer data, including data on asbestos, and appears at present to be a generally adequate model for assessing cancer risk. Fitting equation (4) to data involves estimating the constants in the model for some suitably determined function h(t). This model has been applied to both mesothelioma and lung cancer data on asbestos-exposed workers. The form of h(t) and the values of the constants from those studies will be discussed in the next section. The function g(d)—and thus the cumulative excess incidence function I(t,d)—can be approximated as a linear function of dose in the low-dose range that equals 0 when d = 0. This relationship can be used for extrapolating from high to low doses and has the following form:

$$I(t,d) = cdh(t). \quad (5)$$

This form assumes that there is at least one dose-dependent stage of cancer development. The argument for a linear (with respect to dose) approximation for low-dose exposures has been justified on the basis that the exposure dose d is added to a background level (Hoel, 1980; Peto, 1978). This assumption may not always be justified in application (see Cornfield et al., 1978 and Van Ryzin, 1981), but it should lead to an appropriate upper bound for the committee's risk assessments for asbestos. Furthermore, and more importantly, ruling out a linear dose term for asbestos exposure does not seem justified by the data now available (Nicholson, 1983; Peto, 1982; Schneiderman et al., 1981). Thus, the model adopted for risk assessment in the next three sections of this chapter is based on the cancer mortality incidence calculated by equation (5).

PUBLISHED RISK ASSESSMENTS

This section reviews some published risk assessments for lung cancer and mesothelioma. These assessments helped the committee select a functional form for h(t) for the two diseases and to establish the value of the constant c in equation (5).

Lung Cancer Risk from Nonoccupational Environmental Exposures

The following summary of risk assessments for lung cancer from asbestos exposures is based on data on exposure of worker populations. These data suggest that the function I(t,d) in equation (5) becomes

$$I(t,d) = c^{*}T_0 d I_0(t), \qquad (6)$$

where T_0 is the duration of exposure to asbestos at dose d, $I_0(t)$ is the cumulative mortality incidence for lung cancer up to age t for Chose who have not been exposed to asbestos, and c^{*} is a constant that depends on the cohort under study, but not on dose or age. As used in equation (6) and in the remainder of this section, d is the concentration of fibers in the workplace air, usually measured in fibers/cm^3. Although d is referred to as dose, some authors would call it dose rate and would refer to the product T_0d as (cumulative) dose. Equation (6), derived by Peto (1982), is consistent with his earlier studies of chrysotile workers (Peto, 1978). This equation is also supported by four studies reviewed by Nicholson (1983), who noted that the relative risk of lung cancer deaths for asbestos workers compared to a similar population was linearly related to the accumulated dose years, i.e., fibers/cm^3 x years, or (fibers/cm^3)yr.

In equation (6), the underlying incidence rate $I_0(t)$ is considerably different for smokers and nonsmokers of each sex. Therefore, the risks for each of these groups must be assessed separately. Another consequence of equation (6) is that the relative risk of lung cancer due to asbestos exposure does not depend on age at first exposure.

Thus, lifelong risk of lung cancer resulting from exposure to asbestos can be calculated quite simply by using equation (6). As an example, consider the following calculation given by Peto (1982).

Consider the effect of 10 years of exposure at 1 fiber/cm^3. If we assume that the relative risk for lung cancer among insulation workers increased approximately fourfold [Hammond et al. (1979) reported 4.2 for nonsmokers and 3.9 for smokers] and that this risk is based on a cumulative dose of 600 fibers/cm^3 (20 years at 30 fibers/cm^3), then 10 years of exposure to 1 fiber/cm^3 will increase the relative risk by $4.0 \times 10/600 = 0.067$. Since approximately 15% of lifelong smokers die of lung cancer, this mortality rate will increase to $0.15 \times 1.067 \times 100$, or 16%. Thus, the difference (1%) is the excess due to asbestos as predicted by the equation. Since only 0.5% of nonsmokers die of lung cancer, this would become 0.533% ($0.005 \times 1.067 \times 100$) for an added risk of 0.033% due to asbestos exposure.

Mesothelioma Risk from Nonoccupational Environmental Exposures

The committee reviewed two estimations of mesothelioma risk, one by Peto and his colleagues (Peto, 1982; Peto et al., 1982) and the other by Nicholson (1983). These analyses and their consequences are summarized in this section.

Using the data of Selikoff et al. (1979) on mortality among 17,800 members of the International Association of Heat and Frost Insulators and Asbestos Workers, Peto et al. (1982) showed that the mortality rate from mesothelioma in these workers was dependent on the time since first exposure, but did not depend on the age at first exposure. From this finding, and the application of the multistage theory of carcinogenesis through equation (5), the cumulative incidence function becomes:

$$I(t,d) = cd(t - t_0)^k, \qquad (7)$$

where $t-t_0$ represents time since first exposure at age t_0. For any group of workers exposed at the same dose level d, the product $cd = b$ is a constant depending on the type of asbestos exposure. Equation (7) suggests that the risk for mesothelioma is primarily dependent on the time since first exposure ($t-t_0$). This same phenomenon was noted by Schneiderman et al. (1981) and Nicholson (1983). Fitting equation (7) with $b = cd$ to the data of Selikoff et al. (1979) for men up to age 80 by the method of maximum likelihood estimation resulted in an estimate of $k = 3.2$ with a standard error of $\pm$ 0.36 and $b = 4.37 \times 10^{-8}$. Using this calculation, Peto et al. (1982) estimated the lifelong mesothelioma risk for this worker group to be 15%, 7%, and 3% for age at first exposures of 20, 30, and 40 years, respectively. These figures have been adjusted for other competing causes of death.

Using equation (7) with $k = 3.2$, Peto and colleagues determined that $b \times 10^8$ ranges in value from 2.94 to 5.15 for four other sets of data (see Table 7-1). Using $k = 3.5$, Peto (1982) computed a lifetime mesothelioma rate of I in 100,000 children exposed from age 12 to age 18 (i.e., 6 years of school age), assuming the fiber level was 0.003 fiber/cm^3 (1/1,000 of the exposure of the insulation workers).

TABLE 7-1. Mesothelioma Death Rates in Various Studies and Predictions of Risk[a]

		Corresponding Lifetime Risk (%)[b] by Age at First Exposure (yrs)		
Study Population and Reference	Relative Risk ($b \times 10^8$)	20	30	40
North American insulation workers (mixed exposure) Selikoff et al., 1979	4.37	15	7	3
Factory workers (mixed exposure) Newhouse and Berry, 1976	4.95	17	8	3
Chrysotile textile factory workers Peto, 1980b	2.94	10	5	2
Australian crocidolite miners Hobbs et al., 1980	5.15	17	8	3
U.S. amosite factory workers Seidman et al., 1979	4.91	17	8	3

[a] Adapted from Peto et al. (1982). The death rate at time $t\text{-}t_0$ since first exposure at age t_0 is proportional to b, obtained by fitting equation (7) with k = 3.2.

[b] The calculation of lifetime risk," i.e., the percentage of similarly exposed men who would die of mesothelioma before age 80, is based on an actuarial calculation using 1977 U.S. rates for white males for all causes of death other than mesothelioma inflated by a factor of 1.26, the observed relative risk among insulation workers (Selikoff et al., 1979).

A second risk assessment was done by Nicholson (1983), who criticized the Peto et al. (1982) analysis for fitting equation (7) to only those men who died of mesothelioma up to age 80. By including all insulation workers, he estimated k to be 5.0.

QUANTITATIVE RISK ASSESSMENT FOR NONOCCUPATIONAL ENVIRONMENTAL EXPOSURES

As a starting point for assessing the risk from nonoccupational environmental exposure to asbestiform fibers, the committee adopted equation (6) as representing the cumulative mortality up to age t, which is appropriate for lung cancer induced by a continuous exposure of T_0 years at dose level d in fibers/cm^3. This model implies that any given total dose before time t would have the same effect on the relative risk at time t, regardless of the time at which exposure started or its duration. The model thus ignores a minimum latency period, which might cause the model to overestimate effects, but also ignores the difference between exposures at earlier and later ages, which might cause the model to underestimate effects.

Equation (7) was assumed to be a reasonable representation of the cumulative mortality from mesothelioma up to age t for continuous exposure to asbestos at dose level d in fibers/cm^3 from age t_0 until age t. In this case, latency is implicitly included in the dependence on (t-t_0), because k is greater than 1, but no minimum latency is assumes. These assumptions are supported by the work of Peto (1982), Peto et al. (1982), Nicholson (1983), and Schneiderman et al. (1981), who extensively reviewed the basis for these assumptions by examining the models and their consistency for several observed worker cohorts exposed to ambient concentrations of asbestos fibers. These authors have suggested that asbestos acts as a late-stage carcinogen in producing lung cancer but acts at earlier stages in the development of mesothelioma. Using these models, the committee developed lifetime estimates of risk for lung cancer and mesothelioma mortality from continuous nonoccupational exposures to 0.0004 fibers/cm^3 and for 0.002 fibers/cm^3.

For lung cancer, the committee assessed the risk for four exposure subgroups: male smokers, female smokers, male nonsmokers, and female nonsmokers. For mesothelioma, only one calculation was made, since equation (7) and the supporting data in the papers cited above suggest that mesothelioma mortality does not depend on sex or smoking history, but does depend strongly on age at first exposure.

Lifetime Risk Estimates For Lung Cancer and Mesothelioma

Table 7-2 summarizes lifetime risk estimates for lung cancer and mesothelioma for nonoccupational environmental exposures to 0.0004 fibers/cm^3 (a median level) and 0.002 fibers/cm^3 (a high level). It is assumed this exposure is continuous from birth through a lifetime of 73 years, an approximate average lifetime in the United States. Thus, in equations (6) and (7), $t = 73$ years and $d = 0.0004$ or 0.002. In equation (6), $T_0 = 73$ and in equation (7), $t_0 = 0$ to account for continuous exposure. Because equations (6) and (7) are linear in the dose unit d, one can immediately obtain from Table 7-2 lifetime risks at other continuous (from birth) environmental exposures by multiplying by the appropriate dose factor. For example, lifetime risk estimates at 0.02 fibers/cm^3 are 10 times higher than the estimates at 0.002 fibers/cm^3.

TABLE 7-2. Estimated Individual Lifetime Risks from a Continuous Exposure to Asbestos at 0.0004 Fibers/cm3 (a Median Dose) or 0.002 Fibers/cm3 (a High Dose)[a]

		Estimated Individual Lifetime Risk × 106	
Disease	Exposure Group	Median Exposure (0.0004 fibers/cm^3)	High Exposure (0.002 fibers/cm^3
Lung cancer[b]	Male smoker	64 (0 to 290)[c]	320 (0 to 1,500)
Lung cancer	Female smoker	23 (0 to 110)	120 (0 to 530)
Lung cancer	Male nonsmoker	6 (0 to 22)	29 (0 to 130)
Lung cancer	Female nonsmoker	3 (0 to 13)	15 (0 to 66)
Mesothelioma	All	9 (0 to 350)	46 (0 to 1,700)

[a] Lifetime assumed to be 73 years; exposure occurs from birth. Lung cancer risks are calculated with C* = 1.02 or an excess risk of 2% per (fiber/cm^3)yr, estimated from nine studies with varied results. Mesothelioma risks are calculated with $c = 2.53 \times 10^{-8}$ and $k = 3.2$, estimated from five studies with varied results. See also explanations in text.

[b] Sex differences for lung cancer risk are due to differences in lung cancer background rates associated with smoking patterns, occupational exposures, and other factors.

[c] Range of estimates. The lower limit of 0 is always possible if linear extrapolation overestimates risk. See also text below.

The estimates in Table 7-2 were based on the following five considerations:

- Exposure levels. A mix of indoor and outdoor measured exposure levels was used to select the median value of 0.0004 fibers/cm^3 and the high value of 0.002 fibers/cm^3 as the reference levels.
- Use of the linear model. The models used by the committee all assume low-dose linearity and, as such, produce higher estimates of risk at low doses than would be obtained with other models. However, because the occupational data do not rule out low-dose linearity, the committee believes that these estimates do not unduly overstate the risks.
- Count-mass conversion. The conversion of ambient fiber mass measurements to an equivalent number of fibers was based on measurements

of mass and numbers of fibers in the workplace, The committee realized, however, that the number of fibers in ambient air would be much greater because these fibers tend to be smaller than those in the workplace (see Chapter 4). Depending on the toxicity of small fibers, the risks could be greater or less than those calculated in this chapter. If the presence of long fibers is necessary for a toxic response, risks would be lower.

- Model dependence. The results of the mesochelioma model depend very heavily on the value of k. This accounts for the large range of estimates for mesothelioma. It is assumed that this dependence on k among workers holds for the entire population throughout a lifetime. If the dependence is not as strong (i.e., a lower k value), the lower end of the range would apply. If this dependence is as strong (i.e., a higher k value), the upper bound may be more appropriate.
- Childhood exposure. The models used for extrapolation for both lung cancer and mesothelioma are based on the assumption that a unit dose of exposure (measured as fibers/cm^3 > 5 µm long) in early life is equivalent in its intrinsic carcinogenic potential to a unit dose in later life. If children are more biologically sensitive than the worker group, the risk per unit dose would be increased. Results from studies of exposure to other materials indicate that children are often more sensitive than adults to a given dose, even when expressed as dose/body weight.

The risk estimates and ranges shown in Table 7-2 are those the committee considers most reasonable. Because of the uncertain value of k and the sensitivity of equation (7) to its value, the range of estimates is much larger for mesothelioma than for lung cancer. Two conclusions can be drawn from the estimates in Table 7-2:

- For nonsmokers, the lifetime risk for mesothelioma from non-occupational environmental exposure to asbestos is higher than for lung cancer. For smokers, however, the risks of lung cancer are substantially higher than for mesothelioma, because of the multiplicative interaction of smoking and asbestos exposures.
- Individual lifetime risk estimates for lung cancer from nonoccupational environmental exposures to 0.0004 fibers/cm^3 are much lower than the risks observed for smoking.

The basis for the calculations in Table 7-2 is discussed in detail in the following two subsections.

Calculation of the Lung Cancer Risk Estimates in Table 7-2. Calculating lifetime risk estimates from equation (6) involves the notion of relative risk up to time t, designated here as RR. From equation (6), the RR for lung cancer by age r can be shown as follows:

$$\frac{I(t,d)}{I_0(t)} \tag{8}$$

$$= \frac{\text{cumulative lung cancer mortality by age t at dose d}}{\text{baseline cumulative lung cancer mortality by age t}}$$

$$= c^*(T_0d),$$

where (T_0d) = total dose-years for the exposed group and c^* is a constant that depends on the cohort, For a given study showing an increased relative risk for lung cancer,

$$c^* = (1 + P/100), \tag{9}$$

where P is the percentage increase in lung cancer risk per unit dose [% per (fibers/cm^3)yr]. Schneiderman et al. (1981) presented the values of P for nine different worker cohorts. The results are summarized in Table 7-3.

Values for P in Table 7-3 range from 0.06 (Study 8) to 9.1 (Study 1). The higher value establishes the upper end of the range given in Table 7-2. The zero value for the lower end of the range indicates that the low-dose linear approximation in equation (5) may overstate risk.

The median value for P in the studies shown in Table 7-3 is P = 1.1 (Study 7). This value, rounded upward to 2, was used in obtaining the estimates for lifetime lung cancer risk in Table 7-2. To calculate these estimates, it was necessary to know only the baseline absolute risks for the appropriate subpopulations. The baseline cumulative incidence rates of lung cancer for the four subgroups in Table 7-2 have been estimated by Schneiderman et al. (1981) as follows: male smokers = 0.11; female smokers = 0.04; male nonsmokers = 0.01; and female nonsmokers = 0.005.

Thus, using 2% as a value for P, the lifetime risk of lung cancer for a male smoker is

$$(0.11)(1 + P/100) = (0.11)(1 + 0.02) = 0.1122. \tag{10}$$

The increased lifetime risk attributable to asbestos exposure at 1 fiber/tin^3 for 1 year is 0.0022, i.e., 0.1122-0.1100. At the ambient exposure of 0.0004 fibers/cm^3 assumed in Table 7-2 and for a 73-year lifetime exposure, the increased lifetime risk of lung cancer is 6.42×10^{-5}, i.e., $0.0022 \times 0.0004 \times 73$. Rounding to two significant figures gives the estimate in Table 7-2 for male smokers. The other calculations in that table were derived in a similar fashion.

When describing the use of the percentages given in Table 7-3, Schneiderman et al. (1981) commented that the low percentage increases in risk in Studies 3, 6, 8, and 9 probably resulted from several factors. In Study 3, for example, the subjects were retirees older than 65.

TABLE 7-3. Estimated Increase in Lung Cancer Risk per Unit of Exposure to Asbestos[a]

Study No.	Occupation of Worker Cohort	Asbestos Type	Percent Increase in Lung Cancer Risk per (fibers/cm^3)yr	Reference
1	Insulation manufacturing	Amosite	9.1	Seidman et al., 1979
2	Asbestos product manufacturing	Crocidolite, chrysotile, and amosite	1.3 males 8.4 females	Newhouse and Berry, 1979
3	Asbestos manufacturing	Amosite and chrysotile; some crocidolite	0.3	Henderson and Enterline, 1979
4	Asbestos product manufacturing	Chrysotile; some amosite and crocidolite	1.1	Nicholson et al., 1979
5	Textile production	Chrysotile	5.3	Dement et al., 1982
6	Textile production	Chrysotile	0.07 early employees[b] 0.8 later employees[b]	Peto, 1980
7	Insulation manufacturing	Chrysotile and amosite	1.7	Selikoff et al., 1979
8	Mining and milling	Chrysotile	0.06	McDonald and Liddell 1979
9	Mining and milling	Chrysotile	0.15	Nicholson et al., 1979

[a] Adapted from Table 4 in Schneiderman et al., 1981.

[b] Early employees began work before or during 1950. Later employees began work after 1950.

Schneiderman et al. stated that the investigators may thus have missed asbestos-related deaths occurring at earlier ages. In Study 6, the disease rates for workers employed earlier were lower than those employed later who were followed for shorter periods. The discrepancy has diminished as more data have accumulated. The subjects in Studies 8 and 9 were mining and milling workers whose exposure patterns were quite different from environmental ambient air exposures. There is also some evidence that many lung cancer cases were missed in Studies 8 and 9 because of competing causes of death at earlier ages. Thus, Schneiderman et al. (1981) concluded that the range from 1.1 (Study 4) to 9.1 (Study 1) is the most representative of true values. The value of $P = 2$ used in the calculations in Table 7-2 falls near the bottom of this range, but is within a factor of 5 of the top of the range. If we use $P = 5$, which is the middle of the range, the lung cancer risk estimates in Table 7-2 would be multiplied by a factor of 2.5.

Calculation of Mesothelioma Risk Estimates. To calculate the lifetime risk with equation (7), the numbers c and k must be determined. Then the lifetime risk L at $d = 0.0004$ fibers/cm^3, assuming $t = 73$ and $t_0 = 0$ (continuous exposure from birth to age 73), is

$$L = c(0.0004)(73)^k. \quad (11)$$

To apply this equation, c and k must be estimated from epidemiological studies of occupational exposures to asbestos. Each study must be stratified by duration of exposure ($t-t_0$) to estimate these parameters. Most of the following analysis is similar to that of Peto et al. (1982).

First, let us consider the choice of k. As noted earlier, when Peto et al. (1982) fitted equation (7) to the data of Selikoff et al. (1979), they obtained the equation $I(t,d) = b(t-t_0)^{3.2}$, with $b = 4.37$ and $k = 3.2 \pm 0.36$ (standard error). In equation (11), therefore, we initially use $k = 3.2$. Modifications using different values for k will give the range of estimates for $d = 0.0004$ fibers/cm^3 in Table 7-2. For $d = 0.002$ fibers/cm^3, we replace 0.0004 with 0.002 in equation (11). With $k = 3.2$, Peto et al. (1982) also fitted four other data sets to obtain four values of b in the equation $I(t,d) = b(t-t_0)^{3.2}$. The value of b is specific to each worker cohort and depends on three numbers: d (the average fiber/cm^3 exposure), ℓ (the average length of exposure), and $t-t_0$ (the average time since first exposure). These values are given in Table 7-4. In addition, Table 7-4 contains the estimates of c that are appropriate for equation (7), based on the corresponding estimate of b given by Peto et al. (1982). When exposure is not continuous from time of first exposure (t_0) to the age of observation (t) for these studies, the relationship between b and c changes from $c = b/d$ to

$$\frac{4.56\ b/d}{1 - [1 - \ell/(t-t_0)]^{3.2}} . \quad (12)$$

TABLE 7-4. Estimated Constants for Equations (11) and (12) for Five Studies

Study	b × 10^8	d^a	$\bar{\ell}^a$	$t-t_0^a$	c × 10^8
Selikoff et al., 1979	4.37	15	15	24	1.39
Newhouse and Berry, 1976	4.95	12.5	6	31.5	3.67
Peto, 1980 a,b	2.94	16.5	14	22.5	0.85
Hobbs et al., 1980	5.15	NA[b]	NA	NA	NA
Seidman et al., 1979	4.91	35	1	35	7.22

[a] Estimated from data given in Tables 4 and 10 of Schneiderman et al. (1981), using estimated median values. The product d ℓ from columns 3 and 4 above is the estimated cumulative exposure in (fiber/cm^3)yr of their Table 10.
[b] NA = not available.

The factor 4.56 adjusts from occupational exposures at about 1,920 hours per year to environmental exposures at 8,760 hours per year. Appendix G provides the mathematical basis for equation (12). Table 7-4 gives the values of the constants for each study in which Peto et al. (1982) estimated b.

To obtain the estimates for mesothelioma at the dose of 0.0004 fibers/cm^3 in Table 7-2, equation (11) is used with values for c from Table 7-4 and k = 3.2. In Table 7-2 the lifetime risk for mesothelioma at d = 0.0004 fibers/cm^3 is 9 per million. This is calculated from equation (11) with $c = 2.53 \times 10^{-8}$, the median of the range of the c values in Table 7-4, and k = 3.2. The highest value of the range in Table 7-2 at d = 0.0004 uses equation (11) with $c = 7.22 \times 10^{-8}$, the upper value of c in Table 7-4, and k = 3.8, obtained from $3.2 + 1.65 \times 0.36$. The selection of 3.8 as the value for k is based on an approximate upper 95% confidence limit for the estimate of k. The lower limit is taken as 0, which is always a possible lower limit, especially if the low-dose linear assumption in equation (5) overestimates the individual lifetime risk.

Peto (1982) recommended using a k value of 3.5 for risk assessment purposes. As an example, he estimated that the risk of mesothelioma for children exposed for a 6-year period (ages 12 to 18) at 0.003 fibers/cm^3 would be one in 100,000. Nicholson reviewed additional data, including data on older workers up to age 80, and determined that a k value would be 5. Schneiderman et al. (1981) used $k = 3.0$. For this study, the committee used a value of 3.2. Although neither existing data nor biological theory can provide very much guidance on the value of k, its value is very important in projecting the lifetime risks of mesothelioma from asbestos exposures. Table 7-5 shows how lifetime risk varies from the value of 9 per million for several values of k. Also shown are risk estimates for other values of c. The reader can easily calculate the results for other values of exposure.

Other authors have also estimated the risks of mesotheliomas. Enterline (1983) derived a lifetime risk of 100 per million by using current reported rates of mesothelioma, an assumption about the relative contributions of nonoccupational and occupational asbestos exposures, and other factors. This estimate clearly relates to past exposure to varying levels of asbestos. Schneiderman et al. (1981) estimated lifetime risks for mesothelioma to be between 800 and 5,000 per million for a cumulative exposure of 1 (fiber/cm^3)yr. These estimates correspond to lifetime risks of 23 to 150 per million for 0.0004 fibers/cm^3 for 73 years. As mentioned above, these investigators effectively assumed $k = 3$, but their equivalent c was higher than that used for the corresponding estimates in Tables 7-2 and 7-5.

TABLE 7-5. Sensitivity of Estimates for Lifetime Risks[a] of Mesothelioma to Values of k and c

	Lifetime Risk Estimates × 10^6, Using k Values from Various Studies						
	This Study (low)	Schneiderman et al., 1981	This Study (middle)	Peto et al., 1982 (middle)	This Study (high)	Peto et al., 1982 (high)	Nicholson, 1983
k / c	2.6	3.0	3.2	3.5	3.8	4.0	5.0
0.85×10^{-8}	0.2	1.3	3	11	41	97	7,000
2.53×10^{-8}	0.7	4	9	34	120	290	21,000
7.22×10^{-8}	2	11	26	96	350	820	60,000

[a] All estimates are derived from equation (11), $L = c(0.0004)(73)^k$, where L = lifetime risk at a continuous exposure to 0.0004 fibers/cm^3 for a lifetime of 73 years.

Note: This table demonstrates that the risk estimates are extremely sensitive to changes in the value of k.

The Use of 0.0004 Fibers/cm^3 and 0.002 Fibers/cm^3 as the Median and,. High Nonoccupational Environmental Exposure Levels. The lifetime risk estimates given in Table 7-2 are based on an assumed continuous environmental ambient exposure equivalent to either 0.0004 or 0.002 fibers longer than 5 μm per cm^3 of air breathed. The committee believes that 0.0004 fibers/cm^3 is a reasonable assumption for a median population exposure level and that 0.002 fibers/cm^3 is a reasonable high exposure level (considering only exposures from breathing ambient air continuously). These assumptions are discussed below. The effects of noncontinuous high exposures are discussed later in this chapter.

Table 7-6 summarizes some environmental asbestos sampling data provided by Nicholson (1983). To convert from mass measurements (ng/m^3) of airborne exposures to fiber counts (fibers/cm^3), the committee used the conversion factor of 30 μg/m^3 for 1 fiber/cm^3. (See Chapter 4 of this report, Schneiderman et al., 1981, and Consumer Product Safety Commission, 1983 for further explanation.)

The dose-response data used in the committee's risk estimate were taken from measurements of exposures in the workplace, where the fibers tend to be longer than those in ambient environments not close to major sources of asbestos. As discussed in Chapter 4, there would typically be approximately 2,000 fibers per nanogram in workplace air; in remote areas, however, there would be approximately 70,000 ambient fibers in a nanogram. To convert mass in the workplace to ambient air, the committee used the number of fibers longer than 5 μm that would be found in the workplace when the workplace mass equaled the remote ambient fiber mass. The dose estimate in numbers of fibers would be approximately 35 times greater (70,000/2,000) if the actual sizes of fibers in ambient air were considered. If we assume that all fibers are equally potent, then the risk estimates would be correspondingly higher. On the other hand, fiber size apparently affects fiber potency, but the appropriate adjustment factors for fiber size are not known.

Table 7-6 indicates that median concentrations in outdoor air have ranged from 0.00002 to 0.00075 fibers/cm^3 in several studies (sample sets 1 to 8); their median is approximately 0.00007 fibers/cm^3. The observed median inside rooms without asbestos is 0.00054 (sample set 9). In rooms with asbestos surfaces, the median is 0.0006 fibers/cm^3 (range of medians for sample sets 10 through 14, 0.00006 to 0.00405 fibers/cm^3). If these three medians are weighted by assuming persons spend approximately one-fourth of their time outdoors, five-eighths of their time indoors in uncontaminated rooms, and one-eighth of their time in asbestos-contaminated rooms, a reasonable estimate for a median population exposure is 0.0004 fibers/cm^3.

The committee also used 0.002 fibers/cm^3 for a high value of continuous exposure in its calculations for Table 7-2. This value was obtained by using the median of the 90th percentiles in Table 7-6 for each exposure subcategory. For outdoor air, the median is 0.0003

TABLE 7-6. Summary of Environmental Asbestos Exposure Samples[a]

		Measured Concentration (ng/m³)		Equivalent Concentration (fibers/cm³)[b]		
Sample Sets	No. of Samples	Median	90th Percentile	Median	90th Percentile	Reference
1. Paris air	161	0.7	3.2	0.00002	0.00011	Sabastien et al., 1980
2. Paris (outdoor control)	19	0.7	5.2	0.00002	0.00017	Sebastien et al., 1980
3. Outdoor control samples, for U.S. schools	31	0.9	9.8	0.00003	0.00033	Constant et al., 1982
4. Air of 48 U.S. cities	187	1.6	6.8	0.00005	0.00023	Nicholson, 1971
5. Air of U.S. cities	127	2.3	7.8	0.00008	0.00026	Agency, 1974
6. Air of five U.S. cities (outdoor control sample)	34	6.7	31.9	0.00022	0.00106	Nicholson et al., 1975, 1976
7. New York City air	22	13.7	42.9	0.00046	0.00143	Nicholson et al., 1971
8. Air 0.5 mile (0.8 km) from asbestos spraying	17	22.5	82.6	0.00075	0.00275	Nicholson et al., 1971
9. Air in U.S. schoolrooms without asbestos	31	16.3	72.7	0.00054	0.00242	Constant et al., 1982
10. Air in Paris buildings with asbestos surfaces	135	1.8	32.2	0.00006	0.00107	Sebastien et al., 1980
11. Air in U.S. buildings with cementitious asbestos	28	7.9	19.1	0.00026	0.00064	Nicholson et al., 1975, 1976
12. Air in U.S. buildings with friable asbestos	54	19.2	96.2	0.00064	0.00321	Nicholson et al., 1975, 1976
13. Air in U.S. schoolrooms with asbestos surfaces	54	62.5	550	0.00208	0.01833	Constant et al., 1982
14. Air in U.S. schools with damaged asbestos surfacing materials	27	121.5	465	0.00405	0.01550	Nicholson et al., 1978

[a] Adapted from Nicholson, 1983.

[b] Based on conversion factor of 30 μg/m³ = 1 fiber/cm³.

fibers/cm^3; for indoor uncontaminated air, it is 0.002 fibers/cm^3; and for indoor asbestos-contaminated air, it is 0.003 fibers/cm^3. The same distribution of occupancy over time was used to arrive at the 0.002 fibers/cm^3 figure for a high exposure level.

Risk Assessments For Special Subpopulations

Table 7-2 shows lifetime risk estimates for people who are exposed throughout their lives to levels of either 0.0004 or 0.002 fibers/cm^3 in ambient air. The predominant risk is from mesothelioma, but lung cancers also contribute to the risk, especially for male smokers. For exposure patterns that are different from those assumed, lifetime risks could be higher or lower. The following are three illustrations of how lifetime risks could be derived for such special populations.

Children Exposed in Asbestos-Contaminated Schools. The committee estimated the risk for persons exposed from birth to age 73 years to environmental levels of 0.002 fibers/cm^3 (as assumed in Table 7-2) plus an additional risk from a 10-year exposure (from ages 6 to 16) in an asbestos-contaminated schoolroom for 6 hours daily, 200 days per year, to 0.02 fibers/cm^3 (550 ng/m^3, the 90th percentile in Table 7-6). The equivalent continuous daily 10-year exposure is approximately 0.003 fibers/cm^3, i.e., $0.02 \times (200 \times 6)/(365 \times 24)$. Using equation (6), the lifetime risk of lung cancer for a male who eventually becomes a smoker is $0.003 \times 10 \times 0.0022$, or 66 in a million. This risk represents an approximately 20% addition to his ambient lifetime risk of 320 in a million ($0.002 \times 73 \times 0.0022$), for a total of about 390 in a million. For such an individual, the schoolroom exposure adds relatively more to the risk of mesothelioma, as shown below. Using equations (G4) and (G5) in Appendix G for the lifetime mesothelioma risk, L, at t = 73 for an exposure of $\ell = 10$ years starting at age $t_0 = 6$ at the dose level d, this risk can be calculated from the formula:

$$L = cd\{1-[1 - \ell/(t-t_0)]^k\}(t-t_0)^k$$

, with d = 0.003, $\ell = 10$, $t-t_0 = 73-6 = 67$, and k = 3.2. This lifetime mesothelioma risk becomes

$$L = c(0.003)\{1-[1-(10/67)]^{3.2}\}(67)^{3.2} = 845c.$$

If c is the median value of Table 7-4 (i.e., $c = 2.53 \times 10^{-8}$), the estimated lifetime mesothelioma risk, L, from the 10-year exposure is 21×10^{-6}.

This risk is then added to the background risk of 46×10^{-6} in Table 7-2, giving a lifetime mesothelioma risk for this subpopulation of 67×10^{-6}. If a million people had received such a pattern of exposures, about 67 might be expected to die of mesothelioma. In this example, the contribution to total risk from the schoolrooms is less than that of the lifetime exposure to the lower concentrations of asbestos estimated for the ambient air. However, if the value for k in Equation (7) were higher than 3.2, the significance of the schoolroom exposures would increase because of the stronger dependence on time since first exposure. For example, if k = 3.8, the highest value used in Table 7-2, the lifetime mesothelioma risk would be 910×10^{-6}. If k were less than 3.2, the corresponding lifetime risk for mesothelioma would be less than 67×10^{-6}. These calculations show that childhood exposures to asbestiform fibers might contribute noticeable lifetime mesothelioma risks to those so exposed.

A Female Nonsmoker in a Relatively Asbestos-Free Environment. An example of a person in a low-risk group is a female nonsmoker exposed to an average level of 0.0001 fibers/tin^3. This exposure level would not be too unlikely for a person exposed primarily to rural indoor and outdoor air, since 0.00002 fibers/tin^3 is the lowest median value for all the outdoor city readings in Table 7-6. Then, the calculations in Table 7-2 would lead to a mesothelioma lifetime risk of 2.25×10^{-6} (9×10^{-6} divided by 4) plus a lung cancer lifetime risk of 0.73×10^{-6}. The lifetime individual risk for such a person would be 3×10^{-6} for both types of cancer.

A Male Smoker Living in an Area Contaminated with High Levels of Asbestos Who is Also Exposed to High Indoor Concentrations. As an example of a high-risk person, consider an urban male smoker exposed to 0.003 fibers/cm^3 for one-half the time and 0.018 fibers/cm^3 for the other half. This pattern is based on the assumption that the subject spends one-half of his time in indoor environments with a high asbestos concentration (see sample sets 13 and 14 of Table 7-6) and one-half either in highly contaminated outdoor environments (see sample sets 7 and 8 of Table 7-6) or in indoor environments at the high end of the distribution for rooms that are normally not contaminated with asbestos (see sample set 9 of Table 7-6). Thus, his continuous average exposure would be approximately 0.01 fibers/cm^3, i.e., 0.5(0.003) + 0.5(0.018). Therefore, multiplying the second column of Table 7-2 by a factor of 5 ($0.01 = 5 \times 0.002$) would give the individual lifetime risks for such a person as 1.8×10^{-3} for the two forms of cancer taken together (230×10^{-6} for mesothelioma and $1{,}600 \times 10^{-6}$ for lung cancer). This lifetime risk is the additional incurred risk attributable to the nonoccupational environmental exposure to asbestos and does not include the risk incurred by the smoking itself. The portion of the additional risk attributable to lung cancer is considerably higher than it would be for a nonsmoker experiencing identical asbestos exposures.

COMPARATIVE RISK ASSESSMENT

Methods

The goal of comparative risk assessments is to determine whether the fiber exposure in question presents risks—in terms of total number and severity of effects per year in the United States—that are about the same, considerably more, or considerably less than those assessed quantitatively above. The quantitative assessments made in the earlier part of this chapter were based on exposure to a generalized "asbestos" fiber. Because future exposures to asbestos in the United States will be dominated by chrysotile, risks of lung cancer and mesothelioma from chrysotile inhalation are assumed to be approximately the same as those attributed in the quantitative assessment to "asbestos." However, if at equal doses chrysotile is less hazardous than the other kinds of asbestos, the assumption of equal potency may lead to overstated risk estimates.

These comparative risks are population risks, which combine information about the inherent risks that a given exposure to fibers could pose to an individual and information about the current and projected distribution of exposures over the U.S. population. Unlike the quantitative risk estimates for particular assumed exposure levels, the population risk estimates can easily change along with changing patterns of production and use. Even at a known population risk level, some individuals will receive higher than average exposures and stand at correspondingly greater individual risk, whereas the majority of the population will usually have lower risks.

General Methodological Considerations

The comparative risk assessments in this chapter are based on several factors, such as:

- fiber type

- -asbestos
- -other fibers with some similar properties

- type of effect[1]

- -lung cancer
- -mesothelioma

- route of exposure

- -inhalation
- -ingestion

- source of exposure
- population at risk

- -smokers
- -other special groups (such as schoolchildren)

[1] The committee did not assess fibrosis or nonmalignant pleural disease because functional impairment resulting from such effects would occur much less often than would the cancers at nonoccupational levels of exposures.

Taking the first three of these factors as examples, risk assessment can be visualized as a three-dimensional matrix. As shown in Figure 7-1, the best understood combinations (inhaled chrysotile and crocidolite asbestos for lung cancer and mesothelioma) are in the upper right "cells" of the matrix, and the less understood combinations are successively further from that position to emphasize their "distance" from the state of knowledge necessary for quantitative risk assessment. Additional cells could be added for other combinations.

The following combinations of fiber type, effect, and route of exposure were considered for comparative risk assessments:

chrysotile/gastrointestinal cancer/ingestion
chrysotile/mesothelioma/ingestion
crocidolite/lung cancer/inhalation
crocidolite/mesothelioma/inhalation
other asbestos/all cancers/both routes
fibrous glass/lung cancer/inhalation
fibrous glass/mesothelioma/inhalation
attapulgite/lung cancer/inhalation
attapulgite/mesothelioma/inhalation
mineral wool/lung cancer/inhalation
mineral wool/mesothelioma/inhalation
ceramic fiber/lung cancer/inhalation
ceramic fiber/mesothelioma/inhalation
carbon fiber/lung cancer/inhalation
carbon fiber/mesothelioma/inhalation

The committee's results are expressed in comparison with the chrysotile/lung cancer/inhalation cell, hereafter called the prime cell. Its designation as the prime cell does not imply that it is the cell corresponding to greatest population risk. According to the calculations in the preceding section, if environmental exposures to asbestos in early life are frequent, mesothelioma may prove to be the dominant effect.

Both the comparative scores and the evaluation of the uncertainty in them were made qualitatively rather than quantitatively; the entries are symbols (+, 0, -, a, b, c) rather than numeric. Appendix H describes how the committee went about assigning, combining, and assessing the symbolic codes.

A score sheet for recording judgments about comparative risks is shown in Figure 7-2. Completed sheets for scored cells are included in Appendix H. These sheets are supplied to allow the reader to evaluate the individual judgments or the committee's subjective combination of them.

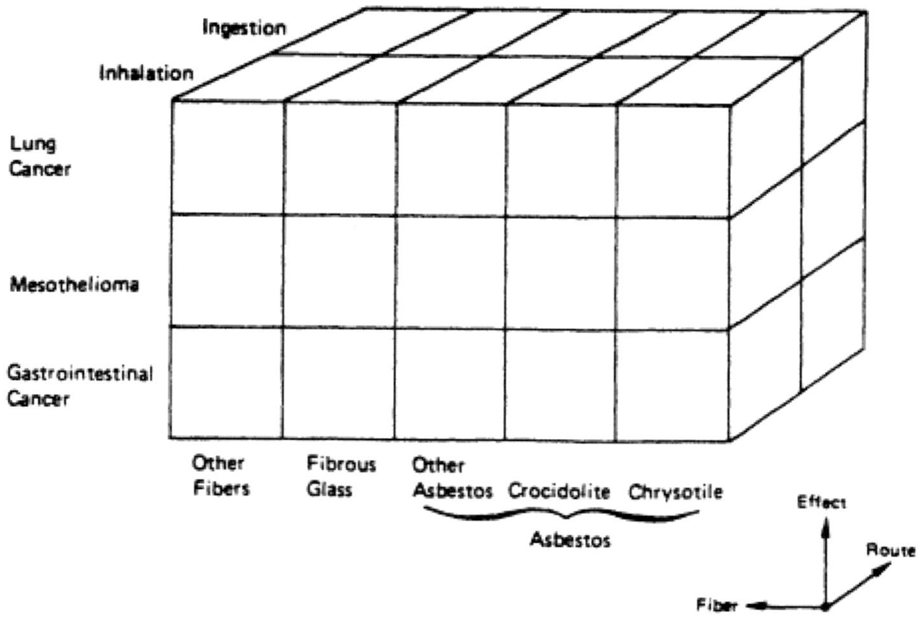

Figure 7-1.
Three-dimensional matrix for conceptualizing the risk assessment problem.

COMPARATIVE RISK ASSESSMENT SCORESHEET

Cell Scored	/	/	
	Fiber	Effect	Route
Scores Comparative with Cell	/	/	
	Fiber	Effect	Route

Exposure Score	Score	Biodisposition	Effects	Score
Production		Fiber Size		Human Studies
Use Pattern		Morphology		Animal Studies
Geography		Chemistry		In-Vitro Studies
Popular ion		Penetration		Synergism
Trends		Stability		Other
Overall risk compared with cell above				
Overall risk compared with prime cell				
Quality of comparative risk assessment				

Figure 7-2.
Score sheet for recording judgments about comparative risks.

Remarks:

Scoring Considerations

Production. If all other factors were equivalent, a greater production volume (or U.S. consumption level, if that is significantly different) would result in a greater level of exposure and a correspondingly greater population risk. If natural occurrence is important, it can be used here as another surrogate for exposure.

Use Pattern. Several concepts are embodied here. All have to do with the degree to which production, consumption, or natural occurrence will lead to actual human exposures. If the fibers are used only in products where they are tightly bound into a matrix, relatively little exposure will occur at least until final disposal, whereas loose fiber use in consumer applications would lead to relatively heavy and immediate exposures. Products such as talcum powder, which are intended for direct human will lead to higher exposures per unit production than those that are not.

Geography. This score applies to the spatial distribution of sources including natural deposits, mills or production facilities, fiber product manufacturing sites, use sites, and disposal sites. Concentrated sources tend to imply higher exposures of fewer people. This classification can also be used as a basis for evaluating such factors as the likelihood of fibers reaching drinking water.

Population. The size of the population at risk determines the extent of the hazard for a given level of individual risk. A type of fiber that yields exposures to many people, such as a constituent of a common consumer product, has more potential for producing adverse health effects than one that affects only a few people, such as a naturally occurring but noncommercial fiber that is present only in selected, sparsely populated regions.

Trends. Exposure is a dynamic process that changes with changes in total production volume, production processes, use patterns, population distribution and habits, and many other factors that do not remain static. Thus, the risk that would apply to a steady state of exposure at current levels can be misleading both for currently observed effects or for future occurrence of effects. The sharp downtrend in asbestos exposures tends to ameliorate the population risks that might otherwise be assessed, whereas new fiber types may present enormously higher exposures in the future than they do at present.

Fiber Size. Two counteracting influences are at work with fiber size. The clearest is their respirability, which declines markedly as fiber diameter increases, becoming essentially zero above 3 or 4 μm. It is likely that length also eventually affects respirability and, especially, transport potential the body. On the other hand, short fibers are probably more easily removed from the body by phagocytes; thinner ones may be more easily dissolved, coated, or gelled by body fluids; and small fibers in general may not act biologically the same as large fibers, which can disturb many cells at once. Furthermore, small fibers may be more likely to be exhaled with the tidal volume and, thus, not retained in the lung. The overall significance of fiber size may therefore be represented as a potency that is greatest for fibers around 0.2 μm diameter and 20 μm in length (Pott, 1978).

Morphology. Whatever the response to fiber size, it seems likely that long, thin fibers that have strength, durability, flexibility, and a high aspect ratio are more likely to cause adverse health effects than are fibers without these characteristics. The curliness of chrysotile fiber bundles may increase their effective aerodynamic diameter, thus decreasing their respirability below that expected on the basis of fiber diameter alone.

Chemistry. Although little is known about the influence of fiber chemistry on potential for health effects, it seems possible that the chemical properties of fibers play some role, especially respect to surface chemistry. Another feature of surface chemistry, i.e., the ability to adsorb carcinogenic substances, is included under "synergism."

Penetration. The ability of a fiber to penetrate to the site where effects are developed, for example, to the pleura or peritoneum in the development of mesothelioma, is clearly important to its potential for causing disease. This category includes all fiber properties that facilitate such penetration. It is closely related to fiber size, morphology, and stability.

Stability. Some experimental evidence suggests that the longer a fiber remains in a tissue, the greater is its opportunity for inducing its biological effects, for example, stimulating cell hyperplasia when a transformed cell is present. In this case, the important factor is not the resistance to translocation but the resistance to chemical or physical degradation such as dissolution or gelling.

Human Studies. This category includes both clinical and epidemiological observations in human populations.

Animal Studies. The demonstration of significant biological effects in a well-designed animal experiment is considered evidence that the test substance has a potential for causing similar effects in humans.

In Vitro Studies. Although the meaningfulness of short-term, in vitro experiments with respect to the effects of fibers is questionable, it is known that asbestos and some other fibers demonstrate some cellular-level effects such as hemolysis. The ability to cause such effects is considered a weak, but not entirely worthless, argument for health effects potential.

Synergism. Information on synergistic effects would markedly affect assessment of comparative risk. The only such information available involves asbestos and cigarette smoking.

Other. This catchall category could be applied to any influence on overall risk, including exposure, biodisposition, and effects. For example, if a particular fiber is found to be more likely than the others to reach young children and if the effect in question is most prevalent in children or if it increases in incidence with time after first exposure as with mesothelioma, then the comparative risk estimate would be increased.

Discussion of Comparative Risks

Table 7-7 summarizes from a different perspective the information in Appendix H.

No cell of the fiber/effect/route matrix approaches the population risk levels associated with the prime cell (chrysotile/lung cancer/inhalation). As noted in the quantitative assessment, the mesothelioma risk from lifetime exposure to asbestos is potentially much greater than the lung cancer risk. Although some researchers question whether chrysotile is as potent as other asbestos varieties in causing mesothelioma, the committee has assumed that even exposure only to chrysotile continously since birth would cause more mesothelioma than lung cancer. Chrysotile has been extensively used in the past and thus also provides a source of in-place exposure. Of the other combinations, the committee believes the ones most worth watching in the near term are fibrous glass and attapulgite for lung cancer by inhalation. The risks for effects of crocidolite and other asbestos varieties are reasonably well understood, and measures taken to reduce occupational exposures in the future may also keep the nonoccupational exposures to a mininum. However, general population exposures to crocidolite already in place could be substantial, especially in connection with its disposal.

The other cells seem to entail significantly less population risk (more than 10 times less) than the prime cell. In several cases, this judgment is based principally on current exposure or biodisposition rather than on definitive evidence that the fibers have low intrinsic health effects potential. For example, both ceramic and carbon fibers can be found in respirable size ranges and may well have Biological properties similar to those of asbestos. However, they are produced in low volumes and are used in limited, generally contained applications. Population risks could become substantial if these facts changed. Most fibrous glass and mineral wool is produced in nonrespirable sizes, and some evidence from epidemiological and animal studies suggests that their biological toxicity is low. Thus, risk levels for these substances are rated low despite the substantial potential for exposure.

TABLE 7-7. Summary of Comparative Risk Assessment

	Compared with Chrysotile/Lung Cancer/Inhalation, Data on the Factor Suggest that Population Risk Should be			
Factor	Higher	Similar	Lower	Much Lower
Production	Fibrous glass Attapulgite		Mineral wool	Crocidolite Other asbestos Carbon fiber Ceramic fiber
Use pattern	Fibrous glass Attapulgite	Other asbestos	Crocidolite Carbon fiber Mineral wool Chryatile/ingestion	Ceramic fiber
Geography	Fibrous glass	Other asbestos Mineral wool Carbon fiber	Crocidolite Attapulgite Ceramic fiber Chrysotile/ingestion	
Population	Fibrous glass Attapulgite	Crocidolite Other asbestos Mineral wool	Carbon fiber Ceramic fiber	
Trends	Fibrous glass Attapulgite Mineral wool Carbon fiber Ceramic fiber	Other asbestos	Crocidolite	
Fiber aize		Crocidolite Other asbestos Carbon fiber Ceramic fiber	Mineral wool	Fibrous glass Attapulgite
Morphology	Crocidolite	All others		
Chemistry	No clear effect of chemistry evident			
Penetration	Crocidolite Other asbestos Attapulgite	Carbon fiber Ceramic fiber	Mineral wool Chrysotile/ingestion	Fibrous glass
Stability	Crocidolite Other asbestos	All others	Fibrous glass	

	Compared with Chrysotile/Lung Cancer/Inhalation, Data on the Factor Suggest that Population Risk Should be			
Facor	Higher	Similar	Lower	Much Lower
Epidemiological studies	Crocidolitte/ mestheliona	Crocidolite/lung cancer Mineral wool	Fibrous glass Ceramic fiber Mineral wool	
Animal studies		Crocidolite Other asbestos	All others	
In Vitro studies[a]	—	—	—	—
Synergism		All others	Fibrous glass	
Other[b]	—	—	—	—
Overall population risk			Chrysotile/ mesothelions/ingestion Crocidolite Attapulgite/lung cancer Fibrous glass	Carbon fiber Ceramic fiber Attapulgite/ mesothelioma Other asbestos/other cancer

[a] Quantitative differences in activity not apparent.

[b] No other factor was sufficiently striking for inclusion.

For any combination of fiber type, effect, and route of exposure not assessed, even for comparative risk, the committee believes either that risks are at most of marginal significance or that there is insufficient information on which to base such a comparison. Most of the combinations fall into the former category. Carcinogenic effects other than lung cancer or mesothelioma constitute examples of the insufficient information category for several fibers.

SUMMARY AND RECOMMENDATIONS

The committee has made quantitative risk assessments for nonoccupational exposures to asbestos and qualitative (or comparative) risk assessments for a variety of asbestiform fibers. Lung cancer and mesothelioma from inhaled materials received the greatest consideration.

For the quantitative risk assessment, a linear model for low dose extrapolation was used. When quantifying risk from nonoccupational exposures, uncertainties are introduced not only by the selection of mathematical models but also because the characteristics of fibrous materials in the ambient environment differ from those in the workplace. By converting mass concentrations measured in the environment to equivalent numbers of fibers in the workplace, the committee assumed a median population exposure of 0.0004 fibers/cm^3 air throughout a 73-year lifetime. Based on this and various other assumptions, the individual lifetime risk for lung cancer was estimated to be between 3 in a million for female nonsmokers and 64 in a million for male smokers, and for mesothelioma it was approximately nine in a million, regardless of smoking habits or sex. However, other assumptions could decrease the risks essentially to zero, or could increase them.

The finding that the risk for mesothelioma is greater than that for lung cancer among nonsmokers is due to the strong dependence of mesothelioma risk on time since first exposure. Thus, a given exposure in childhood markedly increases the lifetime risk of mesothelioma compared with an equivalent dose later. It should be remembered that these risk estimates were based on data obtained from worker cohorts.

Smokers runs a substantially higher risk of malignant disease from asbestos than do nonsmokers; for smokers, lung cancer is a greater risk than mesothelioma.

Studies should be conducted to learn more precisely the dependence of mesothelioma and lung cancer mortality on time since first exposure and on the characteristics of the exposure. Such efforts should include studies in animal models and follow-up studies of occupationally exposed cohorts.

For the comparative risk assessment, population risks (as opposed to individual risks) were considered. The risks were based on three major factors: exposure levels, biodisposition, and evidence of adverse health effects. The potential for exposure was a dominant factor. Thus, risk estimates for substances of equal biological potency may be widely divergent if the populations exposed to them differ greatly. Two points follow from this. First, some individuals may be exposed to high levels of a fiber for which the overall population exposure is low. Second, the overall population risk would change if use patterns change.

Current population risk from exposures to the various substances considered, including fibrous glass, attapulgite, and carbon fibers, appears to be much less than for the risk from asbestos, especially chrysotile. However, further information is needed to evaluate the possible adverse effects of exposures to fine fibrous glass and attapulgite.

REFERENCES

Armitage, P. 1982. The assessment of low-dose carcinogenicity. Biometrics 38 (supplement):119-129.

Armitage, P., and R. Doll. 1961. Stochastic models for carcinogenesis. Pp. 19-38 in Proceedings of the Fourth Berkeley Symposium on Statistics and Probability. Vol. 4. University of California Press, Berkeley.

Babich, H., and D. L. Davis. 1981. Food tolerances and action levels: Do they adequately protect children ? Bio-Science 31:429-438.

Calabrese, E. J. 1978. Pollutants and High-Risk Groups. Wiley-Interscience, New York.

Calabrese, E. J. 1980. Nutrition and Environmental Health. Vol. 1: The Vitamins. Wiley-Interscience, New York.

Constant, Jr., P. C., F. J. Bergman, and G. R. Atkinson. 1982. Airborne asbestos levels in schools. Final Report, Environmental Protection Agency. Midwest Research Institute. Contract 68-01-5915.

Consumer Product Safety Commission. 1983. Report by the Chronic Hazard Advisory Panel on Asbestos. Consumer Product Safety Commission, Washington, D.C.

Cornfield, J., F. Carlborg, and J. Van Ryzin. 1978. Setting tolerances on the basis of mathematical treatment of dose-response data extrapolated to low doses. Pp. 143-164 in G. L. Plaa and W. A. M. Duncan, eds. Proceedings of the First International Congress on Toxicology. Academic Press, New York.

Crump, K. S., D. G. Hoel, C. H. Langley, and R. Peto. 1976. Fundamental carcinogenic processes and their implications for low dose risk assessment. Cancer Res. 36:2973-2979.

Dement, J. J., R. L. Harris, M. J. Symons, and C. Shy. 1982. Estimate of dose-response for respiratory cancer among chrysotile asbestos textile workers. Ann. Occup. Hyg. 26:869-887.

Doull, J., C. D. Klaassen, and M. O. Amdur, eds. 1980. Casarett and Doull's Toxicology: The Basic Science of Poisons. Macmillan, New York. 778 pp.

Enterline, P. E. 1983. Cancer produced by nonoccupational asbestos exposure in the United States. J. Air Pollut. Control Assoc. 33:318-322.

Fishbein, L. 1980. Overview of some aspects of quantitative risk assessment. J. Toxicol. Environ. Health 6:1275-1296.

Food Safety Council. 1980. Proposed System for Food Safety Assessment. Food Safety Council, Washington, D.C.

Goldenthal, E. I. 1971. A compilation of LD_{50} values in newborn and adult animals. Toxicol. Appl. Pharmacol. 18:185-207.

Hammond, E. C., I. J. Selikoff, and H. Seidman. 1979. Asbestos exposure, cigarette smoking and death rates. Ann. N. Y. Acad. Sci. 330:473-490.

Hartley, H. O., and R. Sielken. 1977. Estimation of "safe doses" in carcinogenesis experiments. Biometrics 33:1-30.

Hartley, H. O., H. Tolley, and R. Sielken. 1981. The product form of the hazard rate model in carcinogenic testing. Pp. 185-200 in M. Csorgo, D. A. Dawson, J. N. K. Rao, and E. Saleh, eds. Statistics and Related Topics. North-Holland, Amsterdam.

Henderson, V., and P. E. Enterline. 1979. Asbestos exposure: Factors associated with excess cancer and respiratory mortalilty. Ann. N.Y. Acad. Sci. 330:117-126.

Hobbs, M. S. T., S. D. Woodward, B. Murphy, A. W. Musk, and J. E. Elder. 1980. The incidence of pneumoconiosis, mesothelioma and other respiratory cancer in men engaged in mining and milling crocidolite in Western Australia. Pp. 615-625 in J. C. Wagner, ed. Biological Effects of Mineral Fibres. IARC Scientific Publication No. 30. International Agency for Research on Cancer, Lyon.

Hoel, D. G. 1980. Incorporation of background response in dose-response models. Fed. Proc. 39:73-75.

Hoel, D. G., N. L. Kaplan, and M. W. Anderson. 1983. Implication of non-linear kinetics on risk estimation in carcinogenesis. Science 219:1037.

Interagency Regulatory Liaison Group. 1979. Work Group on Risk Assessment. Scientific bases for identification of potential carcinogens and estimation of risks. J. Natl. Cancer Inst. 63:242.

Kalbfleisch, J. D., and R. L. Prentice. 1980. The Statistical Analysis of Failure Time Data. John Wiley and Sons, New York.

Kalbfleisch, J. D., D. Krewski, and J. Van Ryzin. 1983. Dose response models for time to response toxicity data. Can. J. Statist. 11:25-46.

Klaassen, C. D., and J. Doull. 1980. Evaluation of safety: Toxicologic evaluation. Chapter 2 in J. Doull, C. D. Klaassen, and M. O. Amdur, eds. Casarett and Doull's Toxicology: The Basic Science of Poisons. Macmillan, New York.

Krewski, D., and J. Van Ryzin. 1981. Dose response models for quantal response toxicity data. Pp. 201-231 in M. Csorgo, D. A. Dawson, J. N. K. Rao, and E. Saleh, eds. Statistics and Related Topics. North-Holland, Amsterdam.

McDonald, J. C., and F. D. K. Liddell. 1979. Mortality in Canadian miners and millers exposed to chrysotile. Ann. N. Y. Acad. Sci. 330:1-9.

National Research Council. 1977. Principles and Procedures for Evaluating the Toxicity of Household Substances. A report of the Committee for the Revision of NAS Publication 1138, Assembly of Life Sciences. National Academy of Sciences, Washington, D.C. 130 pp.

National Research Council. 1983. Risk Assessment in the Federal Government: Managing the Process. A report of the Committee on the Institutional Means for Assessment of Risks to Public Health, Commission on Life Sciences. National Academy Press, Washington, D.C. 191 pp.

Newhouse, M. L., and G. Berry. 1976. Predictions of mortality from mesothelial tumours in asbestos factory workers. Br. J. Indus. Med. 33:147-151.

Newhouse, M. C., and G. Berry. 1979. Patterns of disease among long-term asbestos workers in the United Kingdom. Ann. N. Y. Acad. Sci. 330:53-60.

Nicholson, W. J. 1971. Measurement of asbestos in ambient air. National Air Pollution Control Administration. Final Report, Contract CPA 70-92.

Nicholson, W. J. 1978. Control of sprayed asbestos surfaces in school buildings: A feasibility study. Final Report. Contract I-ES-2113. National Institute of Environmental Health Sciences, Research Triangle Park, N.C.

Nicholson, W. J. 1983. Health Effects Update. June 1983. Unpublished draft prepared by W. J. Nicholson, Mt. Sinai School of Medicine, City University of New York. 148 pp.

Nicholson, W. J., A. N. Rohl, and E. F. Ferrand. 1971. Asbestos air pollution in New York City. Pp. 136-139 in H. M. England and W. T. Barry, eds. Proceedings of the Second Clean Air Congress. Academic Press, New York.

Nicholson, W. J., A. N. Rohl, and I. Weisman. 1975. Asbestos contamination of the air in public buildings. EPA-450/3-76-004. Environmental Protection Agency, Research Triangle Park, N.C.

Nicholson, W. J., A. N. Rohl, and I. Weisman. 1976. Asbestos contamination of building air supply systems. Paper 29-6 in Proceedings of the International Conference on Environmental Sensing and Assessment. Institute of Electrical and Electronic Engineers, Vol. II. Institute of Electrical and Electronic Engineers, New York.

Nicholson, W. J., I. J. Selikoff, H. Seidman, R. Lilis, and P. Formby. 1979. Long-term mortality experience of chrysotile miners and millers in Thetford mines, Quebec. Ann. N. Y. Acad. Sci. 330:11-21.

Nicholson, W. J., A. N. Rohl, I. Weisman, and I. J. Selikoff. 1980. Environmental asbestos concentrations in the United States. Pp. 823-827 in J. E. Wagner, ed. Biological Effects of Mineral Fibres. Vol. 2. IARC Scientific Publication No. 30. International Agency for Research on Cancer, Lyon.

Office of Technology Assessment. 1981. Assessment of Technologies for Determining Cancer Risks from the Environment. Office of Technology Assessment, Washington, D.C. 240 pp.

Pelkonen, O., E. H. Kaltiala, T. K. Karmi, and N. T. Karki. 1973. Comparison of activities of drug-metabolizing enzymes in human fetal and adult livers. Clin. Pharmacol. Ther. 14:840-846.

Peto, R. 1978. Carcinogenic effects of chronic exposure to very low levels of toxic substances. Environ. Health Perspect. 22:155-159.

Peto, J. 1980a. Lung cancer mortality in relation to measured dust levels in an asbestos textile factory. Pp. 829-836 in J. C. Wagner, ed. Biological Effects of Mineral Fibres. Vol. 2. IARC Scientific Publication No. 30. International Agency for Research on Cancer, Lyon.

Peto, J. 1980b. The incidence of pleural mesothelioma in chrysotile asbestos textile workers. Pp. 703-711 in J. C. Wagner, ed. Biological Effects of Mineral Fibres. Vol. 2. IARC Scientific Publication No. 30. International Agency for Research on Cancer, Lyon.

Peto, J. 1982. Dose and time relationships for lung cancer and mesothelioma in relation to smoking and asbestos exposure. Presented at the Symposium on Asbestos Carcinogenesis. Feb. 17-19, 1982, in West Berlin. Organized by Bundesgesundheitsamt.

Peto, J., H. Seidman, and I. J. Selikoff. 1982. Mesothelioma mortality in asbestos workers: Implications for models of carcinogenesis and risk assessment. Br. J. Cancer 45:124-135.
Pott, F. 1978. Some aspects on the dosimetry of the carcinogenic potency of asbestos and other fibrous dusts. Staub Reinhalt. Luft 38:486-490.
Rane, A., and E. Ackerman. 1972. Metabolism of ethylmorphine and aniline in human fetal liver. Clin. Pharmacol. Ther. 13:663-670.
Richmond, C. R., P. J. Walsh, and E. D. Copenhaver, eds. 1981. Proceedings of the Third Life Sciences Symposium, Health Risk Analysis, Gatlinburg, Tenn., Oct. 27-30, 1980. Franklin Institute Press, Philadelphia. 438 pp.
Schneiderman, M. A., I. C. Nisbet, and S. M. Brett. 1981. Assessment of risks posed by exposure to low levels of asbestos in the general environment. Prepared for Institut für Wasser, Boden, und Lufthygiene des Bundesgesundheitsamtes. No. 4. Dietrich Reimer Verlag, Berlin.
Sebastien, P., M. A. Billion-Galland, G. Dufour, and J. Bignon. 1980. Measurement of asbestos air pollution inside buildings sprayed with asbestos. EPA 560/13-80-026. Environmental Protection Agency, Washington, D.C.
Seidman, H., I. J. Selikoff, and E. C. Hammond. 1979. Short-term asbestos work exposure and long-term observation. Ann. N.Y. Acad. Sci. 330:61-89.
Selikoff, I. J., E. C. Hammond, and H. Seidman. 1979. Mortality experience of insulation workers in the U.S. and Canada, 1943-1976. Ann. N.Y. Acad. Sci. 330:91-116.
Tager, I. B., S. T. Weiss, A. Munoz, B. Rosner, and F. E. Speizer. 1983. Longitudinal study of the effects of maternal smoking on pulmonary function in children. N. Engl. J. Med. 309:699-703.
U.S. Environmental Protection Agency. 1974. A preliminary report on asbestos in the Duluth, Minnesota area. Office of Technical Analysis. Environmental Protection Agency, Washington, D.C.
Van Ryzin, J. 1980. Quantitative risk assessment. J. Occup. Med. 22:321-326.
Van Ryzin, J. 1981. Discussion: The assessment of low-dose carcinogenicity. Biometrics 38 (suppl. 2):130-139.

Appendix A

Asbestos Exposure and Human Disease. Hallmark Observations and Studies From 1898 to 1979

Disease or Benchmark	Contribution to the Field	References
Bronchitis Phthisis	"Asbestos fiber inhalation in the workplace injurious to the bronchial tubes and lungs." Clinical latency mitigates against establishing a stronger association between work with asbestos fiber and disease, because sick workers leave industry. No mortality data.	Anderson, 1898 (see Greenberg, 1982)
Pulmonary fibrosis	Death due to pulmonary fibrosis (in an asbestos textile worker without tuberculosis). Autopay showed fibrosed lungs and presence of "spicules of asbestos" in pulmonary tissues. When the worker was alive, this sputum contained what was thought to be "asbestos spicules." Fibrosis was believed to be induced by dust. Different work areas had a range of dust conditions.	Murray, 1907 (see Greenberg, 1982)
Asbestosis	Complete histological and gross pathological description of asbestos. Author originated term asbestosis and cited experimental pathology studies indicating that asbestos dust causes fibrosis in the lungs of guinea pigs.	Cooke, 1924
Asbestosis	First major reviews of asbestosis. Detailed clinical, radiological, and pathological descriptions. Cooke noted the presence of "curious bodies" in pulmonary tissues of asbestotics. Asbestosis attack rate high for textile workers spinning Canadian chrysotile.	Cooke, 1927; McDonald, 1927; Oliver, 1927
Asbestosis	"Curious bodies" probably some form of coated fiber. Author recommended the term "asbestosis body."	Cooke, 1929
Asbestosis	Review of asbestosis in Great Britain and other parts of the world. Relationship between asbestosis and tuberculosis discussed. Latency also discussed. Author suggested different forms of fiber may have different biological activities.	Merewether, 1930

Disease or Benchmark	Contribution to the Field	References
Asbestosis	Authors suggested, on the basis of 57 cases they had seen, that tuberculosis increases severity of scarring in asbestotics.	Wood and Gloyne, 1931
Asbestosis	"Constitutional factors" may be important in determining who among the work force is "susceptible to asbestosis."	Gerbis, 1932
Asbestosis	German government issues dictum forbidding all those under the age of 18 from employment in the asbestos industry. Germans followed British Home Office.	Gerbis, 1932
Asbestosis Pleural asbestosis	Author discussed the different physical and chemical properties of the various asbestos types used in commerce (e.g., size, shape, "others") and their possible role in determining the occurrence of disease and the types and patterns of lesions observed. Different kinds and intensities of exposures in industry also described. Geographic differences in occurrence of disease may be related to fiber types and/or genetic factors. Role of mineral contaminants unknown.	Gloyne, 1932
Asbestosis	Mortality data suggested asbestos workers have shortened life expectancies. Greater attack rate in mills may be related to the "ability of the fiber to split longitudinally into fibrils creating respirable dust."	Merewether, 1933, 1934
Asbestosis Lung cancer	Primary lung cancer found at autopsy in two female textile workers with asbestosis.	Gloyne, 1935
Asbestosilicosis Lung cancer	Primary lung cancer in men employed in textile plants in South Carolina. Lungs fibrosed.	Lynch and Smith, 1935
Lung cancer and latency Asbestosis	Author found that the length of elapsed time from the start of asbestos work until the time of death was 15 to 21 years in all six of the cases known to him. In five of the six cases, the tumors developed in the lower lobes of the lung, whereas in the general population lung cancer was most common in the upper lobes. It was well recognized that the more extensive fibrosis in asbestosis was also found in the lower lobes of the lung.	Nordmann, 1938
Asbestosis and lung cancer attack rate	Among 943 cases of fatal silicosis in Great Britain in 1938, 23 lung cancers occurred (2.4%). Among 103 cases of fatal asbestosis for all prior years, 12 lung cancers were found (11.6%). Attack rates appeared to be different, although true incidence was unknown.	Wilson, 1939

Disease or Benchmark	Contribution to the Field	References
Asbestosis Lung cancer Mesothelioma (?)[a] Other cancers (?)	Comparison of autopsy series in general population with 92 asbestotics. Fourteen malignancies in asbestotics (16%), compared with approximately 2% in the "unexposed" general population. Metastases to pleura, peritoneum, and pericardium. Histology much like "sarcomas."	Wedler, 1943
Asbestosis Lung cancer	Prevalence of lung cancer among asbestotics increases with age: 25-34, 4.8%; 35-44, 5.6%; 45-54, 18.9%; 55-64, 25.6%; 65 and older, 23.5%. Latency, dose, and aging not separated as factors in this pattern.	Barnett, 1948
Pneumoconiosis Lung cancer Other cancers and other sites	Compared mortality experience in different "dusty trades" in Great Britain. Age at death for seven silica-exposed groups ranged from 44 to 63 years (lowest in pottery industry). Asbestos trades averaged 36 years (39 for males, 34 for females. Approximately 14% of asbestotics died with lung cancer. Author noted "strikingly" different attack rates in males and females: 19.6% for males, 9.7% for females. Neoplasms at other sites twice as high in asbestotics as compared to other pneumoconiosis groups (about 6%, compared to 3%).	Gloyne, 1951
Lung cancer, occupation, and cigarette smoking	This study provided evidence linking certain occupations (including those involving asbestos exposure) with lung cancer. The study also offered additional evidence associating cigarette smoking with lung cancer.	Breslow et al., 1954
Asbestosis Lung cancer Mesothelioma	Cohort study of textile workers at a plant in Great Britain. Incidence data indicated a standardized mortality ratio (SMR) of almost 14; 11 observed, 0.8 expected for lung cancer in workers employed before "protective standards" of the Asbestos Regulations Act of 1931. Author cautioned that smaller risk in workers employed after 1931 may be an artifact; they may have not yet reached "risk" period because of their short elapsed time after onset of exposure. An endothelioma was observed in a worker.	Doll, 1955

[a] "?" indicates the disease was not diagnosed by name.

Disease or Benchmark	Contribution to the Field	References
Pleural mesothelioma Environmental mesothelioma	Thirty-three cases of pleural mesothelioma reported among miners and millers of crocidolite in the Northwest Cape Province, South Africa. Among the cases were area residents with no known occupational exposure. Histological evidence of asbestosis was not present in all cases.	Wagner et al., 1960
Pleural plaques Environmental stigmata	Pleural fibrosis and calcification—stigmata normally associated with fibrous dust insult—were found in a population living in a region of Finland where anthophyllite asbestos was mined and milled. Ambient asbestos pollution was implicated.	Kiviluoto, 1960
Asbestosis Abdominal tumors Mesothelioma (?)	Abdominal tumors found in asbestotics during autopsy. Ovarian cancers in women and general carcinomatosis (no primary) in men.	Keal, 1960
Asbestos bodies and exposure	Asbestos bodies were found in pulmonary tissues in 26% of 500 consecutive autopsies conducted in the general population of Capetown, South Africa. Use of asbestos by society was questioned in view of the known cancer hazard.	Thomson et al., 1963
Asbestosis Lung cancer Mesothelioma (pleural and peritoneal) Gastrointestinal (GI) cancer	Morbidity and mortality data for insulation workers showed excess cancer and asbestosis accounting for most decreased life expectancy. Malignancies included lung cancer and pleural mesothelioma. There was also peritoneal mesothelioma and an excess of gastrointestinal cancer.	Selikoff et al., 1964
Peritoneal mesothelioma Other cancer (GI)	Peritoneal mesothelioma seen in crocidolite-exposed workers. Other intraabdominal tumors may have been present as well.	Entiknap and Smither, 1964
Mesothelioma	Records in an east-end London hospital showed that a large proportion of the mesotheliomas that occurred were in nonoccupationally exposed persons: residents living within a half mile of an asbestos plant and families of workers.	Newhouse and Thompson, 1965
Mesothelioma Bystander occupational exposure	Mesothelioma observed in shipyard workers whose jobs were not asbestos-related. Most mesotheliomas occurred in bystander populations. Importance of fugitive dust raised.	Harries, 1968

Disease or Benchmark	Contribution to the Field	References
Lung cancer and cigarette smoking	Evidence suggested that cigarette-smoking asbestos workers had a greatly increased risk of developing lung cancer as compared to nonsmoking workmates. The risk appeared to be multiplicative—the product of both smoking and asbestos risks.	Selikoff et al., 1968
Pleural asbestosis Pulmonary asbestosis Household exposures	Radiographic and clinical survey of 678 individuals cohabiting with asbestos workers. Thirty-five percent (239) of them had pleural or pulmonary asbestosis. Questions raised concerning dust on clothing as the vector of the fiber. (In a follow-up study published in 1979, the authors stated that they were ascertaining causes of death among a larger population of household members. Of 550 decedents traced, five deaths were due to pleural mesothelioma.)	Anderson et al., 1976, 1979
Extrapulmonary cancers Multiple cancer in single hosts	SMRs showed slight excesses of cancer of the larynx, buccal cavity, brain, skin, kidney, pancreas, and prostate among 2,271 deaths (168,000 man-years of observation) in a cohort of 17,800 insulation workers in the United States and Canada. Authors reported that 2.1% of the deaths involved multiple primary cancers and that occult malignancies were present at time of death.	Selikoff et al., 1979
Fiber dose, latency, risk	Short-term (1-month) intense exposure to amosite fiber increased lung cancer risk. Latency period inversely related to dose.	Seidman et al., 1979

REFERENCES

Anderson, A. M. 1898. Observations published in H.M. Chief Inspector of Factories and Workshops, Report for the year 1898.

Anderson, H. A., R. Lilis, S. M. Daum, A. S. Fischbein, and I. J. Selikoff. 1976. Household contact asbestos neoplastic risk. Ann. N.Y. Acad. Sci. 271:311.

Anderson, H. A., R. Lilis, S. M. Daum, and I. J. Selikoff. 1979. Asbestosis among household contacts of asbestos factory workers. Ann. N.Y. Acad. Sci. 330:387-400.

Barnett, G. P. 1948. Annual Report of the Chief Inspector of Factories for the year 1946. CMD 7299, Her Majesty's Stationary Office, London. 132 pp.

Breslow, L., L. Hoaglin, G. Rasmussen, and H. Abrams. 1954. Occupations and cigarette smoking as factors in lung cancer. Am. J. Pub. Health 44:171-181.

Cooke, W. E. 1924. Fibrosis of the lungs due to the inhalation of asbestos dust. Br. Med. J. 2:147.

Cooke, W. E. 1927. Pulmonary asbestosis. Br. Med. J. 2:1024-1025.

Cooke, W. E. 1929. Asbestos dust and the curious bodies found in pulmonary asbestosis. Br. Med. J. 2:578-580.

Doll, R. 1955. Mortality from lung cancer in asbestos workers. Br. J. Ind. Med. 12:81-86.

Entiknap, J. B., and W. J. Smither. 1964. Peritoneal tumors in asbestosis. Br. J. Ind. Med. 21:20-31.

Gerbis, U. 1932. Ueber asbestosis der Lungen. Deut. Med. Woch. 58:285-287.

Gloyne, S. R. 1932. The morbid anatomy and histology of asbestosis. Tubercle 14:445-451.

Gloyne, S. R. 1935. Two cases of squamous carcinoma of the lung occurring in asbestosis. Tubercle 17:5-10.

Gloyne, S. R. 1951. Pneumoconiosis. A histological survey of necropsy material in 1,205 cases. Lancet 1:810-814.

Greenberg, M. 1983. Classical syndromes in occupational medicine: The Montague Murray Case. Am. J. Ind. Med. 3:351-356.

Harris, P. G. 1968. Asbestos hazards in naval dockyards. Ann. Occup. Hyg. 11:136.

Kiviluoto, R. 1960. Pleural calcification as a roentgenologic sign of non-occupational endemic anthophyllite asbestos. Acta Radiologica (Supp.) 194:1-67.

Keal, E. E. 1960. Asbestos and abdominal neoplasms. Lancet II:1211-1216.

Lynch, K. M., and W. A. Smith. 1935. Pulmonary asbestosis III. Carcinoma of the lung in asbesto-silicosis. Am. J. Cancer 24:56-64.

McDonald, S. 1927. Histology of pulmonary asbestosis: A review. Br. Med. J. 2:1025-1026.

Merewether, E. R. A. 1930. The occurrence of pulmonary fibrosis and other pulmonary affections in asbestos workers. J. Ind. Hyg. 12:198-222, 239-257.

Merewether, E. R. A. 1933, 1934. A memorandum on asbestosis. Tubercle 15:69-81, 109-118.

Murray, J. M. 1907. Report of the Committee on Compensation for Industrial Diseases. Minutes of Evidence.
Newhouse, M. L., and H. Thompson. 1965. Mesothelioma of pleura and peritoneum following exposure to asbestos in the London area. Br. J. Ind. Med. 22:261.
Nordmann, M. 1938. Der Berufskrebs der Asbesarbeiter. Zeitschrift für Krebsforschung. Vol. 47. 288 pp.
Oliver, T. 1927. Clinical aspects of pulmonary asbestosis. Br. Med. J. 2:1026-1027.
Seidman, H., I. J. Selikoff, and E. C. Hammond. 1979. Short-term asbestos work exposure and long-term observation. Ann. N.Y. Acad. Sci. 330:61-90.
Selikoff, I. J., J. Churg, and E. C. Hammond. 1964. Asbestos exposure and neoplasia. J. Am. Med. Assoc. 188:22-26.
Selikoff, I.J., E.C. Hammond, and J. Churg. 1968. Asbestos exposure, smoking and neoplasia. J. Am. Med. Assoc. 204:104-110.
Selikoff, I. J., E. C. Hammond, and H. Seidman. 1979. Mortality experience of insulation workers in the U.S. and Canada, 1943-1976. Ann. N.Y. Acad. Sci. 330:91-116.
Thomson, J. G., R. O. Kaschula, and R. R. McDonald. 1963. Asbestos as a modern urban hazard. S. Afr. Med. J. 37:77-81.
Wagner, J. C., C. A. Sleggs, and P. Marchand. 1960. Diffuse pleural mesothelioma and asbestos exposure in the Northwestern Cape Province. Br. J. Ind. Med. 17:260-271.
Wedler, H. W. 1943. Asbestose und Lungenkrebs. Deut. Med. Woch. 69:575-576.
Wilson, D. R. 1939. Annual Report of the Chief Inspector of Factories for the year 1938. CMD. 6081. Her Majesty's Stationary Office, London. 133 pp.
Wood, W. B., and S. R. Gloyne. 1931. Pulmonary asbestosis complicated by pulmonary tuberculosis. Lancet II:954-956.

Appendix B

Natural and Synthetic Fibrous Substances and Some of their Known Biological Effects

B-1. COMMERCIAL ASBESTOS (ASBESTIFORM)

Mineral	Mineralogical Category	Pathological Effects Observed in Animals and/or Humans[a]: Fibrosis	Lung Cancer	Meso-thelioma	Comments
Natural:					
Actinolite -tremolite	Chain silicate	+	–	+	Common contaminant of amosite. May contaminate chrysotile and talc deposits. Indirectly linked to human disease. (Mesothelioma among Cyprus chrysotile miners and millers. Pulmonary burden was tremolite, not chrysotile.) (F. D. Pooley, University College, Wales, personal communication, 1979.) Animal data demonstrate pathological activity (Coffin et al., 1982; Cook et al., 1982; Wagner, 1962).
Anthophyllite	Chain silicate	+	+	+	Usually a low quality asbestos. Rarely used in the United States. Present as a contaminant in amosite and in some chrysotile and talc deposits. Data on animals and humans (International Agency for Research on Cancer, 1973). Mesothelioma reported in animals but not in exposed human populations.
Chrysotile	Layer silicate	+	+	+	Most commonly used as asbestos in the United States. Also known as white asbestos. Extensive data in humans and animals (International Agency for Research on Cancer, 1973).
Cummingtonite-grunerite (amosite)	Chain silicate	+	+	+	Common trade name "amosite." Also known as brown asbestos. Used extensively in U.S. shipyards (International Agency for Research on Cancer, 1973). Extensive biological data on humans and animals (Irwig et al., 1979; Seidman et al., 1979).
Riebeckite (crocidolite)	Chain silicate	+	+	+	Also known as blue asbestos. Extensive biological data on humans and animals (International Agency for Research on Cancer, 1973).

[a]"+", pathological effect has been observed in animals and/or humans.
"–", pathological effect has not been observed.

B-2. VARIABLE QUALITY FIBERS (PROBABLY ASBESTIFORM)

		Pathological Effects Observed in Animals and/or Humans[a]			
Mineral	Mineralogical Category	Fibrosis	Lung Cancer	Mesothelioma	Comments
Natural:					
Brucite (nemalite)	Layer hydroxide	+	-	+	Relatively rare. Contaminant of chrysotile deposits. Human contact through chrysotile processing. Experimentally induced fibrosis and mesotheliomas in mice (Pott et al., 1974, 1976; Schnitzer and Pundsack, 1970).
Erionite	Zeolite	+	-	+	Occurs as a mineral constituent of tuffaceous (volcanic ash) deposits. Associated with endemic mesothelioma among residents of Cappadocian Plateau of central Turkey. Pleural plaques and pulmonary fibrosis also reported (Artvinli and Baris, 1979; Baris et al., 1978; Suzuki, 1982).
Palygorskite[b] (attapulgite)	Layer silicate with triple subchain structure	+	-	-	Used as an absorbent in cosmetics, drugs, insecticides. Known under the trade name "attapulgite." Other fibrous variety is Mountain Leather. In experimental systems, shown to be membranolytic (Bignon et al., 1980; Koshi et al., 1968; Pott et al., 1974, 1976; Sakabe et al., 1971; Schnitzer and Pundsack, 1970).
Sepiolite[b]	Layer silicate with triple subchain structure	+	-	-	Not used in the United States. Implicated in pleural plaque development in Bulgaria (Burilkov and Michailova, 1972). Limited animal data suggest biological activity (Pott et al., 1974, 1976; Sakabe et al., 1971). There are no biological data on meerschaum, a variety of sepiolite used in making pipes for smoking.

[a] See first page of Appendix.

[b] May occur in fibrous and nonfibrous forms.

	Pathological Effects Observed in Animals and/or Humans[a]			
Mineral	Fibrosis	Lung Cancer	Mesothelioma	Comments
Synthetic:				
Fine glass fiber (textile quality)	+	+	+	Manufacture of small diameter glass fibers is relatively recent. For data on fibrous glass in humans, see Chapter 5. For animal data, see Appendix E. Information on the fineness of fibrous glass is often not available.
Fine whiskers (e.g., metals, oxides, and carbides)	+	-	+	Some whiskers have fibrous mineral equivalents. Most carbon fibers (so-called graphite whiskers) have a chrysotile type structure. For most whiskers and carbon fibers, there are no biological data.

[a] See first page of Appendix.

B-3. VARIABLE QUALITY FIBERS (POSSIBLY ASBESTIFORM)

Mineral	Mineralogical Category	Comments
Natural:		
Chalcotrichite	Fibrous cuprite	This "mineral" is probably a fibrous variety of cuprite (copper oxide). Rare.
Chlorites	Layer silicates	Many chlorites are known to have probable ashestiform character. They usually crystallise in microscopic scale and are relatively widespread in many metamorphic rocks.
Complex sulfides (e.g., jamesonite and plumosite)		Like other sulfides, these minerals are frequently fibrous. Some have small diameters and are true fibers (Maleev et al., 1972). The minerals are rather rare mineralogical curiosities.
Fibrous quartz, chalcedony	Silica minerals	Most fibrous quartz is nonasbestiform. Like other silica minerals, they are possible inducers of silicosis (Langer, 1978). Fine "glass" fibers were reported to have a quartz (or other silica) structure. There are no biological data on these quartz type fibers.
Glaucophane (rhodesite)	Amphibole	This amphibole occurs occasionally in submicroscopic fibers. The physical character of the fibers is not known. It is possible that they are like other asbestiform amphibole fibers and may have comparable biological activity. Glaucophanes are relatively widespread in certain metamorphic rocks.
Guembelite	Layer silicate	A rare mineral occasionally described as "fibrous."
Halloysite (tubular halloysite)	Layer silicate	In tubular halloysite, the silicate layers are curled up in tubes, as in chrysotile. The average diameter of the tubes is larger than in chrysotile, and most of the halloysite fibers are assused to have diameters larger than respirable size.
Minnesotaite	Layer silicate	There are reports on asbestiform occurrences of minnesotaite (Gruner, 1946). Samples of fibrous minnesotaite examined to date appear to be nonasbestiform.

Mineral	Mineralogical Category	Comments
Natural:		
Mordenite	Zeolite	There are some limited data indicating that this mineral produces fibrosis experimentally (Suzuki, 1982). There are no data on humans. Other zeolites similar to mordenite are relatively rare.
Native elements (e.g., antimony, silver, etc.)		Wirelike fibrous crystals of the native elements, such as silver, are relatively common. Some of the smaller fibers have properties comparable to those of metallic whiskers (Maleev et al., 1972).
Nephrite	Jade of actinolite-tremolite	Electron microscope studies showed that the amphibole (actinolite-tremolite) crystals in nephrite are fibrous and may be asbestiform.
Other amphiboles (e.g., richterite, winchite)		Although there is no information on their biological behavior, their physical properties appear to be similar to those of other asbestiform amphibole fibers. These minerals may occur as contaminants in commercial deposits of other materials, e.g., winchite is a contaminant of some talc deposits.
Pyrolusite	Manganese hydroxide	This mineral occurs relatively commonly in a platy dendritic form in layered sedimentary rocks. It is not known whether any portion of it is asbestiform.
Rutile	Titanium oxide	Asbestiform fibers of rutile have been detected as fine fibrous inclusions in other crystals (e.g., quartz) (Maleev et al., 1972). Asbestiform fibers of rutile are extremely rare.
Sericite, illite	Micas, layer silicates	Sericite has been implicated as a scarring agent in early silicosis studies. Animal data support fibrogenic activity (Cummins, 1936). Human data equivocal due to complex nature of dust exposures. There are no data on their asbestiform character and carcinogenicity.
Sulfide minerals (e.g., sphalerite, millerite)		Sulfide minerals frequently crystallize in a fibrous habit. They are relatively rare and large (filiform). Thus, inhalation exposure to these minerals are not of concern.

Mineral	Mineralogical Category	Comments
Natural:		
Talc (agalite)	Layer silicate	Many talc samples contain asbestiform amphiboles. Some talc is known to be asbestiform and has been linked to excess malignancies in some populations (Kleinfeld et al., 1968).
Tourmaline	Ring silicate	High quality asbestiform fibers were discovered in the Ural Mountains (Tarnovskii et al., 1976) and in Switzerland (Dietrich et al., 1966). They are rare mineralogical curiosities.
Vermiculites	Micalike layer silicates	Vermiculites crystallize in fiberlike crystals. They may be asbestiform. They are widely used in industry as insulators, soil substitutes, and ahsorbents. Vermiculite is considered to be a potentially fibrogenic mineral (Bowes et al., 1977).
Wollastonite, pectolite	Chain silicates	Has been shown to stimulate interferon production in specific cells in vitro (Hahon et al., 1980). Limited human data suggest possible low risk of pneumoconiosis and excess cancers. There is no information on their possible asbestiform properties.
Synthetic:		
Coarse whiskers	Metals and inorganic compounds	Probably larger than respirable size.
Heavier fiber glass and rock wool		Probably larger than respirable size.
Fine steel wool, piano cord		Probably larger than respirable size.

B-4. POOR QUALITY FIBERS (QUESTIONABLY ASBESTIFORM)[c]

Mineral	Examples and Comments
Natural:	
Other chain silicates	Pyroxenes, rhodonite, xonotlite, spodumene
Stilpnomelane	Frequently fibrous, rare layer silicate
Other fibrous zeolites	Natrolite, thomsonite, edingtonite. Commonly fibrous.
Other fibrous silicates	Epidote, chrysocolla
Halides	Fibrous varieties of halite, sylvite
Magnesium-fluorite	Fibrous variety: zamboninite
Aragonite and calcite[d]	Carbonates. Fibrous variety: satin spar
Gypsum[d]	Sulfate. Fibrous variety: satin spar
Epsomite[d]	Frequently fibrous variety: hydrous sulfate
Pyromorphite[d]	Occasionally fibrous variety: phosphate
Other fibrous minerals	Erythrite, atacamite, orpiment, hematite, goethite, siderite, strontianite, alunite, datolite, chalcanthite, melanterite
Natural glass:	
Pele's hair	Natural volcanic glass that forms fibers. Generally diameters too large to be respirable.
Synthetic:	
Steel wool, fine wires, and cords	Not likely to be respirable
Coarse fiber glass and rock wool	Not likely to be respirable (see fine glass fiber, above)

[c] These minerals are often fibrous and may occasionally be ashestiform. Some are water soluble.

[d] Soluble fibers, especially carbonates, sulfates, etc., might tend not to show the pathological effects induced by durable fibers.

REFERENCES

Artvinli, M., and Y. I. Baris. 1979. Malignant mesotheliomas in a small village in the Anatolian region of Turkey: An epidemiological study. J. Natl. Cancer Inst. 63:17-22.

Baris, Y. I., A. A. Sahin, and M. Ozesmi. 1978. An outbreak of pleural mesothelioma and chronic fibrosing pleurisy in the village of Karain Urgup in Anatolia. Thorax 33:181-192.

Bignon, J., P. Sebastien, A. Gaudichet, and M. C. Jaurand. 1980. Biological effects of attapulgite. Pp. 25-27 in J. C. Wagner, ed. Biological Effects of Mineral Fibres. IARC Scientific Pub. No. 30. International Agency for Research on Cancer, Lyon.

Bowes, D. R., A. M. Langer, and A. N. Rohl. 1977. Nature and range of mineral dust in the environment. Trans. R. Soc. London, Ser. A 286:593-610.

Burilkov, T., and L. Michailova. 1972. Über den Sepiolitgehalt des Bodens in Gebieten mit endemischen Pleural-Verkalkungen. Int. Arch. Arbeitsmed. 29:95-101.

Coffin, D. L., L. D. Palekar, and P. Cooke. 1982. Tumorigenesis by a ferroactinolite mineral. Toxicol. Lett. 13:143-150.

Cook, P., L. D. Palekar, and D. L. Coffin. 1982. Interpretation of the carcinogenicity of amosite asbestos and ferroactinolite on the basis of retained fiber dose and characteristics in vivo. Toxicol. Lett. 13:151-158.

Cummins, S. L. 1936. Sericite and silica: Experimental dust lesions in rabbits. Br. J. Exp. Pathol. 18:395-401.

Dietrich, V., F. de Quervain, and H. U. Nissen. 1966. Turmalin-Asbest aus den alpinen Mineralkluften. Schweiz. Mineral. Petrogr. Mitt. 46:695-697.

Gruner, J. W. 1946. The Mineralogy and Geology of the Taconites and Iron Ores of the Mesabi Range, Minnesota. Commission of Iron Range Research Rehabilitation, Minnesota Geological Survey, Minneapolis.

Hahon, N., J. A. Booth., B. A. Boehlecke, and J. A. Merchant. 1980. Enhanced viral interferon induction by the mineral wollastonite. J. Interferon Res. 1:49-60.

International Agency for Research on Cancer. 1973. Biological Effects of Asbestos. P. Bogovski, V. Timbrell, J. C. Gilson, and J. C. Wagner, eds. IARC Scientific Pub. No. 8. International Agency for Research on Cancer, Lyon. 346 pp.

Irwig, L. M., R. S. J. DuToit, G. K. Sluis-Cremer, A. Solomon, R. G. Thomas, P. P H. Hamel, I. Webster, and T. Hastie. 1979. Risk of asbestosis in crocidolite and amosite mines in South Africa. Ann. N. Y. Acad. Sci. 330:35-52.

Kleinfeld, M., J. Mescite, O. Kooyman, and M. H. Zaki. 1968. Mortality among talc miners and millers in New York State. Arch. Environ. Health 14:663-667.

Koshi, R., H. Hayashi, and H. Sakabe. 1968. Cell toxicity and hemolytic action of asbestos dust. Ind. Health (Japan) 6:69-79.

Langer, A. M. 1978. Crystal faces and cleavage planes in quartz as templates in biological processes. Quart. Rev. Biophys. II, 4:543-575.

Maleev, M. N., A. P. Krusilina, and V. N. Rozanckij. 1972. Ultimate strength of naturally fibrous rutile, antimony and jamesonite crystals. (In Russian) C. R. Acad. Bulg. Sci. 25:1085-1088.

Pott, F., F. Huth, and K. H. Friedrichs. 1974. Tumorigenic effect of fibrous dust in experimental animals. Environ. Health Perspect. 9:313-314.

Pott, F., K. H. Friedrichs, and F. Huth. 1976. Ergebnisse aus Tierversuchen zur kanzerogenen Wirkung faserförmiger Staube und ihre Deutung, I. Hinblick auf die Tumor-Entstehung beim Menschen. Zbl. Bakt. Hyg. I. Abt. Orig. B. 162:467-505.

Sakabe, H., K. Koshi, and H. Hayashi. 1971. On the cell toxicity of mineral dust. Pp. 423-434 in W. H. Walton, ed. Inhaled Particles III, Vol. I. Unwin Brothers, Surrey, England.

Schnitzer, R. J., and F. L. Pundsack. 1970. Asbestos hemolysis. Environ. Res. 3:1-13.

Seidman, H., I. J. Selikoff, and E. C. Hammond. 1979. Short-term asbestos work exposure and long-term observation. Ann. N.Y. Acad. Sci. 330:61-90.

Suzuki, Y. 1982. Carcinogenic and fibrogenic effects of zeolites. Preliminary observations. Environ. Res. 27:433-445.

Tarnovskii, G. N., G. M. Kashaeva, V. A. Shirgaeva, and G. G. Afonina. 1976. First discovery of tourmaline asbestos in pegmatites of the USSR. (In Russian). Vopr. Mineral. Geokhim. Pegmat. Vost. Sib.: 54-64.

Wagner, J. C. 1962. Experimental production of mesothelial tumors of the pleura by implantation of dusts in laboratory animals. Nature 196:567-581.

Appendix C

Fiber-Quality Parameters of Selected Asbestos, Whisker, and Glass Fibers

The strength-diameter effect of fine wires and fibers has been discovered and rediscovered several times during the last 250 years. Each time it excited great interest within the scientific community but was soon doubted and finally ignored after a few years. It is difficult to explain the reasons for this cyclical interest in the strength-diameter effect. One reason could be that no satisfactory theory has been developed and experimentally proven. Today, it is possible to observe surface defects and other submicroscopic features, such as the dissolution pattern of fibers, but the surface structure of fine fibrous substances still cannot be determined.

In the early 1800s, Karmarsch (1834) completed an extensive and systematic study on the strength-diameter effect of 18 different metal and alloy wires. In 1859, he derived an equation expressing the relationship between the increasing strength (F) and the decreasing diameter (D) of small-diameter wires. His equation (rephrased by Griffith, 1921) is:

$$F = A + B/D, \qquad \text{(C-1)}$$

where A and B are constants.

The constant A in the Karmarsch equation (C-1) was interpreted by Orowan (1933) as the strength of the internal structure and B as the strength of the surface structure. However, the Karmarsch equation did not satisfy all the more than 100 available strength-diameter measurements. This problem was recently resolved (Zoltai, 1981) by changing the surface area-to-volume ratio (B/D in the Karmarsch equation) to incorporate other features of the surface structure, e.g., the depth of the surface layer, the presence of growth steps (Marsh, 1962), and the effect of longitudinal cleavages (Cook and Gordon, 1964). Thus,

$$\sigma_f = \sigma_i \, (1 + 4K/D)^{1} + 4k/D, \qquad \text{(C-2)}$$

where σ_f is the strength of the fiber, σ_i is its internal strength, and K and k are factors expressing the increased strength of the surface layer over that of the internal structure.

Table C-1 shows the fiber characteristics (internal strength, K and k constants, etc.) of a selected group of natural and synthetic fibers. The values shown in the table illustrate the general characteristics of the examples and the relative magnitudes of the parameters given. Experimental data in reports by various researchers are difficult to compare because they often use different expressions of strength, different methods, and different units of measurement. Further limitations result from inaccurate readings of strength and diameter values from published small-scale graphs.

SIGNIFICANCE OF THE FIBER-QUALITY PARAMETERS

From the measurement of the tensile strength of sets of fibers and from subsequent calculations (using the above equations), one can calculate: (1) the internal strength of the fibers (σ_i) and (2) two constants (K and k), which express the relative increase in the strength of the surface structure. These parameters reflect the differences in the mechanical properties of fibers that grew under different conditions or that were modified by treatment and wear.

The following conclusions about fiber-quality parameters may be relevant to the potential health effects of fibers:

(1) The mechanical properties of fibers are directly related to the common properties of asbestiform fibers. Consequently, the three parameters can be used as numerical indicators of the degree of asbestiform development of fibers.

(2) - The two constants, K and k, must be positive for asbestiform fibers in order to account for their enhanced strength and flexibility.

- The K and k constants must be equal to zero for crystals that have no enhanced strength despite a defect-free surface structure.

- The K and k constants must be negative for cleavage fragments and other fragments whose surfaces are weaker than their internal structure because of the physical damage introduced by fracturing and subsequent processes.

(3) Because of the interdependent nature of the common asbestiform fiber properties, these three parameters may include a direct or indirect measure of the critical physicochemical property or properties that may be primarily responsible for the adverse health effects of asbestiform fibers. However, the nature of relationship between the fiber quality and carcinogenic potential of asbestiform fibers is still unknown.

TABLE C-1. Fiber "Parameters" of Selected Asbestos, Whisker, and Glass Fibers

Material or Fiber	Internal Strength (kg/cm^2)	K	k	Strength at 1 µm diameter (kg/cm^2)	Correlation Coefficient	Range of Diameters (µm)	Number of Fibers	References
Fiberglass:								
Fused silica	9,600	+2.4	-	>10	0.76	2-35	148	Reinkober, 1931
Fused silica	9,500	+1.9	-	82,000	0.74	2-25	23	Reinkober, 1931
Textile fiber	2,850	+9.3	-	115,000	0.99	2.5-18	>200	Anderegg, 1939
Fused silica	2,100	+20	-	175,000	0.85	1.5-10	18	Anderegg, 1939
Textile fiber	2,900	+4.6	-	57,000	0.84	4-11	21	Bateson, 1958
Aluminum-boron silicate	21,500	+0.01	-	22,000	0.97	0.1-1.5	9	Bartenev and Izmailova, 1962
Metal Whiskers:								
Silver	3,400	+1.6	-	25,000	0.37	2.5-11	10	Brenner, 1956
Copper	4,400	+2.2	-	42,000	0.75	2-16	32	Brenner, 1956
Copper	2,600	+2.3	-	27,000	0.69	2-14	43	Bokshtein et al., 1963
Copper	1,250	+12	-	64,000	0.79	3-16	29	Wolff and Coskren, 1965
Iron	6,700	+2.9	-	85,000	0.68	2-15	39	Brenner, 1958
Iron	4,500	+0.8	+0.8	109,000	0.84	2-4	14	Herzog, 1963
Iron	438	0.9	+0.3	14,000	0.89	1-3	9	Weik, 1959
Nickel coated	480	+1.0	+0.4	32,000	0.91	1-2	8	Weik, 1959
Silicon	6,375	+1.9	-	56,000	0.80	1-40	34	Marsh, 1963
Chromium	18,000	+0.3	-	37,000	0.74	0.3-1.2	24	Salkind et al., 1970

Material or Fiber	Internal Strength (kg/cm^2)	K	k	Strength at 1 μm diameter (kg/cm^2)	Correlation Coefficient	Range of Diameters (μm)	Number of Fibers	Reference
Halide Whiskers:								
Lithium fluoride	4,250	+0.4	+0.2	19,000	0.60	0.5-20	32	Fridman and Shpunt, 1963
Potassium chloride	120	+0.7	+0.3	2,250	0.71	1-25	22	Marsh, 1963
Sodium chloride (wet)	90	+0.3	—	200	0.23	3-7	11	Ewald and Folanyi, 1925
Sodium chloride	325	+0.6	+1.7	3,500	0.75	1-25	55	Gyulai, 1954
Sodium chloride	450	+0.5	—	1,400	0.66	1-10	18	Marsh, 1963
Sodium chloride ceramic substrate	250	+0.9	+0.7	7,600	0.84	2-14	42	Gyulai et al., 1961
Sodium chloride oil substrate	170	+1.5	+0.7	60,000	0.84	2-15	27	Gyulai et al., 1961
Sodium chloride alcohol solution	100	+2.9	+1.0	949,000	0.74	3-15	46	Gyulai et al., 1961
Oxide Whiskers:								
Zinc oxide	400	+0.6	+0.3	10,400	0.73	2-40	27	Evans et al., 1964
Dialuminum trioxide	13,000	+2.1	—	123,000	0.70	1.5-15	46	Bayer and Cooper, 1967
Dialuminum trioxide	19,000	+2.1	—	178,000	0.61	1-20	27	Mehan et al., 1965
Dialuminum trioxide	36,000	+0.2	—	100,000	0.39	0.6-38	40	Mehan et al., 1966
Dialuminum trioxide	39,000	+0.6	—	139,000	0.60	0.6-28	33	Soltia, 1967
Dialuminum trioxide	58,000	+0.5	—	150,000	0.63	0.5-5	33	Kelsey and Krock, 1967
Dialuminum trioxide	73,000	+0.3	—	166,000	0.66	1.5-25	29	Bokshtein et al., 1968

Material or Fiber	Internal Strength (kg/cm^2)	K	k	Strength at 1 μm diameter (kg/cm^2)	Correlation Coefficient	Range of Diameters (μm)	Number of Fibers	Reference
Carbon and Carbide Whiskers:								
Grafil A	3,850	+0.9	-	64,000	0.31	7-11	11	Perry et al., 1971
Thornel 50	4,250	+2.4	+0.8	>10	0.40	7-10	36	Jones and Duncan, 1971
PAN Precursor	1,800	+4.6	+1.3	>10	0.41	7-10	36	Jones and Duncan, 1971
Same at 1,000°C	25,400	+0.2	+0.1	61,000	0.40	7-11	82	Jones, 1971
Same at 2,500°C	2,750	+3.8	+1.1	>10	0.41	7-11	37	Jones, 1971
Silicon carbide	4,500	+1.2	+0.4	480,000	0.46	2-5	11	Kirchner and Knoll, 1963
Silicon carbide	9,900	+0.1	+0.2	12,000	0.30	0.2-5	15	Cook, 1970
Silicon carbide	10,100	+0.3	+0.1	34,000	0.49	1-4	20	Cook, 1970
Silicon carbide	72,000	+0.7	-	283,000	0.29	3-55	19	Webb et al., 1966
Silicon carbide	46,500	+1.2	-	264,000	0.54	2-8	34	Noone, 1967
Silicon carbide	47,900	+0.1	-	70,00	0.13	1-6	34	Herzog, 1967
Silicon nitride	8,700	+2.6	-	100,000	0.78	0.7-10	16	Bayer and Cooper, 1967

Material or Fiber	Internal Strength (kg/cm²)	K	k	Strength at 1 µm diameter (kg/cm²)	Correlation Coefficient	Range of Diameters (µm)	Number of Fibers	Reference
Asbestiform Mineral Fibers:								
Chrysotile	2,450	+1.0	+0.1	127,000	0.88	1.5-19	11	Nadgornyi et al., 1965
Crocidolite	6,150	+0.6	-	22,100	0.77	1-24	28	Nadgornyi et al., 1965
Anthophyllite	3,000	+1.5	-	21,000	0.81	0.7-21	31	Nadgornyi et al., 1965
Anthophyllite	670	+0.6	+0.3	8,200	0.92	0.5-6	25	Zoltai, personal communication, 1983
Rutile	14,000	+2.5	-	127,000	0.88	4-56	32	Maleev et al., 1972
Jamesonite	830	+11	-	24,000	0.75	10-105	36	Maleev et al., 1972
Bynthetic Asbestos:								
Magnesium-fluor richterite	1,200	+6.0	-	29,000	0.90	1.5-25	24	Nadgornyi et al., 1965
Same, slow cooled	4,700	+1.0	-	23,000	0.78	1-24	22	Nadgornyi et al., 1965
Lithium-flour amphibole	1,650	+1.8	-	13,200	0.92	1.5-24	27	Nadgornyi et al., 1965
Same, slow cooled	2,150	+3.9	-	35,000	0.92	0.8-15	23	Nadgornyi et al., 1965

REFERENCES

Anderegg, F. O. 1939. Strength of glass fiber. Ind. Eng. Chem. 31: 290-298.

Bartenev, G. M., and L. K. Izmailova. 1962. Defect-free glass fibers. (In Russian) Akad. Nauk. SSSR, Chem. Tech. Sect. 146:196-198.

Bateson, S. 1958. Critical study of the optical properties of glass fibres. J. Appl. Phys. 29:13-21.

Bayer, P. D., and R. E. Cooper. 1967. Size-strength effects in sapphire and silicon nitride whiskers at 20°C. J. Mater. Sci. 2:233-237.

Bokshtein, S. Z., S. T. Koshkin, and I. L. Svotkov. 1963. Tensile testing of filament crystals of copper, nickel and cobalt to failure. Sov. Phys. Solid State 4:1271-1277.

Bokshtein, S. Z., S. T. Koshkin, M. P. Nazarrova, and I. I. Svetlov. 1968. Size effect and anisotropy in the strength of sapphire whiskers at room temperature. Sov. Phys. Solid State 9:1488-1494.

Brenner, S. S. 1956. Tensile strength of whiskers. J. Appl. Phys. 27:1481-1491.

Brenner, S. S. 1958. Growth and properties of whiskers. Science 128: 569-575.

Cook, J. 1970. Mechanical testing of whiskers. Composites (March):176-180.

Cook, J., and J. J. Gordon. 1964. A mechanism for the control of crack propagation in all brittle systems. Proc. R. Soc. London, Ser. A 282:508-518.

Evans, C. C., J. E. Gordon, and D. M. Marsh. 1964. The strength of whiskers of silicon, zinc oxide and phthalocyanine. Proc. R. Soc. London, Ser. A 282:218-220.

Ewald, W., and M. Polanyi. 1925. Plastizität und Festigkeit von Steinsalz unter Wasser. Z. Phys. 31:29-50.

Fridman, V. Y., and A. A. Shpunt. 1963. Investigation of the strength of lithium fluoride crystal fragments. Sov. Phys. Solid State 5:575-579.

Griffith, A. R. 1921. The phenomena of rupture and flow in solids. Phil. Trans. R. Soc. London, Ser. A 221:163-198.

Gyulai, Z. 1954. Festigkeit-und Plastizitäteigenschaften von NaCl Nadelkristallen. Z. Phys. 138:317-321.

Gyulai, Z., E. Hartman, and B. Jeszenszky. 1961. Zerreissfestigkeit-Messungen an NaCl Nadelkristallen (whiskers). Phys. Satue Solidi 1:726-729.

Herzog, J. A. 1963. Strength investigations with unidimensionally grown cyrstalline iron (whisker). Metallurgia 17:7-14.

Herzog, J. A. 1967. Entwicklung und Zukunft in der Whiskerforschung. Jahrb. Wissen. Gesellsch. Luftfahrt. (WGLR)

Jones, B. F. 1971. Further observations concerning the effect of diameter on the fracture strength and Yung's Modulus of carbon and graphite fibers made from polyacrylonitrile. J. Mater. Sci. 6:1225-1227.

Jones, B. F., and R. G. Duncan. 1971. The effect of fiber diameter on the mechanical properties of graphite fibers manufactured from polyacrylonitrile and rayon. J. Mater. Sci. 6:289-293.

Karmarsch, K. 1834. Versuche über die Festigkeit der zu Draht gezogenen Metallen. Jhhrb. Polytech. Inst. Wien 18:57-115.
Karmarsch, K. 1859. Über die absolute Festigkeit der Metalldrähte. Mitt. Gew. Ver. Konigr. Hannover, pp. 137-156.
Kelsey, R. H., and R. H. Krock. 1967. Tension testing alumina whiskers. J. Mater. Sci. 2:146-159.
Kirchner, H. P., and P. Knoll. 1963. Silicon carbide whiskers. J. Am. Ceram. Soc. 46:299-300.
Maleev, M. N., A. P. Krusilina, and V. N. Rosanckij. 1972. Ultimate strength of naturally fibrous rutile, antimony and jamesonite crystals. (In Russian) C. R. Acad. Bulg. Sci. 25:1085-1088.
Marsh, D. M. 1963. Stress concentration at steps on crystal surfaces and their role in fracture. Fracture of Solids, Metal. Society Conference 20. Interscience Publishers, New York.
Mehan, R. L., E. Feingold, and E. Gatti. 1965. Technical Report AFMLTR 65 275, August.
Mehan, R. L., W. H. Sutton, and J. A. Herzog. 1966. A review of measuring the strength of whiskers and their role in reinforcing ductile matrices. AIAA J. 4:1889-1898.
Nadgornyi, E. M., L. F. Grigoreva, and A. P. Ivanor. 1965. The mechanical properties of synthetic fibrous fluoramphiboles and certain forms of natural asbestos. Izv. Akad. Nauk. SSSR Neorg. Mater. 1:1117-1123.
Noone, M. J. 1967. The preparation, structure and mechanical properties of filamentary forms of silicon carbide. Ph.D. Thesis. University of Leeds, United Kingdom.
Orowan, E. 1933. Die erhöhte Festigkeit dünner Fäden, der Joffe-Effekt und verwandte Erscheinungen vom Standpunkt der Griffitschen-Bruchtheorie. Z. Phys. 86:195-213.
Perry, A. J., K. Phillips, and E. de Lamotte. 1971. The mechanical properties of carbon fibres. Fibre Sci. Technol. 3:317-319.
Reinkober, O. 1931. Die Zerreissfestigkeit dünner Quarzfäden. Phys. Zeitschr. 32:243-250.
Salkind, M. J., F. D. Lemkey, and F. D. George. 1970. Whisker composites by eutectic solidification. Chapter 10 in A. P. Levitt, ed. Whisker Technology. Interscience Publishers, New York.
Soltis, P. J. 1967. A new method and technique for tension testing whiskers. J. Mater. Sci. 2:300-324.
Webb, W. W., R. D. Dragsdorff, and W. D. Forgeng. 1957. Dislocations of whiskers. Phys. Rev. 108:498-499.
Webb, W. W., H. D. Bathand, and R. S. Shaffer. 1966. Strength characteristics of whisker crystals, microcrystals and macrocrystals. Chapter 14 in J. J. Purke, N. L. Reed, and V. Weiss, eds. Strengthening Mechanisms. Syracuse University Press, Syracuse, N.Y.
Weik, H. 1959. Whisker structure and tensile strength. J. Appl. Phys. 30:791-792.
Wolff, E. G., and T. D. Coskren. 1965. Growth and morphology of magnesium oxide whiskers. J. Am. Ceram. Soc. 48:279-285.
Zoltai, T. 1981. Amphibole asbestos mineralogy. Pp. 237-278 in D. R. Veblen, ed. Amphiboles and Other Hydrous Pyriboles. MSA Reviews in Mineralogy, 9A. Mineralogical Society of America, Washington, D.C.

Appendix D

Conceptual Model of Fiber Exposure

Because measurement of exposures to all potentially hazardous asbestiform fibers is technically infeasible in some cases and prohibitively expensive in others, indirect methods of estimating exposure must augment the direct measurements. Although the committee did not develop a comprehensive mathematical model of fiber exposure, it did develop a conceptual model of the computations that would be necessary for a full mathematical model of the exposure process. This conceptual model enabled the committee to identify the factors that could be important in determining exposure so that it could seek information in an organized way and attempt to relate the information about one fiber type to that for other fibers to facilitate an analysis of comparative exposure potentials.

Figure D-1 provides a conceptual overview of the calculations that would be necessary to estimate nonoccupational exposures of humans in the absence of direct measurements. The scheme shows four types of information: quantities, factors, units, and operators. A <u>quantity</u> is a calculated numeric value that represents some physical aspect of exposure to asbestiform fibers. A <u>factor</u> is an exogenous (external) input to the calculation, which can be measured or itself calculated outside the system. Without factor inputs, the quantities cannot be calculated. <u>Units</u> are the physical units of measurement for the quantities and factors. An <u>operator</u> is a mathematical manipulation that derives a new quantity from one or more factors and other quantities. For example, the quantity "human intake rate (by inhalation)" is calculated by multiplying (using the multiplication operator on) the quantity "ambient concentration in air" by the factor "breathing rate." In each step, the input quantity is a result of all the previous steps; the factor represents a new, physically important parameter <u>not</u> a result of the previous steps; and the output quantity serves as the input quantity for the next step. In every case, the units of the input quantities and factors must combine correctly under the operator to yield the units of the output quantity.

In this conceptual-level scheme it is not necessary to be able to measure each factor physically, but each must describe a phenomenon of interest and be, at least in principle, estimatable from physically

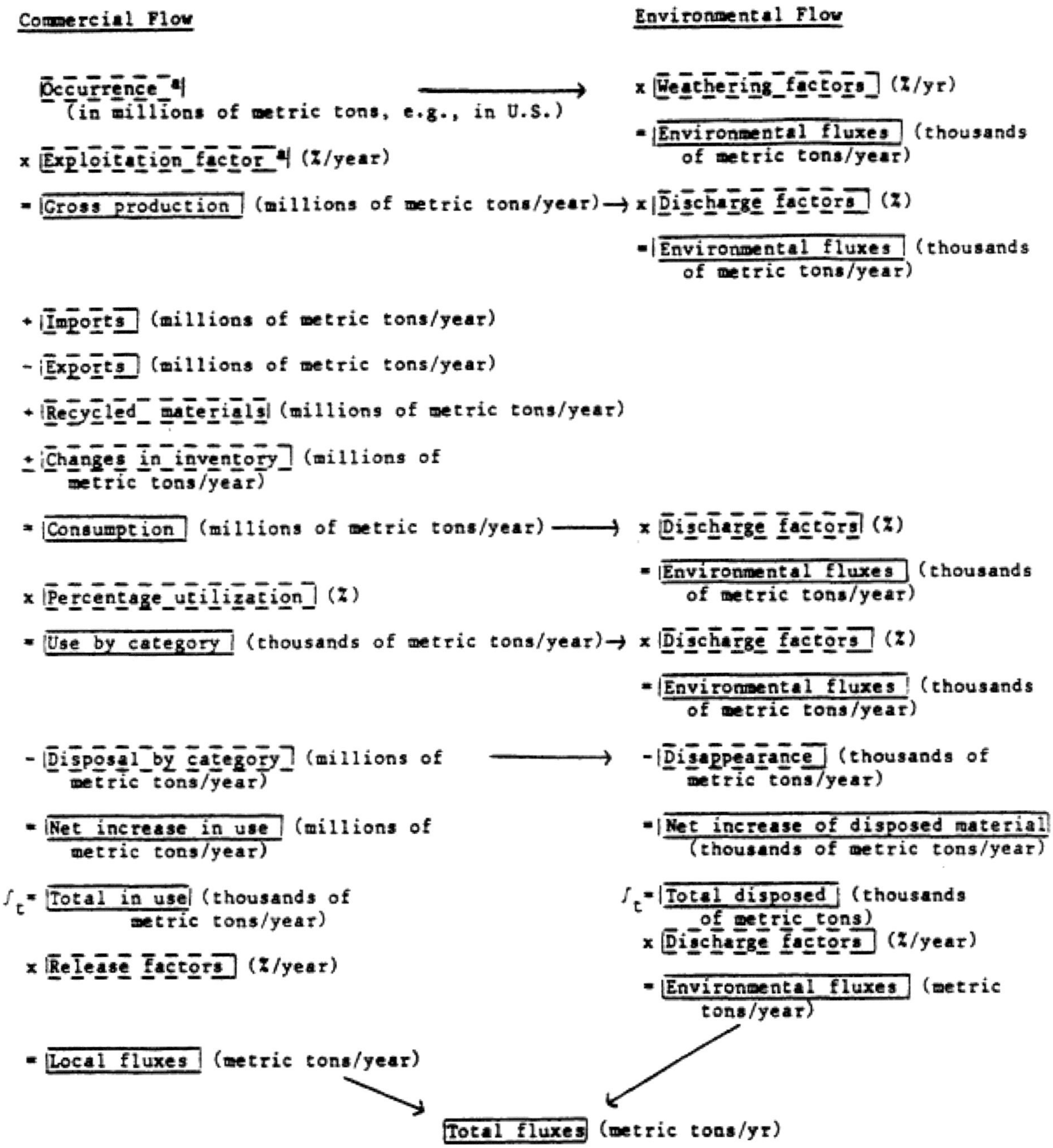
Commercial Flow
Environmental Flow
Occurrence [a]
(in millions of metric tons, e.g., in U.S.)
x Weathering factors (%/yr)
= Environmental fluxes (thousands of metric tons/year)
x Exploitation factor [a] (%/year)
= Gross production (millions of metric tons/year)
x Discharge factors (%)
= Environmental fluxes (thousands of metric tons/year)
+ Imports (millions of metric tons/year)
- Exports (millions of metric tons/year)
+ Recycled materials (millions of metric tons/year)
± Changes in inventory (millions of metric tons/year)
= Consumption (millions of metric tons/year)
x Discharge factors (%)
= Environmental fluxes (thousands of metric tons/year)
x Percentage utilization (%)
= Use by category (thousands of metric tons/year)
x Discharge factors (%)
= Environmental fluxes (thousands of metric tons/year)
- Disposal by category (millions of metric tons/year)
- Disappearance (thousands of metric tons/year)
= Net increase in use (millions of metric tons/year)
= Net increase of disposed material (thousands of metric tons/year)
∫t = Total in use (thousands of metric tons/year)
∫t = Total disposed (thousands of metric tons)
x Discharge factors (%/year)
x Release factors (%/year)
= Environmental fluxes (metric tons/year)
= Local fluxes (metric tons/year)
Total fluxes (metric tons/yr)

[a]Natural materials only.

Figure D-1
General flow of computational logic for estimating exposures to fibers.

Total fluxes (metric tons/year)

− Deposition (metric tons/year)

÷ Dilution factors (m^3/yr; liters/year)

= Ambient concentrations (μg/m^3; μg/liter)

x Conversion factors (fibers/cm^3 per μg/m^3; fibers/ml per μg/liter)

= Fiber concentrations (fibers/cm^3; fibers/ml)

x Breathing, drinking rates (m^3/day, liters/day)

= Human intake rates (fibers/day)

x Biodisposition factors (%/organ)

= Tissue fluxes (fibers/day)

− Disappearance (fibers/day)

= Net tissue increase (fibers/day)

$\int_t$ = Tissue burden (fibers)

x Tissue clearance rate (%/day)

= Disappearance

Key: [solid box] = quantity

[dashed box] = factor

(   ) = unit

⟶ = link from commercial to environmental flow

t = time

Metric ton = 2,205 pounds.

measurable quantities. For example, the "deposition" of fibers on their way from source to exposed humans may not be directly measurable, but the principle can be demonstrated by measuring concentrations of fibers at various distances from known and quantified sources, and then describing the deposition as a function of distance through appropriate computations.

The model sketched in Figure D-1 is intended to apply to virtually any fiber type, but not all of the steps would apply to every type. For example, occurrence (millions of metric tons of fibrous material known or suspected) and weathering (relative rate of loss of such material) would not apply to man-made fibers. Moreover, the commercial flows on the left aide of the scheme would be of dominant importance for some fibers, whereas the environmental flows on the right side would predominate for others. This commercial versus environmental flow distinction is important, as explained for Figure 1-2, because of potential need for controls of both types of flow.

In brief, the factors shown in Figure D-1 take into account the following phenomena:

Occurrence: Geologic occurrence in the United States. In principle, this factor could be measured by the proven and indicated reserves of the mineral, if commercially important, or by a relative abundance figure for others. It can be measured in millions of metric tons.

Weathering: The amount of material in place that might be released into the environment (as either airborne or waterborne particulates) per year. The natural weathering processes may occasionally be enhanced through noncommercial disturbance by humans.

Exploitation: The amount deliberately extracted for use. Should include amount used with and without further processing, for example, the asbestos content of road surfacing aggregates.

Imports, exports: The flows of materials to and from foreign countries. For example, on the basis of relative amounts, asbestos flows from Canada are greater than those resulting from extraction in the United States.

Recycled materials: Fibers suitable for recycling after disposal from first use. This practice does not seem to be very widespread in the industry because of the low cost of original production.

Percentage utilization: Essentially synonymous with "use patterns." Considers percentage of the total consumption in the United States that goes into each use. There may be a chain of uses. For example, asbestos fiber may go into asbestos paper, which in turn is used in insulation for electric appliances. In principle, opportunities for release of asbestos occur both in the manufacture of the paper and in the manufacture of the appliance as well as during use of the appliance.

Disposal: Disposal of fiber products after use. Virtually every fiber product has a finite useful life. Afterward, most of the fibers reach some form of landfill, but some enter air, or possibly water, during demolition. The fibers in landfill then pose a secondary source of potential exposure. Fibers lost from such sites ("disappearance") decrease the inventory there, thus decreasing the rate of accumulation.

Discharge factors: The potential for release into environmental air or water for each process through which the fibers pass. The factors can be expressed as a percentage of throughput (i.e., metric tons released per thousand metric tons processed, multiplied by 100) or as a percentage rate of total inventory (i.e., metric tons discharged per year per metric ton in place, multiplied by 100). Generally, the release is called a "discharge" when associated with a manufacturing process, but a "release" when associated with product use, e.g., when fibers are worn off vinyl asbestos tiles.

Dilution factors: The net effect of all processes that disperse fibers in air or water away from the source. If fibers are released inside a building, the dilution factors are related to the number of air changes per hour and the volume of air in the enclosed space. In ambient air, the factors are used to convert the discharge rate to ambient concentration as a function of distance from the source, wind direction, and other influences. In water, they are used to convert the discharge rates to the concentrations in water supplies. In tap water, the actual concentration may be lower than the calculated concentration because of filtration and settling. In each case, the result of applying a dilution factor is to compute a concentration in a medium of exposure (generally air or water) at a location where people are exposed to these concentrations.

Conversion factors: Factors used to convert measurements to number of fibers per unit volume. Concentration is often measured in terms of mass per unit volume. Conversion factors are used to change these measurements to fibers per unit volume to conform with the usual measurements of dose in dose-response relationships. They are functions of fiber type, releasing activity, distance from point of release, and other considerations.

Breathing and drinking rates: Factors used to convert the exposure doses into the intake doses or dose rates. For example, if a worker breathes air at a rate of 8 m^3 per 8-hour day, then one can calculate the intakes of fibers per day, week, year, or working lifetime from the average concentration in the air of the workplace. For nonoccupational exposures, one must also account for such variations in rates as those occurring between working and other activities (including sleep), between ingestion of water or (in principle) food, between high and low exposure areas, and between adults and children.

Biodisposition factors: Factors used to convert intake rates to dose rates for particular tissues. For example, if one estimates that 30% of the inhaled dose is subsequently swallowed (National Research Council, 1983), then one can calculate the dose entering the gastrointestinal (GI) tract (fibers/unit time) from the inhalation rate (fibers/unit time).

Disappearance: Removal of fibers from tissues. Fibers may disappear from tissues through excretion or through various degradation processes. For example, fibrous glass appears to gel (Klingholz and Steinkopf, 1981), whereas chrysotile separates into finer fibers and fibrils (Jaurand et al., 1977) and shorter fibers may be removed from tissues by macrophages. These processes limit the buildup of fibers in tissue. Formation of ferruginous bodies also may "remove" the fibers making them less biologically active. The dose rate and disappearance rate together determine the buildup of tissue burden of fibers.

SUMMARY

Although the above list does not contain all the factors that define exposure at the tissue level, and although the conceptual model captures neither all their relationships nor the difficulty in measuring some of them, the model does give an idea of the complexity of the exposure of an individual to asbestiform fibers. A further difficulty for risk assessment is to estimate the number of people falling into each category of exposure so that the distribution of exposures over the entire U.S. population can be described.

REFERENCES

Jaurand, M.C., J. Bignon, P. Sebastien, and J. Goni. 1977. Leaching of chrysotile asbestos in human beings: Correlation with in vitro studies using rabbit alveolar macrophages. Environ. Res. 14:245-254.

Klingholz, R., and B. Steinkopf. 1981. The Behavior of Synthetic Mineral Fibers in a Physiological Model Liquid and in Water. Report No. 81-0-08, ISOVER, Grunzweig und Hartman und Glasfaser AG, September 30 (Translated from German).

National Research Council. 1983. Drinking Water and Health. Vol. 5. Report of the Safe Drinking Water Committee, Commission on Life Sciences. National Academy Press, Washington, D.C.

Appendix E

Epidemiological Studies Among Cohorts Exposed To Asbestos

Contents

The references given in these tables can be found on the list for Chapter 5.

TABLE E-1. Studies of Cancer Mortality Among Asbestos-Exposed Occupational Cohorts

Cohort Number	Study Population and Design Characteristics	Exposure Characteristics	Results	Summary of Conclusions and Special Comments	Reference[a]
1	Location: Canada 11,379 workers (10,939 men and 440 women) born between 1891 and 1920 who had worked for at least 1 month in the Asbestos and Thetford, Quebec, mines and mills. Analysis based on deaths, 20 or more years after first employment, occurring from 1951 to 1975. Used internal comparison groups for smoking analysis. Expected numbers of deaths were computed from Province of Quebec death rates. Follow-up to end of 1975 with 90.1% traced Cohort includes 5,302 male employees from Asbestos and 5,637 males from Thetford Mines. Females employed mainly at Asbestos (408, 92.7%).	Chrysotile mining at Asbestos and Thetford Mines in Quebec. Quantitative exposure data expressed as mppcf-years[b] and estimated as cumulative dust exposure during the first 20 years from onset of employment. Smoking histories obtained by questionnaire in 1970 for 99.6% of those alive in the cohort. Questionnaires were returned by 93% of the relatives of subjects who had died after 1950. Mines and mills at Thetford Mines believed to be dustier than those in Asbestos, Quebec. Thetford Mines cohort had longer duration of employment and higher estimated dust exposures.	Results for male deaths from 1951 to 1975, 20 or more years from first exposure. Cause of Death — Obs — Exp — O/E[c] All causes — 3,291 — 2,992 — 1.1 Lung cancer — 230 — 184 — 1.3 Gastrointestinal cancer — 276 — 272.4 — 1.0 Mesothelioma — 10 — --[d] — -- There was also one female death from mesothelioma. Total of 4,463 deaths in men and 84 in women by end of 1975. Gradient of risk for lung cancer by length of service noted; SMR[e] 1.0 for <1 year to 1.6 for >20 years. Gradient of risk for lung cancer by exposure level also noted; SMR 0.9 for <30 mppcf-years to 2.3 for >300 mppcf-years. Overall relatively small increase in risk for lung cancer or other causes of death except for pneumoconiosis (230 deaths obs., SMR 1.3 for lung cancer; 42 deaths obs., SMR 13.6 for pneumoconiosis). Excess gastrointestinal cancer noted for males most heavily exposed, principally at Thetford Mines.	Large cohort for study and excellent data analysis. Gradient of lung cancer risk observed with quantitative exposure level. Nonsmokers had greater increase in risk for lung cancer (relative risk, 10.0), compared to smokers (relative risk, 2.0) when the highest and lowest asbestos exposure groups were compared. No evidence for multiplicative effect of asbestos and smoking. Study results suggest an overall small increase in lung cancer associated with asbestos exposure. Consistent dose-response gradient; SMR 0.9 (low exposure) to 2.3 for highest exposure category observed.	McDonald et al., 1979, 1980

[a]See Chapter 5 reference list.
[b]mppcf = million particles per cubic foot.
[c]O/E = observed deaths/expected deaths.
[d]-- Mesothelioma is usually so infrequent that "expected" values are not used.
[e]SMR = standardized mortality ratio (O/E).

Cohort Number	Study Population and Design Characteristics	Exposure Characteristics	Results	Summary of Conclusions and Special Comments	Reference
2	Location: Canada 544 mine and mill male employees employed during 1961 for at least 20 years in one of four companies mining and milling chrysotile asbestos in Thetford Mines, Quebec. Follow-up to August 1977. Trace complete. Expected numbers of deaths were computed from Canadian national death rates. Cohort represents a subgroup of cohort studied by McDonald *et al.* (1980).	Chrysotile mining and milling workers. Dust measurements after 1969 reviewed, but no quantitative exposure data used in analysis. No smoking information	Cause of Death / Obs. / Exp. / O/E All causes: 178 / 159.9 / 1.1 All cancer: 49 / 36.7 / 1.3 Lung cancer: 28 / 11.1 / 2.5 Gastrointestinal cancer: 10 / 9.5 / 1.1 Mesothelioma: 1 / -- / -- Other cancer sites: 10 / 16.1 / 0.6 Observed deaths based on best available evidence. Canadian national rates used for comparison	Evaluation of best diagnostic evidence vs. death certificate statement indicated that principal difference occurred for asbestosis where 10/24 were assigned to other causes of death. In addition, 7/25 deaths due to lung cancer were assigned on death certificate to other causes. Mesothelioma uncommon in this cohort of miners and millers. Increased risk of lung cancer in these analyses suggests that miners and millers experience about the same excess risk as factory workers and that these excesses are less than those reported for insulators studied by Selikoff *et al.* (1979). Study results indicate a small increase in lung cancer risk occurs as asbestos exposure increases, but lack of quantitative exposure data makes it difficult to evaluate this association.	Nicholson *et al.*, 1979

Cohort Number	Study Population and Design Characteristics	Exposure Characteristics	Results	Summary of Conclusions and Special Comments	Reference
3	Location: Italy 952 males with at least 30 days employment at any time between January 1, 1930, and December 31, 1965. Case-control analysis of lung and laryngeal cancer cases within cohort. Italian national death rates were used to compute expected numbers. Workers employed between 1930 and 1945 who did not survive and for whom vital status could not be ascertained were excluded. Follow-up from 1946 to 1975; 98% traced.	Chrysotile asbestos miners. Quantitative exposure data based on individual work histories and fiber counts since 1969, which were used to create a dust index in fiber-years for each study subject.	Cause of Death / Obs / Exp / O/E: All causes 332 214.4 1.6 All cancer 50 47.0 1.1 Lung cancer 11 10.4 1.1 Gastrointestinal cancer 19 19.3 1.0 Mesothelioma (1)* -- -- Other cancer sites 14 15.4 0.9 Larynx 6 1.9 3.2** *suspected case of pleural mesothelioma. **p≤ .05. Increased relative risks for lung cancer (2.9) and laryngeal cancer (3.3) when case-control groups were compared by exposure level.	Gradient of risk for lung cancer with time since onset of exposure (SMR 0.6 for <20 years vs. 1.2 for >20 years) and calendar time (SMR 0.6 for 1961-1965 vs. 2.1 for 1971-1975). Significantly higher risk noted only for laryngeal cancer. Balangero area of Italy has one of the highest incidences of laryngeal cancer in the world. Thus, use of national mortality rates may have resulted in an overestimation of risk for laryngeal cancer associated with asbestos exposure in this cohort. Two hospital-based case-control studies (Stell and MacGill, 1973; Shettigara and Morgan, 1975) showed a positive association of laryngeal cancer and asbestos exposure.	Rubino *et al.*, 1979a

Cohort Number	Study Population and Design Characteristics	Exposure Characteristics	Results	Summary of Conclusions and Special Comments	Reference
4	Location: Finland All workers employed ≥3 months from January 1, 1936 to July 1, 1967 in two asbestos quarries. 1,092 persons in the cohort; 1.045 traced. Cohort consisted of males and females; specific numbers by sex not provided Follow-up 96% complete by mid-1977. Of the 1,045 employees with follow-up information, 248 died between January 1, 1936 and July 1, 1967. The remaining 763 were interviewed for smoking histories. Cohort first compared to an age and sex-matched control group from the surrounding area (Meurman et al., 1974). A second comparison (Meurman et al., 1979) was made using proportional mortality data for Finland (1958 data for deaths from 1936 to 1967 and 1972 data for deaths from 1968 to 1977).	Anthophyllite asbestos mining. No dust measurements or quantitative exposure data.	248 deaths reported in 1974 report: Cause of Death / Obs. / Exp. / O/E Lung cancer / 21 / 12.6 / 1.7 Gastrointestinal cancer / 7 / 8.0 / 0.9 No mesotheliomas observed 384 deaths reported in 1979 report: Cause of Death / Obs. / Exp. / O/E Lung cancer / 44 / 22.4 / 2.0 Gastrointestinal cancer / 18 / Not estimated O/E for lung cancer in low exposure group was 1.4; for heavily exposed employees, it was 3.3. No meso-theliomas reported. All lung cancer claes occurred among males.	Lung cancer data suggest a dose-response relationship. Cigarette smoking date consistent with an increased risk for lung cancer in combination with asbestos exposure. Group / Relative Risk Nonsmoking, asbestos-exposed / 1.4 Smoking, not asbestos-exposed / 12.0 Smoking, asbestos-exposed / 17.0	Meurman et al., 1974. 1979

Cohort Number	Study Population and Design Characteristics	Exposure Characteristics	Results	Summary of Conclusions and Special Comments	Reference
5	Location: Western Australia	Crocidolite mining and Milling.	Cause of Death / Obs. / Exp. / O/E All causes 526 587.2 0.9 All cancer 60 38.2 1.6 Mesotelioma 26 71.6 0.7 Other cancer sites 51	Lack of gastrointestinal cancer excess is consistent with findings in gas-mask exposure cohorts who processed the crocidolite mined in Australia.	Mobbs et al., 1980
	6,200 males ever employes by Australian Blue Asbestos Company between 1943 and 1966 identified from payroll end other records. Mine closed in 1966.	No dust messurements or quantitative exposure date.			
		No. smoking information.	There were 26 cases of mesothelioma. Rates of mesothelioma increased with duration and intensity of exposure. Interval trots first exposure to diagnosis of mesothelioma ranged from 13.3 to 30.7 years.	Cancer risk considerably lower in subgroup with less than 3 months of employment. Follow-up period for majority of employees is still too short to predict the future incidence of mesothelioma in this cohort	
		Three estimated exposure categories used in analysis:			
	Expected deaths were computed from Australian national death rates.	Heavy occupations in the mine and mill Medium/light occupations; employees with other occupations Occupation unspecified	No excesses of gastrointestinal cancer were observed aft this cohort. Data not reported.		
	Follow-up was 80% complete in 1978.		The lung cancer SMR for heavy exposure jobs was 2.1; SMR for medium/light exposure was 1.1 Overall incidence of pneumoconiosis was 3.5%.		

Cohort Number	Study Population and Design Characteristics	Exposure Characteristics	Results	Summary of Conclusions and Special Comments	Reference
6	Location: United States 1,261 white males employed 1 or more months between January 1, 1940 and December 31, 1965. Expected numbers based on U.S. white male death rate even though mortality rates in county where plant is located were 75% higher than U.S. rates for white males (age-adjusted lung cancer mortality rate per 100,000 white males, 66.5 vs. 37.9). Follow-up through December 31, 1975 for 97.1% of cohort. Minimum follow-up for all subjects was 10 years.	Chrysotile asbestos textile factory workers. Quantitative exposure data based on fiber counts by job and calendar time. Fiber counts (mppcf) converted to filter counts (fibers longer than 5 μm/cm³), with 3 fibers/cm³ equivalent to 1 mppcf for all textile operations except preparation, which used 8 fibers/cm³.	Cause of Death / Obs. / Exp. / O/E All causes: 308 / 205.7 / 1.5 All cancer: 59 / 35.1 / 1.7 Lung cancer: 35 / 11.1 / 3.2 Gastrointestinal cancer: 13 / 9.9 / 1.3 Of 308 deaths, only one due to mesothelioma (peritoneal). Increased risk of nonmalignant respiratory disease (28 obs. vs. 9.5 exp.). Some smoking histories were available to estimate smoking patterns of cohort; 52.4% smokers and 22.3% ex-smokers.	Strong gradient of risk observed with quantitative exposure level for lung cancer and nonmalignant respiratory disease. SMR for lung cancer increased with latency to 7.3 (15 obs. vs. 2.1 exp.) for ≥20 years since initial employment. Statistically significant excess of lung cancer even in cumulative exposure category of less than 10,000 (fibers/cm³)days. On the basis of findings in this study, elevated risks are predicted for lung cancer and nonmalignant respiratory disease at an exposure level considerably lower than those in other studies and at the exposure level of the current OSHA standard (2.0 fibers/cm³). Study shows a strong increase in lung cancer risk associated with increased asbestos exposure, but the significant increase in risk even in the lower exposure categories suggests that the exposures may be underestimated. In addition, the O/E ratios may be too high because an inappropriate comparison group was used.	Dement *et al.*, 1982, 1983b

Cohort Number	Study Population and Design Characteristics	Exposure Characteristics	Results	Summary of Conclusions and Special Comments	Reference
7	Location: United States 933 workers ever employed between 1941 and 1945; 820 with 5 years or more since onset of employment. Additional analysis limited to 582 still alive 20 years after employment began (Selikoff et al., 1980). The 351 excluded were either dead (270), lost to follow-up (42), or had worked elsewhere with asbestos (39). When possible, supplementary information on cause of death was obtained. Expected numbers based on death rates in the State of New Jersey and on death rates in the American Cancer Society's (ACS) prospective study of smokers. The latter study provided rates by smoking status. Follow-up of the study cohort was 100% through 1977.	Amosite asbestos factory in operation from 1941 to 1954. No dust measurement or quantitative exposure data. Smoking histories were obtained in 1961 when surveillance of the population began. Examinations were performed on this group after that date.	Results for 5 years or longer since initial employment (Seidman et al., 1979): Cause of Death — Obs — Exp — O/E All causes — 528 — 407.4 — 1.3 All cancer — 164 — 83.8 — 2.0 Lung cancer — 83 — 22.8 — 3.6 Gastrointestinal cancer — 28 — 22.7 — 1.2 Mesothelioma — 14 — -- — -- Results for 20 years or longer since initial employment (Selikoff et al., 1980): Cause of Death — Obs — Exp — O/E All causes — 304 — 158.6 — 1.9 All cancer — 103 — 33.4 — 3.1 Lung cancer — 52 — 10.1 — 5.1 Gastrointestinal cancer — 15 — 7.2 — 2.1 Mesothelioma — 14 — -- — -- Larynx cancer — 3 — 1.6 — 1.9 Kidney cancer — 2 — 0.8 — 2.5 The SMR for all causes of mortality increased 120% when adjusted for smoking on the basis of ACS rates. Excess deaths from nonmalignant respiratory disease also occurred in these workers (29/4.7). Seven pleural and seven peritoneal mesotheliomas were observed.	Cohort represents a somewhat unique study group having had very short intense work exposures, followed by a long period of observation. Long follow-up and exclusion of persons observed less than 20 years will tend to yield higher risk estimates than would other study conditions. Approximately 5% of original cohort lost to follow-up. A clear multiplicative effect of smoking and asbestos was observed. No exposure information available. Study results suggest a very large increase in lung cancer risk associated with asbestos exposure, but exposure estimates are questionable.	Seidman et al., 1979 Selikoff et al., 1972, 1980

Cohort Number	Study Population and Design Characteristics	Exposure Characteristics	Results	Summary of Conclusions and Special Comments	Reference
8 21	Location: United Kingdom 4,600 males with at least 30 days employment between April 1, 1933 and May 31, 1964. 922 females first employed between January 1, 1936 and December 1, 1942. Expected numbers based on national death rates in United Kingdom and Wales. Follow-up through December 31, 1975 (Newhouse and Berry, 1979) Male follow-up was 93%. Female follow-up was 77%. 1,368 male insulation workers analyzed separately.	East London asbestos factory opened in 1913 and closed in 1968. Produced asbestos textiles and insulation materials. Crocidolite asbestos used until the late 1950s; chrysotile and amosite also used. No dust measurements or quantitative exposure data. Smoking histories obtained on workers alive in 1971.	Male deaths: Cause of Deaths: / Obs / Exp / O/E All causes / 545 / 438.0 / 1.2 Lung cancer / 103 / 43.2 / 2.4 Gastrointestinal cancer / 40 / 34.0 / 1.2 Mesothelioma / 46 / -- / -- Other cancer sites / 38 / 27.4 / 1.4 Male Cohort: SMR of 5.4 for lung cancer in severely exposed workers with >2 years employment (54/10.4) and 2.4 for those low to moderately exposed (31/12.8). Risk increased with duration of follow-up and severity of exposure (1979). 19 pleural and 27 peritoneal mesotheliomas observed. Female deaths: Cause of Death / Obs / Exp / O/E All causes / 200 / 118 / 1.7 Lung cancer / 27 / 3.2 / 8.4 Gastrointestinal cancer / 20 / 10.2 / 2.0 Mesothelioma / 21 / -- / -- Female Cohort: SMR for lung cancer, 6.0 (3/0.5) in low to moderately exposed group; 7.9 (15/1.9) and 26.3 (21/0.8) in the severely exposed groups with <2 years and >2 years of employment, respectively. An apparent excess of breast (6/2.1) and ovarian (3/0.7) cancer was observed in the severely exposed group. Thirteen pleural and seven peritoneal mesotheliomas observed (one of unknown origin).	In female cohort, 23% was lost to follow-up, but results were consistent with those in males. Dust levels in low to moderately exposed group were estimated to be 5-10 fibers/cm^3; in the severely exposed group, 20 fibers/cm^3 or greater. After 1946, plant-wide levels were generally lower but probably in excess of 2 fibers/cm^3. A survey of smoking habits in 1971 indicated that 74% of males and 73% of females smoked. Estimates from population surveys would have predicted 66% and 53%, respectively. There were no smoking data on workers in the mortality analysis. The authors believed that smoking did not account for more than 10% to 20% of the excess lung cancer. Approximately 10% of all deaths among males and females were due to mesothelioma.	Newhouse and Berry, 1979 Newhouse *et al.*, 1972 Newhouse, 1969

Cohort Number	Study Population and Design Characteristics	Exposure Characteristics	Results				Summary of Conclusions and Special Comments	References
9, 22	Location: United Kingdom All employees ever employed in a factory that produced friction materials.	Chrysotile with short periods of crocidolite use.	Mortality 10 years after first exposure for men (N = 7,474):				No gradient of risk observed with quantitative exposure level.	Newhouse et al., 1982
		Factory founded in 1898.	Cause of Death	Obs.	Exp.	O/E		Berry and Newhouse, 1983
	13,460 workers (male and female) employed in 1941 or any time later. Case-control analysis within cohort for mesothetioma cases and for lung and Rastrointestinal cases.	Quantitative exposure data bleed on dust measurements and work histories. Exposures simulated for earlier periods.	All causes Lung cancer Gastrointestinal cancer Mesothelioma Other cancer Other causes	1,339 143 103 8 77 1,008	1,362 139 107 88 1,027	0.9 1.0 1.0 0.9 1.0	No evidence of excess mortality due to cancer of any site, except mesothelioma, even when examined by duration of exposure, duration of employment, or period of initial employment. Nine of 10 mesothelioma cases were employed during one or both periods when crocidolite was used.	
			For women (N = 3,708):					
			Cause of Death	Obs	Exp.	O/E		
	Expected numbers were based on notional rates for males and females in the United Kingdom Follow-up was 99% through 1979.		All causes Lung cancer Gastrointestinal cancer Mesothelioma Other cancer Other causes	299 6 29 2 51 211	328 11.3 27 60 229	0.9 0.5 1.1 0.9 0.9	Of the mesothelioma cases, 80% worked with crocidolite compared to 8% of controls No increased risk of lung cancer or gastrointestinal cancer associated with either duration or cumulative exposure in case-control analysis.	
			One of the men certified as pleural mesothelioma (age 50) had worked at factory for 2 weeks (at age 29) in 1960.					

Cohort Number	Study Population and Design Characteristics	Exposure Characteristics	Results				Summary of Conclusions and Special Comments	References
10	Location: United Kingdom	Workers processed raw asbestos fibers into finished textile product. Duties involved fiberizing, carding, spinning, weaving, and plaiting.	Cause of Death	Obs.	Exp.	O/E	Asbestos workers employed 20 years or more in "scheduled areas" experienced a notably higher risk of lung cancer.	Doll, 1955 (same cohort studied by Pets <u>et al</u>., 1977)
			All causes	39	15.4	2.5		
			Lung cancer	11*	0.8	13.8		
			Other respiratory and cardiovascular diseases	20**	7.6	2.6		
			Other cancer	4	2.3	0.9		
	113 males employed in an asbestos textile factory in northern England. Employed prior to 1933 for 20 years Follow-up from 1922. Male population of England and Wales used for comparison group. Follow-up was 100% through 1953.	Predominantly chrysotile, possibly small amounts of crocidolite. "Scheduled areas" where processes conducted were classified as dusty in the Asbestos Industry Regulations of 1931. Exposure before 1933 considered higher, since national regulations introduced in 1931 to control asbestos dust became effective by end of 1932.	*All with mention of asbestosis **14 with mention of asbestosis.				Increase of both as and lung cancer abated with decreased time of exposure to pre-1933 conditions. Overall tenfold increase in lung cancer; increased risk before 1933 estimated as twentyfold. All cases of tuns cancer confirmed histologically and associated with asbestosis.	

Cohort Number	Study Population and Design Characteristics	Exposure Characteristics	Results	Summary of Conclusions and Special Comments	Reference
10	Location: United Kingdom Total of 878 males and females (538 males and 220 females employed after 1932). 256 males employed before to 1933 (136 included in the 538 above). Groups studied: Group / No. / Sex / Duration of Exposure (yrs) Total / Before 1933 1 / 57 / M / >20 / >10 2 / 63 / M / ≥20 / <10 3 / 136 / M / ≥20 / None 4 / 538* / M / 10–19 / None 5 / 220 / F / ≥10 / None *Including 136 men in Group 3 before they had worked for 20 years in "scheduled areas." Follow-up from 1936 to June 1966 for five exposure groups defined by total duration of exposure, by duration of exposure before 1933, and by sex. Follow-up information not obtained for all men and women ever employed.	Asbestos textile factory in northern England (same as that studied by Doll, 1955). Dust records not available until 1951. Pre-1933 exposures considered highest. Numerous changes in process made in 1932 and through the 1940s and 1950s.	Exposure Group 4 (N = 538) Cause of Death / Obs. / Exp. / O/E All causes / 23 / 16.2 / 1.4 Cancer of the lung and pleura / 6 / 6.4 / 0.9 Other neoplasms / 4 / 9.1 / 0.4	Effect of reduced post-1932 exposures evaluated. Results for Groups 1 and 2 with pre-1933 exposure similar to those of Doll (1955), in that tenfold increase in risk of lung cancer for group 1 (12.0 obs. vs. 1.2 exp.), threefold increase for Group 2 (5 obs. vs. 1.6 exp.). Twofold increase in cancer of other sites observed only for Group 1 (5 obs. vs. 2.6 exp.). Slight increase in risk of lung cancer for Group 3 (2 vs. 1.35) and Group 5 (2 vs. 0.24), but none in Group 4 (6 vs. 6.4). Reduced dust levels associated with decreased risk of lung cancer. Four of the five mesotheliomas observed were identified among necropsies of employees <10 years. Duration of exposure for mesothelioma cases ranged from 7 months to 23 years.	Knox et al., 1968 (same cohort studied by Peto et al., 1977)

Cohort Number	Study Population and Design Characteristics	Exposure Characteristics	Results	Summary of Conclusions and Special Comments	Reference
10	*Location:* United Kingdom. 822 males and 284 females 822 males and 284 females *employed* ≥*10 years in* "scheduled area" by end of 1972. *Five exposure groups defined* by total duration of exposure, by duration of exposure before 1933, and by sex. Groups studied: Group / No. / Sex / Length of Exposure (yrs) Total / Before 1933 1 / 69 / M / ≥20 / ≥10 2 / 74 / M / ≥20 / <10 3 / 263 / M / ≥20 / None 4 / 679* / M / 10-19 / None 5 / 284 / F / ≥10 / None *Including 263 men in group 3 before they had worked for 20 years in "scheduled areas." Expected numbers of deaths were computed from national death rates in England and Wales. Follow-up from 1933 to 1974. (2% of workers could not be traced.)	*Asbestos textile factory in* Rochdale in northern England (see also Doll, 1955; Knox et al., *1968*). Dust levels reduced by 50% *to 80% by 1957; 1951 mean* dust level 10.8 fibers/cm^3; 1972 mean dust level 2.9 fibers/cm^3. No information available for smoking.	Cause of Death / Obs. / Exp. / O/E All causes / 317 / 248.6 / 1.3 Lung cancer / 51 / 23.8 / 2.1 Gastrointestinal cancer / 16 / 15.7 / 1.0 Mesothelioma / 10* / -- / -- Exposure Group 4 (N = 679) Cause of Death / Obs. / Exp. / O/E All causes / 127 / 123 / 1.0 Lung cancer / 24** / 12.8 / 1.9 Other cancer / 11 / 17.8 / 0.6 Exposure Group 5 (N = 284) Cause of Death / Obs. / Exp. / O/E All causes / 24 / 23.7 / 1.0 Lung cancer / 3** / 0.9 / 3.3 Other cancer / 6 / 7.6 / 0.8 *10 pleural mesotheliomas observed (nine males and one female). **Includes two mesotheliomas in Group 4 and 1 mesothelioma in Group 5.	Effect of reduced post-1932 dust levels evaluated. Results for Groups 1 and 2 similar to those of Knox et al. (1968) for lung cancer and cancer of other sites. Approximately twofold increase in lung cancer for Group 3 (9 obs. vs. 5-6 exp.) and no increase for cancer of other sites (6 obs. vs. 6.6 exp.). Twofold increase in lung cancer for Group 4 (24 vs. 12.8); Group 5 had threefold increase (3 vs. 0.9). No increase in gastrointestinal cancer for all groups combined (16 obs. vs. 15.7 exp.).	Peto et al., 1977

Cohort Number	Study Population and Design Characteristics	Exposure Characteristics	Results	Summary of Conclusions and Special Comments	Reference
10	Location: United Kingdom 679 males employed in 1933 or later and exposed for 10 years by end of 1972; 255 of them employed since 1950. Two exposure groups defined by duration and time of exposure: 1933-1950 1951-1972 Expected numbers of deaths derived from national death rates in England and Wales. Follow-up from 1943 to 1978; 94% of the cohort has been traced.	Asbestos factory in Rochdale in northern England (same as Doll, 1955; Knox *et al.*, 1968; Peto, 1977).	Group 1 (Total Group) Cause of Death / Obs. / Exp. / O/E Lung cancer: 28 / 18.6 / 1.5 Other cancer: 24 / 25.1 / 0.9 Group 2 (Total Group) Cause of Death / Obs. / Exp. / O/E Lung cancer: 12 / 4.6 / 2.6 Other cancer: 5 / 5.8 / 0.9 Both Groups Cause of Death / Obs. / Exp. / O/E Gastrointestinal cancer: 14 / 12.6 / 1.1 Eight lung cancer deaths (1.62 exp.) for post-1950 employees with >20 years since first exposure.	Risk of lung cancer 20 years after exposure in post-1950 workers was 4.9 (8 obs. vs. 1.6 exp.), significantly higher than in workers initially exposed 1933-1950 (22 obs. vs. 13.8 exp.) Estimated relative risk of 2 to 3 for lung cancer among men with cumulative exposure of 200-300 (fibers/cm^3)(yr.). Inability of static sample measurements to identify those at high risk suggests that ambient level may not be the primary source of inhaled fibers and that certain workplace practices may constitute the major source of risk. Dose-response analyses based on static measurements may be misleading. Higher lung cancer ratios for post-1950 exposed males suggest possible importance of smoking. No clear-cut gradient in risk of lung cancer associated with increased exposure, suggesting that exposure estimate may be imprecise.	Peto, 1980 (same cohort studied by Peto *et al.*, 1977)

Cohort Number	Study Population and Design Characteristics	Exposure Characteristics	Results				Summary of Conclusions and Special Comments	References
			Cause of Death	Obs.	Exp.	O/E		
10	Location: United Kingdom	Same as those reported by Doll (1955), Knox et al., (1968, and Peto et al., (1977).	Cohort 1: Lung cancer (Mesothelioma)	13 (2)	1.6	8.1	No association of risks for mesothelioma with age per se but rather, with time lapsed since exposure	Peto, 1980a (same cohort as Peto et al., 1977)
	567 wen first employed in asbestos textile factory before 1951; 143 before 1933.		Cohort 2: Lung cancer (Mesothelioma)	7 (5)	3.5	2.0	Risk of mesothelioma does not appear to have been much higher among men initially very heavily exposed.	
	Three cohorts defined		Cohort 3: Lung cancer (Mesothelioma)	22 (7)	13.9	1.6		
	1.	69 men with >20 years of exposure and >10 years before 1933.						In Cohort 1, 47% of deaths (31/66) were from asbestosis; in cohort 3, 13% (26/201) of deaths were from asbestosis.
	2.	76 men with >20 years of exposure end <10 years before 1933.						
	3.	424 men with >10 years of exposure between 1933 and 1950.						
	Follow-up through 1978.							

Cohort Number	Study Population and Design Characteristics	Exposure Characteristics	Results	Summary of Conclusions and Special Comments	Reference
11	Location: United States Asbestos products workers. All men employed by company who retired between 1941 and 1967 and lived at least to age 65. The cohort was refined to include 1,345 retired males who had been employed as production, maintenance, and service employees for asbestos company. Later follow-up of 1,075 males. U.S. male death rates were used to compute expected numbers of deaths. Follow-up initially through 1969 (Enterline and Henderson, 1973); subsequently, through 1973 (Henderson and Enterline, 1979). Lost to follow-up not specified.	Chrysotile only and chrysotile and crocidolite mixed. Quantitative exposure data based on cumulative exposure at time of retirement (mppcf-y).	Cause of Death / Obs. / O/E: All causes 781 1.2 Cancer 173 1.6 Lung cancer 63 2.7 Gastrointestinal cancer 55 1.4 Mesothelioma (5) -- Other cancer 55 1.2 Respiratory disease 68 1.7 Asbestosis 19 NA Respiratory cancer (SMR), by type of asbestos Type of Asbestos / No.* / Obs. / O/E: Amosite 58 4 3.6 Chrysotile 754 40 2.5 Amosite and chrysotile 98 4 1.8 Chrysotile and crocidolite 209 12 4.6 Asbestos-cement pipe (chrysotile and crocidolite) 83 11 5.8 Five mesothelioma deaths observed in cohort, of which three occurred during 1970–1973. *Number of men exposed.	Respiratory cancer risk increased as quantitative exposure level increased. SMR for lowest exposure level, 2.0; SMR 7.8 for highest exposure level. Effects of asbestos exposure with respect to lung cancer risk continued well past the termination of exposure. Increased risks differed by type of asbestos exposure (SMR for chrysotile only 2.5 vs. 5 for crocidolite and chrysotile mixed). Of the mesothelioma cases reported from hospitals around New Jersey plant, 41/58 had record of employment at plant but only two were eligible for study cohort as defined. The study population of retirees are "survivors," and mortality experience may not reflect actual risks associated with asbestos exposure. Most likely, risks were underestimated.	Henderson and Enterline, 1979 Enterline, 1965 Enterline and Kendrick, 1967 Enterline and Henderson, 1973

Cohort Number	Study Population and Design Characteristics	Exposure Characteristics	Results	Summary of Conclusions and Special Comments	Reference
12	Location: United States 5,645 white and black male workers employed for at least one continuous month before January 1, 1970 in either of two asbestos-cement building materials plants in New Orleans, Louisiana. Workers in the five dust categories analyzed did not differ by length of follow-up, age at initial exposure, and year of initial exposure. Death rates for males in the United States and in Louisiana separately were used to compute expected deaths. Minimum 20 years of follow-up to December 31, 1974. Approximately 75% of cohort traced.	Predominant fiber chrysotile, but crocidolite used in some areas. Some amosite. Asbestos-cement manufacturing. Both plants opened in early 1920s. Quantitative exposure data based on dust measurements (mppcf) and work histories to establish cumulative dose estimate (mppcf-yr) for initial 20 years of employment.	Cause of Death / Obs. / Exp. / O/E All causes 601 890.1 0.7 All cancer 120 156.6 0.8 Lung cancer 51(2) 49.2 1.0 Gastrointestinal cancer 25 50.1 0.5 Mesothelioma 2 -- -- O/E ratios not higher in any exposure subgroup for any cause except respiratory tract cancer, in two highest exposure groups. Respiratory Tract Cancer / Obs. / Exp. / O/E Exposure Group ≤10 mppcf-yr 19 25.7 0.8 11 - 50 8 11.4 0.7 51 - 100 1 3.8 0.3 101 - 200 9 3.1 2.9 >200 14 6.2 2.3 Respiratory Tract Cancer / Obs. / Exp. / O/E High Exposure No crocidolite 8 4.4 1.8 Crocidolite intermittent 5 1.4 3.6 Steady crocidolite 7 2.9 2.4	Risk increased more steeply with increased quantitative exposure than with increased duration of employment. Excess mortality for lung cancer observed only for groups with moderate and high cumulative exposure (SMR 2.9 and 2.3). No detectable excess risk of lung cancer in persons employed for less than 2 years or with low exposure. Risk appears high for two subgroups exposed to crocidolite, but only in the high exposure group (> 200 mppcf-yr). No increased risk observed for gastrointestinal cancer in any subgroup. Two pleural mesotheliomas observed (one employed less than 1 year and one for 14 years). No increased risk of respiratory cancer for exposures below 100 mppcf-yr. Some deaths may have been missed due to low tracing rate (approximately 75%).	Hughes and Weill, 1980 Weill et al., 1979

Cohort Number	Study Population and Design Characteristics	Exposure Characteristics	Results	Summary of Conclusions and Special Comments	Reference
13	Location: Canada 328 employees of Ontario asbestos-cement factory hired before 1960 end employed for a minimum of 9 years. 3.2% (11) of cohort excluded, since exposures could not be classified. Three subgroups analyzed: 186 production workers (P), 55 maintenance workers (H), end 87 workers in rock wool/fiberglass operations (C) (unexposed to asbestos). Death rates for the Province of Ontario were used to compute expected numbers of deaths. Follow-up to October 31, 1980. Follow-up of 96% of cohort.	Asbestos-cement workers. Factory opened in 1948. Chrysotile and crocidolite used in pipe manufacturing process; chrysotile only in other areas. Quantitative exposure data base on duet measurements and work histories to determine cumulative dose measure (fibers/cm^3)/yr. Smoking histories obtained for 70% of cohort. The 186 production workers ranked on basis of 18-year cumulative exposure and into three groups: A, B, and C, representing different exposure levels.	Production and Maintenance Groups Cause of Death / Obs. / Exp. / O/E All causes / 72 / 42.5 / 1.7 All cancer / 36 / 9.9 / 3.6 Lung cancer / 20 / 3.1 / 6.1 Gastrointestinal / 4 / 2.5 / 1.6 cancer / 11 / — / — Mesothelioma Of the 58 deaths among production workers, 10 were mesotheliomas (five pleural and five peritoneal). One mesothelioma death among maintenance workers. All 11 deaths exposed to both crocidolite and chrysotile. Number and Rotes of Death Among Production Workers No. of Deaths (Rate/1,000 man-years)* by Cumulative Exposure exposure. Exposure Group Cause of Death / A Lowest / B / C Highest Mesothelioma / 1(1.9) / / 6(11.9) Lung cancer / 5(13.6) / / 6(11.9) Gastrointestinal cancer / 0(0.0) / / 3(6.0) *Rates standardized to age distribution of Group C.	No increased risk for lung cancer observed with increased quantitative No association of mesothelioma with smoking, but strong association with exposure level in production workers. High increased risk of lung cancer associated with asbestos exposure, but the lack of increased risk with increasing exposure suggests that exposure estimates may be imprecise.	Finkelstein, 1983

Cohort Number	Study Population and Design Characteristics	Exposure Characteristics	Results				Summary of Conclusions and Special Comments	Reference
14	Location: Denmark	Asbestos-cement workers. The major exposure was to chrysotile, but crocidolite and amosite were used in small amounts in later years.	Cause of Death All cancer 167 151.1 1.1	The excess lung cancer is consistent with an asbestos effect, although it is confounded by cigarette smoking. Lung cancer Gastrointestinal cancer Mesothelioma	Obs. 47 59 3 Other cancer sites: Larynx Prostate Stomach 5 14 14	Exp. 27.8 49.3 — 2.9 7.7 9.2	O/E 1.7 1.2 — 1.7 1.8 1.5	Clemmesen and Hjalgrim-Jenson, 1981
	6,372 males ever employed in three asbestos-cement factories between 1944 and 1976. Subjects were considered exposed if they had ever handled asbestos products (N = 5,686). 646 subjects were clerical and administrative personnel without known exposure.	No dust measurements or quantitative exposure data, although some estimates of fiber concentration were presented.					No data were presented quantifying exposure or permitting assessment of risk by type of asbestos exposure.	
		No smoking data were available for the study subjects, although s survey in one of the three pleats indicated that a higher proportion of markers were smokers than would be expected in the general population.	Mortality was not reported. Standardized incidence ratios (SIRs) for all cancer were 1.1 (167/151.1) in exposed and 1.0 (20/20.6) in the unexposed groups. The SIR in the unexposed group for respiratory cancer was 0.9.				Excess of laryngeal cancer is statistically significant.	
	Incident cases were drawn from company files and compared to expected numbers derived from the Danish Cancer Registry. Follow-up was apparently 100% through 1976.							

Cohort Number	Study Population and Design Characteristics	Exposure Characteristics	Results	Summary of Conclusions and Special Comments	Reference
14	Location: United States Union members in New York City and metropolitan New Jersey. Subjects included 632 who seers union members on December 31, 1942 and 890 who joined the unions between 1943 and 1962. Mortality study limited to the 632 members in the cohort with the earlier members. All members of this cohort had at least 20 years of follow-up. Expected numbers of deaths in the mortality study were based on U.S. male death rates. Smoking rates were obtained from the American Cancer Society prospective study of cigarette smoking. Follow-up of the early cohort was 100% as of December 31, 1962 (Selikoff et al., 1964).	Asbestos insulation workers (New York and New Jersey). No dust measurements or quantitative exposure data. Smoking information obtained from interview of 370 men from the early-member cohort who were alive as of January 1, 1963. This cohort was followed until April 30, 1967.	Cause of Death / Obs. / Exp. / O/E All causes / 478 / 328.9 / 1.5 All cancer / 210 / 51.0 / 3.7 Lung cancer / 93 / 13.3 / 7.0 Gastrointestinal cancer / 43 / 15.0 / 2.9 Mesothelioma / 38 / — / — Other cancer sites: / 6 / 2.8 / 2.1 Larynx / 2 / 1.3 / 1.5 Kidney Early Cohort (Selikoff et al., 1964, 1979): For the 632 workers in the union at the end of 1942, mortality from all causes was elevated (253/196.2). There was a threefold excess of cancer (95/31.4), mostly contributed by cancer of the lung (42/6.0) and gastrointestinal tract (29/9.7). Later-Member Cohort (Selikoff et al., 1979): SMR for all causes was 1.0 (62/64.6); the all cancer SMR was 2.0 (20/10.1); 82% of the person-years were in the groups observed less than 20 years. Of the 38 mesotheliomas observed, 11 were pleural and 27 were peritoneal.	The study subjects worked in a number of different industries, including shipbuilding. The smoking analysis (Selikoff et al., 1968) suggested an interaction between cigarette smoking and asbestos exposure, but the large risk estimates were based on very small expected numbers. Cancers of the lung and gastrointestinal tract were not excessive until after at least 20 years of follow-up. The later-member cohort reflects postwar conditions. No dose-response inference possible because of the lack of exposure data.	Selikoff et al., 1964, 1968, 1979

Cohort Number	Study Population and Design Characteristics	Exposure Characteristics	Results				Summary of Conclusions and Special Comments	Reference
16	Location: United States 17,800 workers listed as members of 120 local unions within the United States and Canada on January l, 1967. Expected numbers computed from U.S. white male death rates and the American Cancer Society study of cigarette smokers. Follow-up through December 31, 1976.	Insulation workers union. No dust measurements or quantitative exposure data. Smoking date were obtained from questionnaires mailed to 12,051 men with at least 20 years of follow-up. The rate of response was 68%.	Cause of Death	Obs.	Exp.	O/E	Risk estimates for overall mortality were lower than in other studies by the same authors, because this cohort included individuals with varying periods of follow-up. The smoking data were based on relatively stable rates and show a consistent multiplicative effect. Study results indicate a high increase in risk of lung cancer associated with asbestos exposure, but the lack of exposure data makes it difficult to show a dose-response relationship.	Selikoff et al., 1979 Hammond et al., 1979
			All causes	2,271	1,658.9	1.4		
			All cancer	922	319.2	2.9		
			Lung cancer	429	105.6	4.1		
			Gastrointestinal cancer	94	59.4	1.6		
			Mesothelioma	175	—	—		
			Other cancer sites:	25	14.8	1.7		
			Larynx, pharynx, and buccal cavity	18	8.1	2.2		
			Kidney					
			More than 50% of the excess cancer was due to cancer of the lung (429/105.6). A tenfold risk of lung cancer was assocciated with smoking in both exposed and unexposed groups; a fivefold risk for asbestos exposure in both smokers and nonsmokers. Ex-smokers had substantially lover lung cancer rates than did current smokers.					

Cohort Number	Study Population and Design Characteristics	Exposure Characteristics	Results				Summary of Conclusions and Special Comments	Reference
17	Location: Northern Ireland All men listed as insulators and pipe coverers on 1940 lists of trade union membership. A total of 170 subjects (Elves and Simpson, 1977). Expected deaths were derived from death rates for Northern Ireland. The cohort received periodic biannual examinations since 1970, and yes under surveillance through 1975. Follow-up was 95% complete (Elmes and Simpson, 1977).	Belfast insulation workers. No dust measurements or quantitative exposure data. Smoking data were unavailable for 46 workers. All but five of the remaining 124 were smokers. Exposed to three of the main commercial types of asbestos: chrysotile, amosite, and crocidolite.	Cause of Death (Elmes and Simpson, 1977) All causes All cancer Lung cancer Gastreintestinal cancer Mesothelioma *Estimated from data. SMR for all causes of mortality was more than 3 for 1950-1964, but only half that after 1965. Cause of Death (Elmes and Simpson, 1971) All causes All cancer Respiratory cancer Gastrointestinal cancer	Obs. 120 65 35 13 13 Obs. 98 45 28 15	Exp. (58.9)* (9.5)* 5.0 2.2 — Exp. 37.7 6.8 1.6 —	O/E 2.2* 6.8* 7.0 5.9 — O/E 2.6 6.6 17.5 —	Gastrointestinal cancer risk peaked before 1960 and then returned to background levels. Risk of bronchial cancer and mesothelioma remained high in 1975 (Elmes and Simpson, 1977). Although no data are presented, the text states that no difference in risk was apparent in workers first hired before 1933 and those hired after 1933. Surveillance of the study population resulted in more complete ascertainment of deaths than in the comparison population, thus biasing risk estimates upward. Risk estimates (O/E) in this cohort unusually high, although cohort had a long period of follow-up No information available on type of asbestos exposure or dust measurements. Too few nonsmokers to show the significance of smoking.	Elmes and Simpson, 1971, 1977

Cohort Number	Study Population and Design Characteristics	Exposure Characteristics	Results	Summary of Conclusions and Special Comments	Reference
18	Location: United Kingdom All employees (6,292 men) at the Royal Navy dockyard employed on January 1, 1947 were identified from payroll records. Death rates for England and Hales Mere used to compute deaths. Estimates of death rates for southwest Britain were used to adjust O/E ratios, since these rates were believed to be less than those for England. Successfully traced 96.6% of cohort to 1978.	Industrial dockyard workers in Devonport, United Kingdom. No dust measurements or quantitative exposure data. No smoking information.	Mortality data on 6,076 men. Cause of Death / Exp. / O/E / Adj. O/E All causes / 1,081.2 / 0.9 / 1.0 All cancer / 282.1 / 0.9 / 1.0 Lung cancer / 119.7 / 0.7 / 0.8 Gastrointestinal cancer / 83.3 / 0.8 / 0.8 Mesothelioma / 0.5 / 64.0 / 77.0	Exposure to asbestos was greatest in the 19500 and diminished throughout the 1960s. Thus, the mortality effects may not yet be apparent, especially for mesothelioma. No quantitative exposure data. No smoking data. Study cohort is relatively young (average age 57 years) and should be followed for an additional 20 to 25 years.	Rossiter and Coles, 1980

Cohort Number	Study Population and Design Characteristics	Exposure Characteristics	Results	Summary of Conclusions and Special Comments	Reference
19	Location: Italy All active or retired dockyard workers as of January 1, 1960 (N = 2,190) and all men who worked in the shipyards from January 1, 1960 to June 30, 1975 (N = 2,074). The mortality rates for the city of Genoa were used as one comparison group, A cohort of hospital workers was used as a second com-comparison group. Follow-up through 1975. No data on losses to follow-up.	Shipyard workers in Genoa. No dust measurements or quantitative exposure data. No smoking data reported The cohort may also have been exposed to paints, paint strippers, polyaromatic hydrocarbons, and halogenated hydrocarbons. No data reported on duration or time of employment. Mortality data analyzed by 20 job categories.	Cause of Death / Obs. / Exp. / O/E All causes / 1,070 / 853.7 / 1.3* All cancer / 305 / 212.8 / 1.4* Lung cancer / 123 / 54.9 / 2.2* Gastrointestinal cancer / 74 / 58.6 / 1.3 Mesothelioma / NA** / — / — Other cancer sites: / 15 / 7.7 / 1.9* Larynx / 29 / 14.7 / 2.0* Kidney *p < 0.01. **Mesothelioma deaths were not reported separately. Comparison group was the male population of Genoa. Significant increases in lung cancer deaths observed for seven job categories: carpenters (8/3.0), metallurgical workers (16/6.9), iron-smiths (21/8.1), fitters (9/3.4), electricians (6/2.1), stakers (16/4.3), and insulation workers (5/0.9).	Data were reported for 20 different occupational categories. Insulation workers were most highly exposed group and at highest risk for getting pleural mesothelioma and lung cancer. No quantitative information on levels of dust exposure. No smoking information	Puntoni et al., 1979

Cohort Number	Study Population and Design Characteristics	Exposure Characteristics	Results	Summary of Conclusions and Special Comments	Reference
20	Location: United Kingdom All persons on a salary list were included in the cohort. N = 951 females. Expected numbers based on national rates in the United Kingdom. Follow-up 61% complete through 1975; 578 female gas-mask workers successfully traced through medical records.	Gas-mask factory workers exposed to asbestos. No dust measurements or quantitative exposure data. Predominant exposure was to crocidolite from Western Australia (military gas masks), although chrysotile was used for a few months. No smoking data. Asbestos content of postmortem lung tissue examined in relationship to length and type of dust exposure.	Cause of Death / Obs. / Exp. / O/E All causes / 166 / NA / NA All cancer / 74 / 66.0 / 1.1 Lung cancer / 12 / 6.3 / 1.9 Gastrointestinal / 10 / 20.3 / 0.5 cancer / 17 / — / — Mesothelioma All lung cancer and mesothelioma cases were either In the crocidolite exposure group (727 persons) or both crocidolite and chrysotile exposure group (99 persons). No cases occurred in the group exposed only to chrysotile (102). An additional 12 cases (1 was male) of mesothelioma were found among persons who had apparently worked at the factory, Of the total of 29 cases, 22 were pleural and 7 were peritoneal.	Risk of mesothelioma and lung cancer was confined to the crocidolite-exposed subjects. Losses to follow-up may have reduced the magnitude of the risks observed. In general, no constant relationship between fiber count In tissue specimens and duration of exposure. Data were presented on fiber type, but no quantitative exposure information was available. Mesothelioma risk was strongly associated with duration of exposure, whereas a dose-response relationship was not observed for lung cancer. Method of tracing would increase probability of identifying women who had died or developed malignant disease and would tend to overestimate risks in this cohort.	Jones et al., 1980

Cohort Number	Study Population and Design Characteristics	Exposure Characteristics	Results	Summary of Conclusions and Special Comments	Reference
23	Location: United Kingdom The cohort use identified from a list of all female residents of Leyland, Preston, and Blackburn in 1939. These Mere the three locations where gas masks were manufactured. The lists were derived from the National Health Service Central Resister, and all women whose record indicated service in the manufacture of gas masks were included. 435 women from Leyland and 322 from Preston were involved in manufacture of military gas masks. 570 women from Blackburn made civilian gas masks. Deaths from January 1, 1951 to June 30, 1980 Mere included. Expected numbers of deaths Mere computed from national death rates in England and Wales. Follow-up through June 1980 was 100%.	Gas mask manufacturing workers. No dust measurements or quantitative exposure data. No smoking data. The Leyland (L) and Preston (P) cohorts Mere exposed predominantly to crocidolite but Included a brief exposure to chrysotile. The Blackburn (B) cohort was exposed ex-elusively to chrysotile.	Cause of Death All Locations — Obs. / Exp. / O/E All causes — 396 / 313 / 1.3 All cancer — 110 / 95 / 1.2 Lung cancer — 22 / 11.0 / 2.0 Gastrointestinal cancer — NA / NA / NA Mesothelioma — 6 / — / — Other cancer sites: Ovary — 17 / 7.8 / 2.2 Results by Location, Preston (P), Leyland (L), and Blackburn (B): <u>Deaths from All Causes</u> <u>Location</u> — <u>Obs.</u> / <u>Exp.</u> / <u>O/E</u> P + L — 219 / 185 / 1.2 B — 177 / 128 / 1.4 <u>All Cancer</u> — 66 / 54 / 1.2 P + L — 44 / 41 / 1.1 B — 15 / 6.2 / 2.4 <u>Lung Cancer</u> — 7 / 4.8 / 1.5 P + L B Five deaths at the P + L locations were due to mesothelioma, whereas only one was observed in B. A statistically significant excess of ovarian cancer was present in the P + L cohort (12/4.4) but not in the B cohort (5/3.4).	All cancer and tuns cancer rates were higher in the crocidolite exposure groups. Blackburn cancer rates (chrysotile exposure) Mere slightly above background. Association of ovarian cancer and asbestos exposure consistent with report of Newhouse et al. (1972).	Acheson et al., 1982

TABLE E-2. Respiratory Morbidity Studies of Asbestos-Exposed Populations[a]

Study Population	Fiber Types	Study Design	Summary of Important Findings	References
1,117 Insulation workers	Chrysotile and amosite	Cross-sectional; no external controls	50% Prevalence of pulmonary fibrosis. Increasing prevalence of all chest film changes with employment duration, increasing to 90% prevalence at >30 years.	Selikoff et al., 1965
Persons in central Finland	Anthophyllite and tremolite	Case series	Pleural calcification observed in persons only secondarily exposed to asbestos. Pleural changes unrelated to lung cancer mortality.	Kiviluoto, 1960, 1965, 1979
1,117 Insulation workers	Chrysotile and amosite	Cross-sectional; no external controls	Pleural calcification showed Increasing prevalence, reaching 57.9% among those with 40 years since first exposure. Pleural fibrosis occurred earlier than calcifications; 50% of cases were bilateral.	Selikoff, 1965
1,015 Chrysotile miners and millers	Chrysotile	Cross-sectional; no external controls	Shortness of breath increased with estimated cumulative dust exposure, but there was little correlation with bronchitis.	McDonald et al., 1972
1,015 Chrysotile miners and millers	Chrysotile	Cross-sectional; us external controls	FVC[b] found to decrease with estimated cumulative dust exposure in smokers and nonsmokers. Same trends seen in FEV_1.[c] Obstructive impairment seen in high exposure group. Few trends in diffusing capacity.	Becklake et al., 1972

[a] Adapted from Dement et al., in press.
[b] FVC = Forced vital capacity, the maximum total volume of air that can be expired in one breath.
[c] FEV_1 = Forced expiratory volume, the maximum volume of air that can be expired in one second. Note: Both FVC and FEV_1 are measures of lung function.

Study Population	Fiber Types	Study Design	Summary of Important Findings	References
5,083 Miners and millers with chest films	Chrysotile	Mortality follow-up	Increased mortality observed for those with parenchymal changes but not in those with only pleural changes; 32 deaths observed due to all respiratory disease vs. eight expected.	McDonald et al., 1974
267 Miners and millers with chest films	Chrysotile	Prospective follow-up	During 20-year period, the following cumulative incidence was reported: small opacities, 16%; pleural thickening, 5.3%; pleural calcification, 5.3%; obliteration of costophrenic angle, 7.3%.	Liddell et al., 1977
100 Asbestos textile workers	Unknown	Cross-sectional; no external controls	Overall prevalence of fibrosis, 36%; 24% prevalence in nonsmokers and 40% in smokers. None of the 11 nonsmokers with exposures less than 20 years had fibrosis.	Weiss, 1971
290 Asbestos textile workers	Mixed	Cross-sectional; no external controls	Basal rales used as early disease marker; 1% risk estimated for a working lifetime of 50 years at 2 fibers/cm^3.	British Occupational Hygiene Society. 1968
1,287 Asbestos textile workers	Mixed	Cross-sectional; no external controls	Prevalence of pulmonary fibrosis was zero for 0-9 years of exposure, but up to 40.5% after 30-39 years of exposure. Pleural fibrosis prevalence was 1.6% in the 0-9-year group and 50% in the 40-49-year group.	Lewinsohn, 1972

Study Population	Fiber Types	Study Design	Summary of Important Findings	References
379 Asbestos textile workers	Mixed	Prospective follow-up	"Possible" asbestosis in 6.6% of workers after 16 years of follow-up and an average exposure of 5 fibers/cm^3. Cumulative exposure for 1% incidence of "possible asbestosis" for 40 years employment estimated to be 55 (fibers/cm^3)yr.	Berry et al., 1979
908 Asbestos-cement workers	Mixed	Cross-sectional; no external controls	Overall prevalence of small, rounded opacities (ILO category, 1/0[d] or greater) was 3.1%; prevalence of small irregular opacities was 2.5%. Reduced FEV_1 and other measures of lung function were found in those with x-ray abnormalities.	Weill et al., 1973
859 Asbestos-cement workers	Mixed	Cross-sectional; no external controls	Prevalence of small, rounded, and irregular opacities was 4% in lowest exposure group and 30% in highest. Pleural changes were 11% in lowest exposure group and 30% in highest. FVC and FEV_1 were reduced in those with x-ray changes.	Weill et al., 1975
98 Workers age 40 or over in two plants	Chrysotile and amosite	Cross-sectional; no external controls	Prevalence of profusion (1/1 ILO) was 17.5% in chrysotile workers and 16.5% in mixed-fiber workers. Pleural thickening prevalence was 17.5% in chrysotile workers and 35.4% in mixed-fiber workers. Smoking found to be significant factor in those exposed to amosite.	Weiss and Theodos, 1978

[d] Part of the classification system devised by the International Labor Organization (ILO) for x-ray changes seen in pneumoconioses. See Selikoff and Lee, 1978.

Study Population	Fiber Types	Study Design	Summary of Important Findings	References
1,287 Asbestos textile workers	Mixed	Cross-sectional; no external controls	Prevalence of pulmonary fibrosis was zero after 0-9 years of exposure, and up to 40.5% after 30-39 years of exposure. Pleural fibrosis prevalence was 1.6% in the 0-9-year group and 50% in the 60-49-year group.	Lewinsohn, 1972
485 Miners and millers	Chrysotile	Cross-sectional; no external controls	Prevalence of all radiographic abnormalities was 10%. Pleural changes seen in 3% of all workers, Prevalence of abnormalities among those employed less than 5 years was 5%; 3% were parenchymal changes (profusion ≥/0).	Selikoff et al., 1977
204 Asbestos-cement workers	Mixed	Prospective follow-up, 1970-1976	Progression of small opacities dependent upon both average and Cumulative exposure. Lung function declines were associated with smoking and cumulative exposure. Pleural abnormalities progressed more as a function of time with little association with additional exposure.	Jones et al., 1980
Household contacts of factory workers	Amosite	Cross-sectional; age-and sex-matched controls	Prevalence of x-ray abnormalities was 35.9%, compared to a 4.6% prevalence in control group. Pleural abnormalities more prevalent than parenchymal changes.	Anderson et al., 1979

Study Population	Fiber Types	Study Design	Summary of Important Findings	References
121 Talc miners and millers	Anthophyllite and tremolite	Cross-sectional; external comparison populations	The prevalence of pleural abnormalities in talc workers with more than 15 years employment was greater than in comparison populations. Decreases in FEV_1 and FVC were associated with duration of employment and with dust exposure.	Gamble et al., 1979
1,801 Miners and millers with chest x-rays	Crocidolite and amosite	Cross-sectional; no external controls	Prevalence of pleural changes increased from 2.5% for workers with less than 1 year employment to 33.6% for workers employed 15 or more years. Parenchymal changes (>1/0 ILO) found in 2.3% of workers employed less than I year and 26.7% of workers employed more than 15 years.	Irwig et al., 1979
119 Asbestos workers referred to Pneumoconiosis Medical Panel	Mixed	Prospective follow-up	One-third of workers followed for 6 years (2/7) showed disease progression after 6 years of follow-up and no further asbestos exposure. Progression frequency higher among those with profusion >1/1 or 1/2 ILO. Among s larger study group of 123 subjects with minimal or no pulmonary fibrosis, 10 subjects, or 8.1%, died of of pleural mesothelioma during follow-up.	Gregor et al., 1979
56 Retired chrysotile miners and millers surviving > 3 years	Chrysotile	Prospective follow-up	Of persons with abnormal films (profusion >1/0 ILO), 39% showed progression after an average follow-up of 8 years. Of workers with normal initial films, 7.9% developed radiographic changes.	Rubino et al., 1979b

Study Population	Fiber Types	Study Design	Summary of, Important Findings	References
101 Shipyard pipe coverers and 95 controls	Mixed	Cross-sectional with further follow-up; matched controls	Prevalence of asbestosis 11 times greater in exposed than in controls. Asbestosis evident after cumulative exposures of 60 mppcf-yr.	Murphy et al., 1971, 1978
1,185 Block mine workers in the Cape crocidolite mines—current and former employees	Crocidolite	Cross-sectional study of radiographic findings with follow-back for lung cancer and mesothelioma	In this group with limited exposure (68% worked 5 years or less, and 69% started work no more than 20 years ago); 8.9% had only category ≥/0 ILO small opacities; 17.7% had pleural thickening or calcification; 7.3% had both.	Tolent et al., 1980
185 Maintenance workers in chemical plants and 137 oil refinery workers	Mixed	Cross-sectional studies of radiographic and pulmonary function	In chemical plant workers, there were small irregular opacities in 24%, only pleural thickening in 10%, and only calcification in 4%, for a total of 38% with radiographic findings consistent with asbestos exposure. In oil refinery workers, 23% had small irregular opacities, and more than 25% had evidence of pleural thickening or calcification. Thus, 40% showed radiographic findings consistent with asbestos exposure.	Lilis et al., 1980

[e] mppcf-yr = million particles per cubic foot times years worked. It is s measure of cumulative exposure.

Study Population	Fiber Types	Study Design	Summary of important Findings	References
513 Factory workers with exposure to vermiculite contaminated with tremolite	Tremolite	Cross-sectional study utilizing standard American Thoracic Society respiratory questionnaire, pulmonary function testing. and cheat radiography	In 4.4%, there were pleural or parenchymal abnormalities (2.2% had only costophrenic angle blunting). Those with radiographic findings had 3 times the fiber-year exposure as matched controls.	Lockey et al., 1982
266 Current and former railroad workers with at least 2 years of exposure before 1950 (steam locomotive era)	Mixed	Cross-sectional study utilizing standard-questionnaire and chest radiography (posterior-anterior, right, and left obliques)	80% had less than 10 years of asbestos exposure. 2% had radiographic evidence of asbestosis and 20% had one, or more pleural changes.	Sepulveda and Merchant, 1983

Appendix F

Effects of Administering Asbestiform Fibers to Animals

Contents

The references given on these tables can be found on the list for Chapter 6.

TABLE F-1. Respiratory Tract Tumors in Rodents after Inhalation of Asbestos and Other Asbestiform Fibers

Fiber Type[a]	Concentration (mg/m^3 air)[b]	(No. of Tumors/No. of Animals) or % Tumors	Animal	Latency (months)	Tumor Types	References
CH, CR, AM	10 2, 5	CH (15/50), CR (1/40), AM (2/43) CH (9/42), CR (3/43), control (0/20)	Rat	12-29	Adenoma, carcinoma, mesothelioma	Davis et al., 1978
CH, CR, AM	48	CH (3/54), CR (7/50), AM (3/61)	Rat	6-24	Papilloma, carcinoma, fibrosarcoma, mesothelioma	Reeves, 1976
CH, CR, AM	50	CH (3/69), CR (4/69), AM (3/69), control (0/12)	Rat	24	Carcinoma, fibrosarcoma, mesothelioma	Reeves et al., 1974
CH, CR, AM	48	CH (5/40), CR (2/31), AM (0/40)	Rat	33	Adenoma, carcinoma	Reeves et al., 1971
CH, CR, AM	10	CH (104/281), CR (55/141), AM (38/146), control (7/126)	Rat	3-24	Adenoma, carcinoma, mesothelioma	Wagner et al., 1974
AM, FG (fine), Fybex (>5 µm length), PKT	Experiment 1. AM (0.3), FG (0.4), PKT (0.07), Fybex (0.08) (3 months) Experiment 2. Fybex (0.04, 0.08, 0.37) (3 months)	Experiment 1. AM (3/16), FG (2/19), PKT (0/20), Fybex (1/21) in rats; Fybex (1/12) in hamsters Experiment 2. Fybex, 0.08 mg (3/25), Fybex, 0.37 mg (1/19) in rats; Fybex, 0.08 mg (1/13), Fybex, 0.37 mg (2/16) in hamsters	Rat, guinea pig, hamster	21-27	Adenoma, carcinoma, mesothelioma	Lee et al., 1981
Alumina (med. length, 35-62 µm; diam., 1-5 µm) vs. CH (UICC)	Cumulative exposure = 7,000 (alumina); 14,000 (CH)	Alumina = 0/60 CH = 5/38	Rat	21.5	Adenoma, squamous cell, adenocarcinoma	Piggott et al., 1981

Fiber Type[a]	Concentration (mg/m³ air)[b]	(No. of Tumors/No. of Animals) or % Tumors	Animal	Latency (months)	Tumor Types	References
CH, GW, RW, GMF	10 (3, 12 months)	CH (12/48), GW (1/48), RW (2/48), GMF (1/48)	Rat	17-33	Adenoma, adenocarcinoma	Wagner et al., 1982a
CASG	10 (1 year)	8/48	Rat	12-33	Adenoma, carcinoma, malignant histiocytoma	Davis et al., 1982
Pulverized asbestos pipe	85 (7 months)	6/34 in rats; 0/35 in controls; 0 in hamsters	Rat, hamster	14-29	Carcinoma	Leong, 1978
CH (UICC)	10.9 (2 hours/ day, 5 day/week for 95 days)	92%; 10% in controls	Mouse	12-18	Adenocarcinoma, mesothelioma	Bozelka et al., 1983
FG[c] insulation	In shavings for 30 days	5/12; 0 in controls	Mouse	3	Bronchogenic, septal cell	Morrison et al., 1981

[a] CH = chrysotile, AM = amosite, PKT = pigmentary potassium titanate, Fybex = potassium octatitanate, FG = fibrous glass, CASG = ceramic aluminum silicate glass fiber, GW = glass wool, RW = rock wool, GMF = microfiber.
[b] Mean airborne mass of fibers.
[c] Data from Schepers and Delahant (1955) and Schepers et al. (1958) on guinea pigs, rate, rabbits, and monkeys; Moorman (in press) on rata and monkeys; and Gross et al. (1970, 1974) on rate after exposure to glass fibers were negative and not included here.

TABLE F-2. Tumors in Rodents After Inhalation or Intratracheal Instillation of Asbestos in Combination with Other Chemicals

	No. of Tumors/No. of Animals					
Mode of Administration	Chrysotile	Agent Alone	Combination	Tumor Types	Animal	References
Inhalation	10/41	0/39 (NaOH)[a]	15/31 (+ NaOH)	Carcinoma, fibrosarcoma, mesothelioma	Rat	Gross et al., 1967
	5/51	12/51 (smoke)	9/51 (+ smoke)	Adenoma, papilloma, carcinoma	Rat	Wehner et al., 1975
	0/46	ND[b]	0/16 (+ smoke) 0/21 (+ BP)[c]	ND	Rat	Shabad et al., 1974
Intratracheal instillation	ND	8/37 (BP)	18/35 (+ BP)	Adenoma, papilloma, carcinoma	Hamster	Smith et al., 1968a
	0/17	10/34 (BP)	24/31 (+ BP)	Adenoma, papilloma, carcinoma	Hamster	Smith et al., 1968a
	0/49	0/19 (BP)	6/11 (+ BP mixed) 6/21 (+ BP adsorbed)	Adenoma, carcinoma, reticulosarcoma, mesothelioma	Rat	Pylev sad Shabad, 1973
	0/10	4/10 (BP)	15/10[d] (+ BP)	Papilloma, carcinoma	Hamster	Miller et al., 1965

[a] Sodium hydroxide (NaOH) was instilled intratracheally.
[b] ND = no details siren in report.
[c] BP = Benzo(a)pyrene.
[d] Animals developed multiple tumors.

TABLE F-3. Mesotheliomas in Rodents Appearing After injection of Asbestiform Fibers

Mode of Administration	Dose (mg)	(No. of Tumors/No. of Animals) or % Tumors, by Fiber[a] Exposure	Animal	Latency (months)	References
Intrapleural or Intrathoracic	40, 1 time CR = 1, 10, 40 on glass pledget	CH (15/30), AM (15/30), CR (14/30), milled CR (8/30), FG (1-25 μm diam., 1/30), FG (0.06-3 μm diam., 4/60, CR (at 1 mg, 2/40; at 10 mg, 11/40, pledget alone (0/40)	Rat	12 (earliest)	Stanton and Wrench, 1972
	40 on glass pledget	17 samples of FG tested; greatest tumor incidence observed for FG >8 μ length, <1.5 μm diam.	Rat	12	Stanton et al., 1977
	40, 1 time	CR, CH, FG, aluminum oxide all <5 μm diam., >50% tumors	Rat	12 (earliest)	Stanton and Layard, 1978
	40, 1 time	Most fibers ≤0.25 μm diam., >8 μm length were tumorigenic, but induction also observed for fibers ≤ 1.5 μm diam., >4 μm length; 72 experiments	Rat	12	Stanton et al., 1981
	20, 1 time	AM (38/96); CR (61/96); CH (55/96); silica (50/96). Tumors were histiocytic reticulum cell sarcomas	Rat	12 (earliest)	Wagner and Berry, 1969
	0.5, 1, 2, 4, 8 (SFCH, CR); rest, 20, 1 time	Dose response: tumors observed with SFCH, CH, milled CH, AM, AN, CR, brucite ceramic fiber, barium sulfate, FG, glass powder, aluminum oxide. Tumors were induced with nonfibrous materials, but more were seen with fibers > 10 μm length, < μm diam.	Rat	11-33	Wagner et al., 1973
	20, 1 time	TR A (0/31), TR B (0/48), TR C (14/47), SFCH (20/32), CR (2/32), control (0/55)	Rat	18 (average)	Wagner et al., 1982b

Mode of Administration	Dose (mg)	(No. of Tumors/ No. of Animals) or % Tumors, by Fiber[a] Exposure	Animal	Latency (months)	References
Intrapleural or Intrathoracic (Cont.)	20, 1 time	RW without resin (2/48), RW (3/48), SW (0/48), GW (1/48), GMF (4/48) CH (6/48), control (0/24)	Rat	ND[b]	Wagner et al., 1982a
	1:15 suspension in 1 ml	CH (3/34), CR (4/34), AM (5/34)	Rat	13-20	Donna, 1970
	50, 1 time (rat), 25, 1 time (hamster)	CH, AM, CR - all hammer-milled, compared with metal-free and with heated samples. Only heating diminished tumors. Fewer and different tumor types with hamster	Rat, hamster	13 vs 7.75 (earliest)	Gross and Harley, 1973
	20, 1 time	CH (12/32); leached (≤50% initial Mg^{++}), (13/32); leached (≤90% initial Mg^{++}), (2/32)	Rat	23 (average)	Morgan et al., 1977
	20, 1 time	CH (45%); leached (0-3%); CR (54%); JM 104 FG (13%). Leached fibers were shorter, thicker, and there were fever per unit weight	Rat	10-19	Monchaux et al., 1981
	1, 10, 25	CR at 1 mg (2/50), CR at 10 mg (10/50), AM at 10 mg (3/50), CH at 1 mg (0/50), CH at 10 mg (4/50), CH at 25 mg (9/50), AM at 1 mg (0/50), AM at 10 mg (4/50), talc at 25 mg (0/50), control (0/100), milled CH at 25 mg (<0.37 μm length, <0.07 μm diam., 0/150), fibrous nemalite at 25 mg (0/50), silicon dioxide at 10 mg (4/40), FG (50 μm diam., 0/50)	Hamster	5 (earliest)	Smith and Hubert, 1974

Mode of Administration	Dose (mg)	(No. of Tumors/No. of Animals) or % Tumors by Fiber[a] Exposure	Animal	Latency (months)	References
Intrapleural or Intrathoracic (cont.)	25, 1 time	Group 1: FG 0.1 µm diam., 82% >20 µm length (5/60); Group 2: FG (0.3 µm diam., 46% >20 µm length (2/60); Group 3: FG (1.23 µm diam., 34% >20 µm (2/60). None in three groups of FG where 21% >10 µm length.	Hamster	Group 1: 9.5 Group 2: 13.5 Group 3: 17.8	Smith et al., 1980b
	25, 1 time	CASG, majority was particulate (3/32)	Rat	12-33	Davis et al., 1982
Intraperitoneal	10, 1 time	CH (50%), erionite (60%), nonfibrous mordenite (0)	Mouse	CH (9-16) ER (8-22)	Suzuki, 1982
	50, 1 time	CH (0/30), CR (4/30), AM (2/30); all milled <1 µm length (0/30)	Rat	12 (average)	Klosterkotter and Robock, 1970
	25, 3 times	Attapulgite (24/34)	Rat	PA (mean = 12	Pott et al., 1976
	25, 4 times	CH (40%), milled CH (40%)	Rat	CH = 7 milled CH = 13 (earliest)	Pott et al., 1972
	25, 3-4 times	CH (37.5%), FG (57.5%), nemalite (62.5%), attapulgite (65%), gypsum (5%). Nonfibrous analogs did not Induce tumors; gypsum dissolved rapidly in tissues	Rat	6.5-12	Pott et al., 1974
	6.25, 25, 100 (1 time)	CH at 6.25 mg (17/40), CH at 25 mg (19/40), CH at 100 mg (16/40); 100 mg, brucite > FG > CH	Rat	17	Pott and Friedrichs, 1972

Mode of Administration	Dose (mg)	(No. of Tumors/No. of Animals) or % Tumors by Fiber[a] Exposure	Animal	Latency (months)	References
Intraperitoneal (cont.)	0.5, 2, 5, 10	Diversity of mineral fibers ≤20 μm diam., <0.25 μm length; GF induction of tumors reduced with hydrogen chloride and NaOH treatment	Rat	ND	Pott et al., 1982
Subcutaneous Injection	60 divided doses	Controls (0/15); extracted CR (l/14) and AM (1/15); CR (6/17), AM (7/13), CH (2/12)	Mouse	10 (earliest)	Roe et al., 1967

[a] CH - chrysotile, CR = crocidolite, AM = amosite, FG = fibrous glass, CASG = ceramic aluminum silicate glass fiber, GF = glass fiber, SFCH = superfine chrysotile, RW = rock wool, SW = slag wool, GW = glass wool, GMF = glass microfibers, TR A = tremolite (small number of fibers >8 μm length, <1.5 μm diam), TR B = tremolite (no fibers >8 μm length, <1.5 μm diam.), TR C = tremolite (greater number of fibers >8 μm length, <1.5 μm diam.).

[b] ND = No details given in report.

TABLE F-4. Development of Fibrosis in Animals After Inhalation, Intratracheal Instillation, or Pleural Injection of Asbestos and other Asbestiform Fibers

Mode of Administration	Fiber Type[a]	Concentration (mg/m^3)[b]	Animal	Latency (months)	Observations	References
Inhalation	Long CH, ball-milled CH	ND[c]	Rat, guinea pig, rabbit	ND ND	Fibrous reaction (ND) more pronounced with long fiber	Gardner, 1942
Inhalation, instillation	GW 20-50 µm length and short fibers	ND	Guinea pig	ND	No fibrosis	Schepers and Delahant, 1955
Inhalation, injection	CH, CR, AN, AM, TR, brucite, all long (20-50 µm) vs. short (<5 µm)	ND ≤3 years	Rat, guinea pig, mouse, cat, dog	16 (guinea pig) 14 (cat)	Fibrous reaction: guinea pig > rabbit = cat = rat > mouse and dog. Long CR fibers: fibrosis; long AM, CR, brucite peribronchiolitis; long TR → bronchiolar fibrosis; AN → no fibrosis; no fibrosis with short fibers	Vorwald et al., 1951
Inhalation	CH	86 (average)	Rat	ND	Multifocal fibrosis	Gross et al., 1967
Intrapleural	CH (untreated, at 400, 600, 800, and 1,000°C); auto brake-lining dust	10	Mouse	6 months	Fibrosis related inversely to heating; auto dust → little fibrosis	Davis and Coniami, 1973
Inhalation	CASG	10 (1 year)	Rat	6-32	Alveolitis, then PIF[d]	Davis et al., 1982
Inhalation	CH, CR, AM	10	Rat	24	PIF with CH (longer fibers)	Davis et al., 1978
Combined inhalation and instillation	FG (0.5 µm diam., 5-20 µm length)	100 24 months	Rat, hamster	Not applicable	Mild macrophage infiltration without fibrosis	Gross et al., 1970, 1974
Inhalation	CH, CR, AM	50	Rat, guinea ND pig, mouse	ND	Multifocal fibrosis; mice did not develop with CH exposure	Reeves et al., 1976

Mode of Administration	Fiber Type[a]	Content ration (mg/m³)[b]	Animal	Latency (months)	Observations	References
Pleural injection	FG	ND	Mouse	ND	Fibers >5 μm caused adhesions between chest wall and lung; fibers <5 μm produced focal granulomas	Davis, 1976
Instillation	Sized CR, CH, FG, synthetic fluoro-amphibole	3-25, 2-6 times	Guinea pig	24	Minimal peribronchiolar fibrosis only with fibers >10 μm length	Kuschner and Wright, 1976
Inhalation	FG (only 15% generally <10 μm length)	42, 6 hours/ day, 5 day/ week for 90 days	Rat, hamster, guinea pig	3	Alveolar proteinosis disappearing at 1 year	Lee et al., 1979
Inhalation	AM, FG (fine), Fybex, PKT	I = 0.039, 0.082, 0.37 II = 0.079	Rat, hamster, guinea pig	18-27	PIF in rats related to dosage, less prominent in guinea pig and hamster. AM >Fybex >PKT; FG not fibrogenic	Lee et al., 1981
Inhalation	CH A, CH B, CR, AM, AN	10	Rat	24	CH A = AN >CH B = CR >AM, Widespread PIF	Wagner et al., 1974
Inhalation	CH, GW, RW, GMF	10 (3 and 12 months)	Rat	3 (earliest)	CH >GMF >RW >GW; severity increasing with time	Wagner et al., 1982a
Inhalation	Alumina (Saffil)	Cumulative exposure, 7,000 mg/m³, 35 hour/week for 86 weeks	Rat	ND	No fibrosis, although observed with Rhodesian chrysotile	Piggott et al., 1981
Intraperitoneal	Erionite, mordenite	10	Mouse	4-7	Fibrosis more severe with erionite	Suzuki et al., 1980
Instillation	CH	2, 128	Sheep	12	Alveolitis at 128 mg	Begin et al., 1982

Mode of Administration	Fiber Types	Concentration (mg/m^3)[b]	Animal	Latency (months)	Observations	References
Inhalation	FG (˜0.45 µm diam., some >10 µm)	0.3, 3	Hamster, rat	ND ND	No fibrosis	Smith et al., 1982
Inhalation	FG 4-6 µm diam., >20 µm length; 0.05-3.5 µm diam., >10 µm length; <3.5 µm diam., >10 and <10 µm length	5, 15, for 18 and 20 months	Monkey, rat		No fibrosis	Moorman, in press
Inhalation	CH	10.9, 2 hours/ House day, 5 days/week for 75 days	Mouse	12	Diffuse focal interstitial fibrosis	Bozelka et al., in press
Intratracheal	TiP	2, 10, 50 mg/kg. 1 time	Rat, hamster	17	Nodular fibrosis in rats at 10 and 50 mg; no fibrosis in hamsters	Gross et al., 1977

[a] CH = chrysotile; CR = crocidolite; AN = anthophyllite; AM = amosite; FG = fibrous glass; Fybex = potassium octatitanate; PKT = pigmentary potassium titanate; TR = tremolite; GW = glass wool; CASG = ceramic aluminum silicate glass; CH A = UICC chrysotile A; CH B = UICC chrysotile B; TiP = titanium phosphate.

[b] Applies to inhalation exposures. Dose expressed differently for other types of exposure.

[c] ND = No details given in report.

[d] PIF = pulmonary interstitial fibrosis.

Appendix G

Development of Some Equations Used for Quantitative Risk Assessment

This appendix develops the equations necessary for arriving at the cohort-specific adjustment to calculate c in equation (12) of Chapter 7 from the values of the constant b in Table 7-1. The method of calculating the risk of mesothelioma mortality at age t for an exposure starting at age t_0 is also given. In addition, justification is provided for the calculations in Chapter 7 that are used to determine the contribution to lifetime risk resulting from an exposure beginning at t_0.

To begin, the instantaneous mortality (or hazard) function at age u for an exposure of dose level D incurred at age v is defined as follows:

$$i(u,v,D) = aD(u-v)^{k-2}, \quad u \geq v, \tag{G1}$$

where $a \geq 0$ and $k \geq 2$ are specified constants. D is the constant exposure level (concentration) over the period of exposure. By contrast, d in Chapter 7 and later in this appendix is the equivalent average continuous exposure level from time of first exposure until the time that all exposure ceases. It will become apparent from the following development that this equation for the instantaneous hazard from a brief constant exposure was selected to be consistent with equation 7 in Chapter 7. The hazard function i(u,v,D) means that the probability of death in the short time interval (u,u + Δu) of length u from an exposure to dose D at prior time v is given by i (u,v,D)(Δu). If this is the case, then the cumulative mortality (i.e., cumulative hazard) up to time t from the exposure D starting at time v is given by

$$I(t,v,D) = \int_v^t i(u,v,D)du \tag{G2}$$

= sum of instantaneous hazards from time v to t.

Now consider the case of a continuous exposure of length ℓ| starting at t_0, where exposure occurs during the time interval from t_0 to $t_0 + \ell$. If one now calculates the cumulative mortality (hazard) at age t, it becomes

$$I(t,t_0,\ell,D) = \int_{t_0}^{t_0+\ell} I(t,v,D)dv \qquad (G3)$$

$$= \int_{t_0}^{t_0+\ell} \int_{v}^{t} i(u,v,D)dudv$$

= sum of the instantaneous hazards of all u and v so that $v \leq u \leq t$ and $t_0 \leq v \leq t_0 + \ell$.

Using i(u,v,D) as given in equation (G1), one can calculate the integrals in equation (G3) as follows:

$$I(t,t_0,\ell,D) = b(t-t_0)^k, \qquad (G4)$$

with

$$b = cD\{1-[1-\ell/(t-t_0)]^k\}, \qquad (G5)$$

where c = a/k(k-1).

Note that equation (G4) is in the form given by Peto et al. (1982), who estimated k as 3.2. The corresponding values of b for various worker cohorts are given in Table 7-1. Equation (G5) gives the correction term to obtain c in equation (12) with d = (0.219)D = D/4.56. The choice of d = (0.219)D is justified as follows: equations (G1), (G4), and (GS) all assume a continuous daily exposure to dose D. Assuming a worker is employed 240 days per year at 8 hours per day, a rough estimate of a continuous 24-hour exposure to dose d based on an 8-hour workday exposure D is given by d = (0.219)D, since

$$0.219 = \frac{8 \times 240}{24 \times 365}.$$

Equation (12) in Chapter 7 is based on this adjustment to convert workday 8-hour exposures to daily 24-hour exposures along with the adjustment shown in equation (G5) for a partial exposure of length ℓ from t_0 to $t_0 + \ell$, as compared to a continuous exposure t_0 to t, i.e., of duration $(t-t_0)$. If $\ell = t - t_0$, equation (G4) can be simplified to equation (7) with D replacing d.

Equations (G4) and (G5) also provide the framework for the risk assessments in Chapter 7, which are based on partial exposures at levels higher than the assumed environmental level d = 0.002 fibers/cm^3.

REFERENCE

Peto, J., H. Seidman, and I. J. Selikoff. 1982. Mesothelioma mortality in asbestos workers: Implications for models of carcinogenesis and risk assessment. Br. J. Cancer 45:124-135.

Appendix H

Comparative Risk Assessment Score Sheets

The score sheets on the following pages contain the committee's assessments of the comparative risks posed by various combinations of fiber type, route of exposure, and health effects that were not tractable for quantitative risk assessment. Each assessment is made in comparison with the "prime cell" for chrysotile inhalation leading to lung cancer. The comparisons are expressed in terms of population risk, which takes into account recent and projected exposure patterns for the U.S. population. Individual risks for persons with higher than average exposures could easily be as great or greater than those from moderate exposures 'to chrysotile. Comparative population risks would change if unanticipated changes in use levels or patterns affected exposure distributions.

The results are expressed in a +/-system. The 0 means that the risks (number and severity of effects) are about the same as those for the prime cell, + and ++ mean that they are greater or substantially greater, -and — mean that they are less and much less, and so on. A blank means that even comparative risk assessment was untenable given the data available. Thus, the quantitative risk assessment suggested that for lifetime exposures to asbestos in ambient air, mesothelioma risks could easily exceed lung cancer risks by more than a factor of 10, which would result in a comparative risk score for mesothelioma of ++. With respect to the prime cell, all comparative risks have been judged to be either-or—, meaning that they are less or much less important than for the prime cell, even though some of the indicators of risk are positive or more strongly negative.

To determine the comparative risks for each cell, the committee combined scores for several factors related to the potential for causing health effects; each was scored by the same +/-system for comparison with the characteristics of the reference cell. The factors considered fell under three major categories: exposure, biodisposition, and effects.

EXPOSURE

- total production level (metric tons/yr) or surrogate measurement (e.g., level of occurrence in nature)
- use pattern (e.g., dispersive or contained, matrix-bound or unbound, or accidental exposure of humans)
- geographic distribution of sources
- numbers of exposed people
- trends in production and use (e.g., increasing production or diversification of use)

BIODISPOSITION

- fiber size (e.g., length and diameter)
- fiber morphology (e.g., aspect ratio)
- fiber chemistry
- penetration characteristics (e.g., in lung or other target tissue)
- stability in tissue (e.g., solubility, gelling, and fibril formation)

EFFECTS

- epidemiological observations
- observations in animals
- in vitro observations
- synergism (known or hypothesized)
- other considerations (e.g., susceptible populations or theory of action)

The committee's evaluations were based on the following scoring conventions:

0: Within a factor of about 2 of the corresponding values for the prime cell (in the sense of its effect on the total number and severity of effects); for example, if production were between 0.5 and 2.0 times that of chrysotile, the score would be 0.

\+ or-: Between 2 and 10 times the corresponding value or between 0.1 and 0.5 times that value, respectively.

++ or —: Between 10 and 100 times the corresponding value or between 0.01 and 0.1 times that value, respectively, and so on.

Blank: A blank entry means that there is no basis for judgment; in further considerations, it is assumed to be equivalent to 0.

The committee also attempted to provide a sense of the quality of these judgments. The following code was used for this purpose:

a: reasonable assurance that comparative risk is in the direction indicated and approximately of the correct magnitude (e.g., if the risk compared with the prime cell was shown as "—", then it is probable, although not assured, that the effects are less than 0.1 times the effects for the prime cell)

b: comparative risk is probably in the direction indicated, but the level is in great doubt

c: comparative risk is highly uncertain due to paucity of information; this does not mean that the committee believes that the cell is very likely to provide as much risk as the prime cell, only that there is little information assuring a lower risk

COMPAPATIVE RISK ASSESSMENT SCORE SHEET

Cell Scored	Chrysotile	/	GI Cancer	/	Ingestion
	Fiber		Effect		Route
Scores Compared with Cell	Chrysotile	/	Lung Cancer	/	Inhalation
	Fiber		Effect		Route
Exposure	Score	Biodisposition	Score	Effects	Score
Production	0	Fiber Size	0	Human Studies	-
Use Pattern	-	Morphology	0	Animal Studies	-
Geography	-	Chemistry	0	In-Vitro Studies	-
Population	0	Penetration	-	Synergism	-
Trends	0	Stability	0	Other	
Overall risk compared with cell above			-		
Overall risk compared with prime cell			-		
Quality of comparative risk assessment			b		

Remarks:
Even though asbestos uses are more likely to result in air pollution than water pollution, chrysotile enters the water supply from natural as well as human sources (e.g., asbestos-cement water pipe) and the total number of fibers ingested could be greater than the number inhaled. Most is probably excreted rapidly, but the amount that moves into the body is not known. Both epidemiological and animal studies have generally yielded "negative" results, but the epidemiological studies have been too insensitive to detect relatively small effects.

COMPAPATIVE RISK ASSESSMENT SCORE SHEET

Cell Scored	Chrysotile	/	Mesothelioma	/	Ingestion
	Fiber		Effect		Route
Scores Compared with Cell	Chrysotile	/	Mesothelioma	/	Inhalation
Fiber		Effect		Route	
Exposure	Score	Biodisposition	Score	Effects	Score
Production	0	Fiber Size	0	Human Studies	-
Use Pattern	0	Morphology	0	Animal Studies	0
Geography	0	Chemistry	0	In-Vitro Studies	
Population	0	Penetration	-	Synergism	
Trends	0	Stability	0	Other	
Overall risk compared with cell above			-		
Overall risk compared with prime cell			-		
Quality of comparative risk assessment			a		

Remarks:
It is not known whether peritoneal mesothelioma results from ingested asbestos, inhaled asbestos, or both. What little epidemiological information exists does not demonstrate an increased mesothelioma risk associated with ingested asbestos. Ingested asbestos is more likely to be excreted rapidly than is inhaled asbestos.

COMPAPATIVE RISK ASSESSMENT SCORE SHEET

Cell Scored	Crocidolite	/	Lung Cancer	/	Inhalation
	Fiber		Effect		Route
Scores Compared with Cell	Chrysotile	/	Lung Cancer	/	Inhalation
	Fiber		Effect		Route
Exposure	Score	Biodisposition	Score	Effects	Score
Production	—	Fiber Size	0	Human Studies	0
Use Pattern	-	Morphology	+	Animal Studies	0
Geography	-	Chemistry	0	In-Vitro Studies	0
Population	0	Penetration	+	Synergism	0
Trends	-	Stability	+	Other	
Overall risk compared with cell above			-		
Overall risk compared with prime cell			-		
Quality of comparative risk assessment			a		

Remarks:

Crocidolite use has been on the decline and confined to well-contained applications. In the United States, its use is already less than one-tenth that of chrysotile, and its occurrence is also low with respect to chrysotile. On the other hand, many investigators believe that equal exposures to crocidolite and chrysotile will result in more cancer from the former, possibly from crocidolite's greater ability to penetrate to the lung and its greater stability once there, rather than from a fundamental difference in potency at the site. Thus, the lower risk assessment is due almost entirely to much lower likelihood of significant nonoccupational exposures.

COMPAPATIVE RISK ASSESSMENT SCORE SHEET

Cell Scored	Crocidolite	/	Mesothelioma	/	Inhalation
	Fiber		Effect		Route
Scores Compared with Cell	Chrysotile	/	Mesothelioma	/	Inhalation
	Fiber		Effect		Route
Exposure	Score	Biodisposition	Score	Effects	Score
Production	—	Fiber Size	0	Human Studies	+
Use Pattern	-	Morphology	+	Animal Studies	0
Geography	-	Chemistry	0	In-Vitro Studies	0
Population	0	Penetration	+	Synergism	0
Trends	-	Stability	+	Other	
Overall risk compared with cell above			-		
Overall risk compared with prime cell			-		
Quality of comparative risk assessment			a		

Remarks:
As with lung cancer, crocidolite appears to be more effective for the same exposures, but current lower exposures and decreasing trends significantly reduce the risk for crocidolite.

COMPAPATIVE RISK ASSESSMENT SCORE SHEET

Cell Scored	Other Asbestos	/	All	/	Both
	Fiber		Effect		Route
Scores Compared with Cell	Chrysotile	/	Lung Cancer	/	Inhalation
	Fiber		Effect		Route
Exposure	Score	Biodisposition	Score	Effects	Score
Production		Fiber Size	0	Human Studies	+
Use Pattern	0	Morphology	0	Animal Studies	0
Geography	0	Chemistry		In-Vitro Studies	0
Population		Penetration	+	Synergism	
Trends		Stability	+	Other	
Overall risk compared with cell above			—		
Overall risk compared with prime cell			—		
Quality of comparative risk assessment			b		

Remarks:
Most other forms of asbestos have been shown to cause cancers if introduced into the lung in sufficient quantity. Like crocidolite, most amphiboles appear to penetrate to the lung and remain there more easily than chrysotile. None of the other asbestos fibers are used to a great extent in commerce, so their exposure potential is associated with their natural occurrence or contamination of other products such as talc.

COMPAPATIVE RISK ASSESSMENT SCORE SHEET

Cell Scored	Fibrous Glass	/	Lung Cancer	/	Inhalation
	Fiber		Effect		Route
Scores Compared with Cell	Chrysotile	/	Lung Cancer	/	Inhalation
	Fiber		Effect		Route
Exposure	Score	Biodisposition	Score	Effects	Score
Production	+	Fiber Size	—	Human Studies	-
Use Pattern	+	Morphology	0	Animal Studies	-
Geography	+	Chemistry		In-Vitro Studies	-
Population	+	Penetration	—	Synergism	-
Trends	+	Stability	-	Other	
Overall risk compared with cell above			-		
Overall risk compared with prime cell			-		
Quality of comparative risk assessment			b		

Remarks:
Fibrous glass is produced in large quantities and is used widely, although much of it is in fibers larger than respirable size. Most of the population has opportunities for exposure, and the trends are toward increased production and at least level production of fine fiber. Most of the indicators for biological activity point toward lower risk. Evidence from human studies suggests lower, although not necessarily zero, risk of lung cancer. The latency period may not have fully elapsed, but considerations of fiber size distributions and the gelling of glass in tissue also suggest lower risk. Overall, the population risk appears lower despite higher exposure levels.

COMPAPATIVE RISK ASSESSMENT SCORE SHEET

Cell Scored	Fibrous Glass	/	Mesothelioma	/	Inhalation
	Fiber		Effect		Route
Scores Compared with Cell	Chrysotile	/	Mesothelioma	/	Inhalation
	Fiber		Effect		Route
Exposure	Score	Biodisposition	Score	Effects	Score
Production	+	Fiber Size	—	Human Studies	-
Use Pattern	+	Morphology	0	Animal Studies	0
Geography	+	Chemistry		In-Vitro Studies	-
Population	+	Penetration	—	Synergism	-
Trends	+	Stability	-	Other	
Overall risk compared with cell above			-		
Overall risk compared with prime cell			-		
Quality of comparative risk assessment			b		

Remarks:
Epidemiological studies suggest that the association of a mesothelioma with fibrous glass is weaker than it is for lung cancer. but animal experiments have demonstrated the induction of mesothelioma with implanted material.

COMPAPATIVE RISK ASSESSMENT SCORE SHEET

Cell Scored	Attapulgite	/	Lung Cancer	/	Inhalation
	Fiber		Effect		Route
Scores Compared with Cell	Chrysotile	/	Lung Cancer	/	Inhalation
	Fiber		Effect		Route
Exposure	Score	Biodisposition	Score	Effects	Score
Production	+	Fiber Size	—	Human Studies	
Use Pattern	+	Morphology	0	Animal Studies	-
Geography	-	Chemistry		In-Vitro Studies	
Population	+	Penetration	+	Synergism	
Trends	+	Stability		Other	
Overall risk compared with cell above			-		
Overall risk compared with prime cell			-		
Quality of comparative risk assessment			c		

Remarks:
Except for its extremely localized occurrence, attapulgite is more likely to lead to exposures than is chrysotile asbestos. The short, fine fibers are also likely to reach the lung but are cleared rapidly. Evidence is being collected on attapulgite miners, but no positive results have been obtained to date. Positive animal evidence suggesting biological activity is sparse. Overall, the risk is probably less than for chrysotile, but the support for that statement is weak.

COMPAPATIVE RISK ASSESSMENT SCORE SHEET

Cell Scored	Mineral Wool	/	Lung Cancer	/	Inhalation
	Fiber		Effect		Route
Scores Compared with Cell	Chrysotile	/	Lung Cancer	/	Inhalation
	Fiber		Effect		Route
Exposure	Score	Biodisposition	Score	Effects	Score
Production	-	Fiber Size	-	Human Studies	0
Use Pattern	-	Morphology	0	Animal Studies	-
Geography	0	Chemistry		In-Vitro Studies	
Population	0	Penetration	-	Synergism	
Trends	+	Stability		Other	
Overall risk compared with cell above			—		
Overall risk compared with prime cell			—		
Quality of comparative risk assessment			b		

Remarks:
Mineral wools—both slag wool and rock wool—are not produced in as high a volume as asbestos, but neither is their production on the decline. They are used somewhat less widely than asbestos, but probably in forms that are more easily obtainable. Average fiber size is somewhat thicker. Scanty results from studies in occupational cohorts and animals suggest that mineral wool is no more potent than asbestos, and probably less.

COMPAPATIVE RISK ASSESSMENT SCORE SHEET

Cell Scored	Mineral Wool	/	Mesothelioma	/	Inhalation
	Fiber		Effect		Route
Scores Compared with Cell	Chrysotile	/	Mesothelioma	/	Inhalation
	Fiber		Effect		Route
Exposure	Score	Biodisposition	Score	Effects	Score
Production	-	Fiber Size	-	Human Studies	0
Use Pattern	-	Morphology	0	Animal Studies	0
Geography	0	Chemistry		In-Vitro Studies	
Population	0	Penetration	-	Synergism	
Trends	+	Stability		Other	
Overall risk compared with cell above			—		
Overall risk compared with prime cell			—		
Quality of comparative risk assessment			b		

Remarks:
See remarks for lung cancer on previous page.

COMPAPATIVE RISK ASSESSMENT SCORE SHEET

Cell Scored	Attapulgite	/	Mesothelioma	/	Inhalation
	Fiber		Effect		Route
Scores Compared with Cell	Chrysotile	/	Mesothelioma	/	Inhalation
	Fiber		Effect		Route
Exposure	Score	Biodisposition	Score	Effects	Score
Production	+	Fiber Size	—	Human Studies	
Use Pattern	+	Morphology	0	Animal Studies	0
Geography	-	Chemistry		In-Vitro Studies	
Population	+	Penetration	+	Synergism	
Trends	+	Stability		Other	
Overall risk compared with cell above			-		
Overall risk compared with prime cell			—		
Quality of comparative risk assessment			c		

Remarks:
See remarks for lung cancer on previous page.

COMPAPATIVE RISK ASSESSMENT SCORE SHEET

Cell Scored	Ceramic Fiber	/	Lung Cancer	/	Inhalation
	Fiber		Effect		Route
Scores Compared with Cell	Chrysotile	/	Lung Cancer	/	Inhalation
	Fiber		Effect		Route
Exposure	Score	Biodisposition	Score	Effects	Score
Production	—	Fiber Size	0	Human Studies	
Use Pattern	—	Morphology	0	Animal Studies	-
Geography	-	Chemistry		In-Vitro Studies	
Population	-	Penetration	0	Synergism	
Trends	++	Stability		Other	
Overall risk compared with cell above			—		
Overall risk compared with prime cell			—		
Quality of comparative risk assessment			b		

Remarks:
Most of the assessment is based on current production and very limited uses. Fibers are respirable in size but are often well contained, and only a few major sources are likely to provide significant exposures. Little information is available on biological effects.

COMPAPATIVE RISK ASSESSMENT SCORE SHEET

Cell Scored	Ceramic Fiber	/	Mesothelioma	/	Inhalation
	Fiber		Effect		Route
Scores Compared with Cell	Chrysotile	/	Mesothelioma	/	Inhalation
	Fiber		Effect		Route
Exposure	Score	Biodisposition	Score	Effects	Score
Production	—	Fiber Size	0	Human Studies	-
Use Pattern	—	Morphology	0	Animal Studies	0
Geography	-	Chemistry		In-Vitro Studies	
Population	-	Penetration	0	Synergism	
Trends	++	Stability		Other	
Overall risk compared with cell above			—		
Overall risk compared with prime cell			—		
Quality of comparative risk assessment			c		

Remarks:
See remarks on previous page.

COMPAPATIVE RISK ASSESSMENT SCORE SHEET

Cell Scored	Carbon Fiber	/	Lung Cancer	/	Inhalation
	Fiber		Effect		Route
Scores Compared with Cell	Chrysotile	/	Lung Cancer	/	Inhalation
	Fiber		Effect		Route
Exposure	Score	Biodisposition	Score	Effects	Score
Production		Fiber Size	0	Human Studies	
Use Pattern	-	Morphology	0	Animal Studies	
Geography		Chemistry		In-Vitro Studies	
Population	-	Penetration	0	Synergism	
Trends	+++	Stability		Other	
Overall risk compared with cell above			—		
Overall risk compared with prime cell			—		
Quality of comparative risk assessment			c		

Remarks:
Assessment is based almost entirely on consideration of the currently low exposure levels.

COMPAPATIVE RISK ASSESSMENT SCORE SHEET

Cell Scored	Carbon Fiber	/	Mesothelioma	/	Inhalation
	Fiber		Effect		Route
Scores Compared with Cell	Chrysotile	/	Mesothelioma	/	Inhalation
	Fiber		Effect		Route
Exposure	Score	Biodisposition	Score	Effects	Score
Production		Fiber Size	0	Human Studies	
Use Pattern	-	Morphology	0	Animal Studies	
Geography		Chemistry		In-Vitro Studies	
Population	-	Penetration	0	Synergism	
Trends	+++	Stability		Other	
Overall risk compared with cell above			—		
Overall risk compared with prime cell			—		
Quality of comparative risk assessment			c		

Remarks:
See remarks for lung cancer on previous page.

Appendix I

Background Information on Members of the Committee on Nonoccupational Health Risks of Asbestiform Fibers

LESTER BRESLOW, committee chairman, is Dean Emeritus and Professor of Public Health, School of Public Health, University of California at Los Angeles. His work has been devoted mainly to the epidemiology of chronic disease. He is a member of the Institute of Medicine and has served as an adviser on health matters to the World Health Organization and to several federal agencies.

RICHARD R. BATES is Senior Staff Scientist, Health Effects Institute, Cambridge, Massachusetts. Previously, he served as Associate Commissioner for Science of the Food and Drug Administration and Assistant to the Director for Risk Assessment at the National Institute of Environmental Health Sciences. He has extensive knowledge in the fields of risk assessment and experimental pathology and has concentrated his research on chemical carcinogenesis and toxicology. Dr. Bates is a member of the American Association of Pathologists, the American Association for Cancer Research, and the Society of Toxicology.

HENRIK H. BENDIXEN is Professor of Anesthesiology and Chairman of the Department of Anesthesiology at Columbia University in New York City. His research interests include respiratory failure and other aspects of intensive care medicine. In addition to serving on National Research Council committees studying shock and the toxicity of anesthetic agents, he has been a member of various committees of the National Institutes of Health. He is a past president of the Society of Critical Care Medicine and a member of the Institute of Medicine.

STEPHEN L. BROWN is an independent consultant specializing in chemical risk assessment and related problems. His contributions include the development of techniques for estimating human exposure to chemicals and other biologically significant agents, application of systems analysis techniques to chemical risk assessment, and priority-setting for both testing and regulating hazardous substances. He was previously Director of the Center for Health and Environmental Research at SRI International.

PATRICIA A. BUFFLER is Professor of Epidemiology and Associate Dean for Research at the University of Texas Health Science Center at the

School of Public Health in Houston. Her research interests include occupational and environmental epidemiology, with special emphasis on cancer, pulmonary diseases, and reproductive disorders. She is past Chairman of the American Public Health Association Epidemiology Section and is currently on the Board of Directors of the American College of Epidemiology.

ARTHUR M. LANGER is an Associate Professor and the Associate Director of the Environmental Sciences Laboratory at the Mount Sinai School of Medicine. His research interests have included development of analytical techniques for microparticles, measurement and characterization of asbestos fiber in human tissues, and determination of physicochemical properties of mineral dusts that impart biological activity. In addition to serving on many governmental advisory committees, he has acted as consultant to the International Agency for Research on Cancer of the World Health Organization and to the Norwegian and South African governments on subjects related to asbestos exposure and health effects.

JEREMIAH LYNCH is the Industrial Hygiene Manager of the Exxon Chemical Company. Mr. Lynch previously worked at the National Institute for Occupational Safety and Health of the U.S. Public Health Service, where he conducted research in asbestos measurement, exposure monitoring strategy, and engineering control technology. He is a past Chairman of the American Conference of Governmental Industrial Hygienists and is active in U.S. and international occupational health groups.

JAMES A. MERCHANT is Professor in the Department of Preventive Medicine and Environmental Health and the Department of Internal Medicine at the University of Iowa. Before assuming his present position, he was Director of the Appalachian Laboratory for Occupational Safety and Health and the Division of Respiratory Disease Studies at West Virginia University. His research interests include occupational lung diseases, epidemiology, and pulmonary medicine.

RICHARD R. MONSON is Professor of Epidemiology and Director of the Occupational Health Program at the Harvard School of Public Health. His research interests include mortality studies of occupational groups as well as cancer epidemiology in general. Dr. Monson served on the National Research Council Committee on Amines.

BROOKE T. MOSSMAN is Assistant Professor of Pathology at the University of Vermont College of Medicine. She conducts research on cellular mechanisms of asbestos-induced injury and disease, with particular interest in asbestos-associated carcinogenesis. Dr. Mossman has served as a consultant to the National Science Foundation, the National Cancer Institute, the Environmental Protection Agency, and the National Institute of Environmental Health Sciences.

JAMES E. TROSKO is Professor of Pediatrics and Human Development and Associate Director of the Division of Human Genetics, Genetic Toxicology, Endocrinology, and Oncology in the College of Human Medicine, Michigan State University. As a molecular geneticist, Dr. Trosko's research in radiation biology at Oak Ridge National Laboratory included studies on DNA damage, DNA repair mechanisms, and in vitro mutation studies in human and other mammalian cells. He also has conducted extensive research in chemical carcinogenesis. Currently, his research activities include both theoretical and mechanistic studies of initiators and promoters of carcinogenesis. He has served on many academic, governmental, and National Research Council committees and has participated in several symposia concerned with the multiple disease potentials of genotoxic and nongenotoxic agents.

JOHN VAN RYZIN is Professor in the Division of Biostatistics and Department of Statistics at Columbia University and Senior Mathematician at Brookhaven National Laboratory. His research interests include quantitative methods of risk assessment and statistical methodologies for analysis of toxicological and survival data. Dr. Van Ryzin has served as a consultant or reviewer to the Environmental Protection Agency, the Food and Drug Administration, the Office of Technology Assessment, the National Toxicology Program, and the Food Safety Council.

TIBOR ZOLTAI has been on the faculty of the Department of Geology and Geophysics at the University of Minnesota since 1959. His expertise lies in the areas of applied geology, mineralogy, and crystallography. Among his major scientific interests are the crystal chemistry, crystal structure and physical properties of minerals, as well as the nature and properties of asbestiform fibers.